Ultrasonography
of the Eye and Orbit

Per aspera ad astra.

ANONYMOUS

Four things come not back:
the spoken word;
the sped arrow;
time past;
the neglected opportunity.

OMAR IBN AL-HALIF

Ultrasonography of the Eye and Orbit

D. JACKSON COLEMAN, M.D.
Assistant Professor of Clinical Ophthalmology
College of Physicians and Surgeons
Columbia University, New York, New York

FREDERIC L. LIZZI, Eng.Sc.D.
Riverside Research Institute
New York, New York

ROBERT L. JACK, M.D., Med.Sc.D.
Department of Ophthalmology
Stanford University School of Medicine
Palo Alto, California
Palo Alto Retinal Group, Menlo Park, California

LEA & FEBIGER · 1977 · PHILADELPHIA

Library of Congress Cataloging in Publication Data

Coleman, D. Jackson, 1934–
    Ultrasonography of the eye and orbit.

    Bibliography: p.
    Includes index.
    1. Ultrasonics in ophthalmology. 2. Diagnosis, Ultrasonic.
I. Lizzi, Frederic., 1942–   joint author. II. Jack, Robert Lionel,
1943–   joint author. III. Title. [DNLM: 1. Eye diseases—
Diagnosis. 2. Orbit. 3. Ultrasonics—Diagnostic use. WW143
C692u]
RE79.U4C64 1975   617.7′1   74-31002
ISBN 0-8121-0498-6

Published in Great Britain by Henry Kimpton Publishers, London

PRINTED IN THE UNITED STATES OF AMERICA

*This book is dedicated to our wives and families
for their understanding and forbearance.*

Preface

THE medical use of ultrasound, in only a score of years, has reached the point where it is now universally regarded as an essential means of soft tissue examination in the eye and the orbit as well as in many other areas of the body. As utilized in ophthalmology, ultrasound both complements and surpasses the capabilities of other diagnostic techniques in the evaluation of abnormalities, particularly those produced by ocular and orbital tumors, vitreous hemorrhages, trauma and foreign bodies. Ultrasound, by providing this increased diagnostic potential, has modified the treatment of many ophthalmic problems. In this book, we will attempt to summarize our own experience regarding ultrasonic evaluation of the eye and orbit.

Ultrasonic evaluation is a rapidly expanding field in which both techniques and equipment are subject to constant modification and refinement. Thus alternate diagnostic systems are available, based on immersion or contact B-scan techniques or A-scan tissue quantification methods. Our techniques, developed over the past ten years during the evaluation of approximately 7,000 patients, are presented here.

There are three modes of ultrasonic display, A-, B-, and M-modes. This terminology is often confusing, but dates back to an alphabet system devised for radar display modes during World War II. The displays were often called "scans," i.e. A-scan, B-scan, C-scan or M-scan. Since the word "scan" implies a sweeping or scanning motion of the transducer (a feature used for most B-scan types of presentation), the terminology became potentially redundant (e.g. a B-scan scan). In an effort to correct this, the American Institute of Ultrasound in Medicine recommended the word "mode" to describe the display. While most ultrasonographers use the terms A-mode, B-scan mode or M-mode, and we usually follow this convention, we may on occasion revert to A-scan, B-scan or M-scan, mostly for convenience in describing the scanned B-mode which comprises a major part of our description of pathology.

Each of the display modes will be described in detail, as will the electronic means of producing them. Basically, the A-mode, sometimes called "time-amplitude" ultrasound since the height or amplitude of returned echoes is shown in real time, contains all of the echo information provided from any single tissue aspect. This type of display can be used alone, with experience, to diagnose ocular problems, but most observers prefer to use the two-dimensional format of the scanned B-mode, sometimes called "scanned, intensity-modulated ultrasound." In this technique, the amplitude of the echoes is used to modulate the brightness of corresponding dots on the oscilloscope screen. A scanning movement of the transducer, when mechanically and electronically slaved to the display, causes the dots to blend into a two-dimensional cross section or tomogram of the tissue. If the brightness of the dots can be shown well, the B-scan will have good gray scale. Most oscilloscopes cannot provide the gray scale or amplitude variation seen on the A-mode, so that color or isometric displays or concurrent A-mode must be used to provide the full range of these amplitude variations or "acoustic signatures" of tissues.

Regardless of the ultrasonic system used, a basic understanding of the principles of ultrasound is essential to those who use this technique in diagnosis. The first two chapters of this book will be devoted to the principles of ultrasonic energy, its application and display. This material will be presented in a narrative fashion, and complex mathematical equations will be kept to a minimum. The third chapter will deal with the application of these principles to the biometry of the eye, an area where optimal resolution is requisite. Chapters IV, V, and VI will deal with ocular and orbital diagnosis, using a wide assortment of illustrations to demonstrate observations—our own and those of others—that we have found helpful in measuring and evaluating normal and abnormal tissues.

D. JACKSON COLEMAN, M.D.

New York, New York   FREDERIC L. LIZZI, Eng.Sc.D.
Palo Alto, California   ROBERT L. JACK, M.D., Med.Sc.D.

Acknowledgments

THE work of many investigators has been helpful in forming our techniques and classifications. We owe much to co-workers at Riverside Research Institute (RRI) who have helped to design our equipment, and particularly to Louis Katz who has contributed greatly to advances in the state of the art in ultrasonography. We would especially like to acknowledge the able assistance of our laboratory staff. Mary Smith has been indispensable in all phases of writing, editing and producing this book, as well as in supervising the clinical laboratory and assisting in all aspects of patient management. Louise Franzen has helped to scan most of the patients, managed the research laboratory and collated the bibliographies and tables. Emil Bethke has illustrated the ultrasonograms with skill and patience, making the actual photographs of the scans more easily understood. Margaret Cubberly has provided capable photographic assistance. Heinz Rosskothen, our machinist and instrument maker, has designed and fabricated many parts necessary for the maintenance of our equipment. Kurt Weil of RRI has assisted greatly in technical design of the equipment. In the early stages of research, Benson Carlin provided consultative expertise. We also wish to acknowledge the talented assistance of Mary Vickery, William Lewis and James Danella of RRI in the preparation of this manuscript.

We are indebted to Dr. Richard Dallow of the Massachusetts Eye and Ear Infirmary for contributions to the text and to the illustrations. Dr. Dallow's insights as both ultrasonographer and orbital surgeon are particularly valuable.

We wish to thank those of our colleagues, pioneers in the field of ophthalmic ultrasound, who have shared their experience with us and who have graciously provided some illustrations: Drs. Edward Purnell, Gilbert Baum, Karl Ossoinig and Nathaniel Bronson. We thank the American Journal of Ophthalmology and the Archives of Ophthalmology for allowing us to reproduce numerous figures used to illustrate this book.

We thank the many colleagues who have referred patients to us, and who have provided follow-up evaluations vital in determining the usefulness of our methods. Drs. A. G. DeVoe, Algernon Reese, Ira Jones, Robert Ellsworth, and Stephen Trokel have been particularly helpful and encouraging.

Our research has been supported by the National Institute of Neurological Diseases and Blindness and by the National Eye Institute, to which we are profoundly grateful. We are also appreciative of the support of Fight-for-Sight, Inc., the National Council to Combat Blindness.

Last but not least, we wish to thank Thomas Colaiezzi and Rosemary Pattison of Lea & Febiger, whose skill, assistance and encouragement have brought this book to publication.

D.J.C.
F.L.L.
R.L.J.

Contents

CHAPTER I

Physics of Ultrasound

Physics
of Ultrasound

SINCE its first application[1] to ophthalmology in 1956, ultrasound has emerged as an important clinical modality for the diagnosis of a broad spectrum of ocular and orbital abnormalities. Its increasing acceptance within the medical community stems from its ability to provide highly detailed cross-sectional images of ocular and orbital morphology in a rapid, noninvasive manner that poses no significant threat of tissue damage. In addition to providing tissue maps with high accuracy and resolution, ultrasonic systems also convey information about several tissue properties that have been used to identify disease or injury with a high degree of confidence. The use of ultrasound in diagnosis and biometry requires knowledge of its physical nature and the phenomena associated with its propagation.

Ultrasound is an acoustic wave consisting of compressions and rarefactions that can propagate within fluid and solid substances. By definition, an ultrasonic wave exhibits frequencies above 20 KHz* and differs from a sonic wave only because these high frequencies render it inaudible. Because it is a wave, ultrasound can be directed, focused, and reflected according to the same principles that govern these phenomena with other waves such as light. The high frequencies (typically 10 MHz) and small wavelengths

---

*KHz denotes kilohertz or one thousand cycles per second; MHz denotes megahertz or one million cycles per second.

3

(e.g., 150 microns [μ]) available with ultrasound can provide the detailed resolution required for ocular examinations.

The most effective use of ultrasound in examining soft tissue is realized through reflective ("pulse-echo") systems analogous to those used in radar and sonar. This approach allows examination within a thin "slice" through tissue structures as opposed to the compression of tissue data into one plane obtained with X-rays. In pulse-echo ultrasonic systems a short burst of ultrasonic energy is generated by a piezoelectric transducer; it traverses a well-defined path in the eye at a known speed and undergoes partial reflection at tissue boundaries which present abrupt changes in acoustic properties. These reflections, or echoes, return to the transducer where they are electrically detected and displayed in graphic form (A-scan). Alternatively, if the transducer is scanned across the eye, an image (B-scan) of the scanned ocular and orbital structures can be constructed from the echoes.

A- and B-scan results depict acoustic tissue reflectivity as modified by other acoustic properties (e.g., absorption). Acoustic properties are determined by factors that include the surface roughness, density, rigidity, and textural homogeneity of the examined tissue structures. Careful interpretation in terms of several such tissue characteristics has led to highly reliable detection and identification of soft tissue entities. The application of systematic interpretation plans detailed in subsequent chapters requires an understanding of the basic physical principles applying to ultrasound. These principles are reviewed in this chapter, which describes how ultrasound is generated and detected, how it is reflected and absorbed in tissue, and the factors which influence the resolution which can be achieved in examining the eye and orbit. (Comprehensive texts treating the physics of ultrasound are listed at the end of the chapter as *Additional References.*)

Generation and Detection of Ultrasound

The key element in any ultrasonic system is a piezoelectric transducer which is used both to generate an ultrasonic wave from an applied voltage signal and to detect ultrasonic echoes returning from within the eye. A transducer unit consists of a thin, disk-shaped crystal of piezoelectric material such as quartz, a backing section and, usually, an acoustic lens (Fig. I-1) which focuses the generated ultrasonic beam. The entire unit is commonly referred to as the transducer, although this term most correctly applies only to the piezoelectric element; common usage is accepted in this text. In

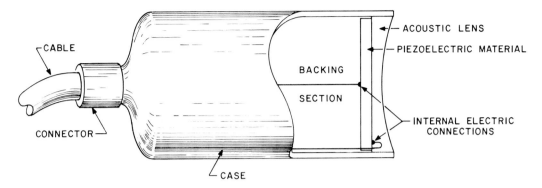

FIG. I-1. Cutaway view of transducer.

clinical systems, transducers are immersed in a saline solution which contacts the eye; the saline solution affords a useful transmission path to and from the eye and is needed because air absorbs high-frequency ultrasound at an extremely high rate. (In some systems, the transducer is held in direct contact with the globe.)

The actual generation and detection of ultrasound take place in the piezoelectric material. The molecular configuration of a simple piezoelectric crystal is shown schematically in Figure I-2. The molecules exhibit net charge polarizations which are forced into alignment by the crystalline structure so that effective positive charge centers are oriented in the same direction. Ultrasonic waves are generated when a voltage is applied across external electrodes plated on the crystal surfaces. The molecules tend to be stretched or shortened depending on whether the voltage polarity causes

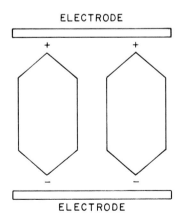

UNEXCITED CONFIGURATION

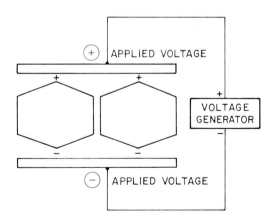

EXCITED CONFIGURATION (CONTRACTION)

FIG. I-2. Schematic representations of molecular configuration in a piezoelectric material illustrating contraction induced by an applied voltage.

attraction or repulsion of the nearest charge centers. Because of these molecular effects, the overall crystal thickness is altered to a degree proportional to the amplitude of the applied voltage. When the polarity of the applied voltage is rapidly varied, the crystal executes rapid expansions and contractions which constitute ultrasonic vibrations.

On the other hand, if the crystal is compressed and expanded by an impinging ultrasonic wave, variations in molecular charge separation induce a voltage difference across the two electrodes. The amplitude of the generated voltage is proportional to that of the ultrasonic wave. This voltage is readily displayed on an oscilloscope enabling ultrasonic echoes to be detected as they return from the eye.

In the past, piezoelectric transducers were most often fabricated from precisely oriented cuts of quartz crystals which can require excitation voltages exceeding 1,000 volts. Now, most transducers are fabricated from more sensitive materials, including lithium sulfate and ceramics such as lead-zirconate-titanate (PZT), that require about 200 volts for excitation and can detect extremely small ultrasonic signals containing only microwatts of power. Some of these materials must be "poled" before they can be used in transducers. In this process, piezoelectric domains are brought into alignment by applying large constant voltages at elevated temperatures. Once this alignment is achieved, these materials can generate and detect ultrasound in a manner similar to that described above.

A piezoelectric crystal responds most actively to ultrasonic waves and voltage signals that have frequencies near its resonant frequency. This frequency is determined by the crystal thickness, increasing as the crystal is made thinner. Resonance effects can lead to prolonged series of ultrasonic vibrations which are suppressed by using backing sections. As discussed in subsequent sections, backing sections and acoustic lenses are required for high-resolution tissue examinations.

Propagation of Ultrasound

When a piezoelectric transducer is immersed in a fluid and electrically excited, its vibrations generate an ultrasonic wave of compression and rarefaction that propagates through the fluid. These waves, termed longitudinal or compressional ultrasonic waves, are the type used in medical systems. They propagate through soft tissues in the same manner as they propagate through fluids.

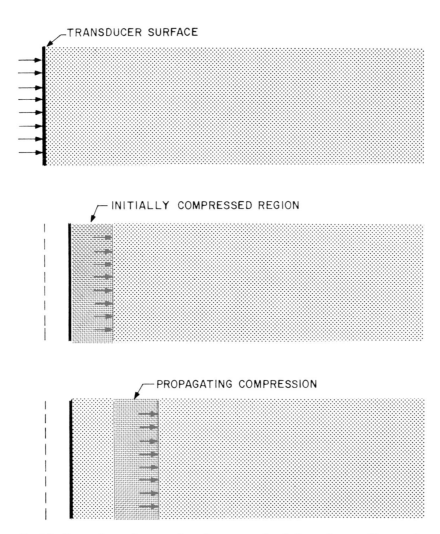

FIG. I-3. Generation and propagation of a compressional ultrasonic wave. The wave is generated by a small extension of a transducer surface into a fluid.

Ultrasonic propagation is illustrated in Figure I-3, where a voltage pulse causes a piezoelectric transducer to undergo a small rapid expansion. Extension of the front transducer surface initially compresses the adjacent fluid layer, raising its density and pressure. Increased molecular collisions in this compressed region eventually couple the elevated density and pressure to the next fluid layer while the initially compressed region returns to its original state. Thus, the compression passes from the first layer to the second and, in the same manner, continually propagates to more distant regions in the fluid. Similar phenomena occur when the transducer contracts rather than expands. In this case, rarefaction characterized by lowered fluid pressure and density propagates away from the transducer.

TABLE I-1. Ultrasonic Propagation Velocities

Substance	Velocity (m/sec)	Temperature (°C)	Reference
Water	1524	37°	2
Aqueous humor	1532	37°	3
Lens	1641	37°	3
Vitreous humor	1532	37°	3
Fat	1476	24°	4
Cataractous lens	1629	37°	5
Sclera	1630	22°	6
Cornea	1550	22°	6

Induced compression and rarefaction disturbances travel through a substance at a speed (velocity of propagation) that is determined by the density and compressibility of that substance. In materials with low compressibilities, such as metals, compression rapidly passes from layer to layer and large propagation velocities are encountered (e.g., 6,000 m/sec). In contrast, materials that are more readily compressed, such as fluids and tissues, exhibit low velocities (e.g., 1,524 m/sec in water). As shown in Table I-1, ocular tissues exhibit propagation velocities close to that of water. The largest velocity is exhibited by the lens. Propagation velocities are temperature dependent; near 37° C, the lenticular velocity increases by 2 m/sec for a 1°-C temperature increase.

In medical systems, brief excitation voltages are used and the transducer surface vibrates back and forth several times at a rate equal to its resonant frequency (e.g., 10 MHz). This series of vibrations generates several contiguous regions of compression and rarefaction that propagate with the above velocity, as shown in Figure I-4. These regions travel together as an ultrasonic pulse and cause roughly sinusoidal variations in density and pressure as they traverse the eye. Clinical systems utilize only small transducer motions (total excursions under one micron) and only small, imperceptible and innocuous pressure variations are produced within the eye and orbit.

Sinusoidal pulses manifest a wavelength which, as in optics, is an important determinant of many operational parameters including resolution. The wavelength, Λ, is the distance over which the pressure perturbation undergoes one complete cycle. Wavelength is determined by the frequency, f, of transducer vibrations and the propagation velocity, c, of the medium;

$$\Lambda = c/f.$$

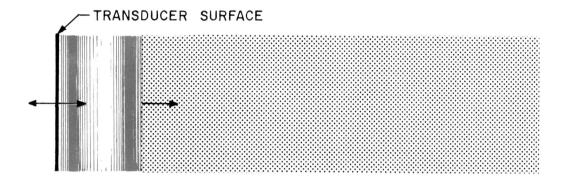

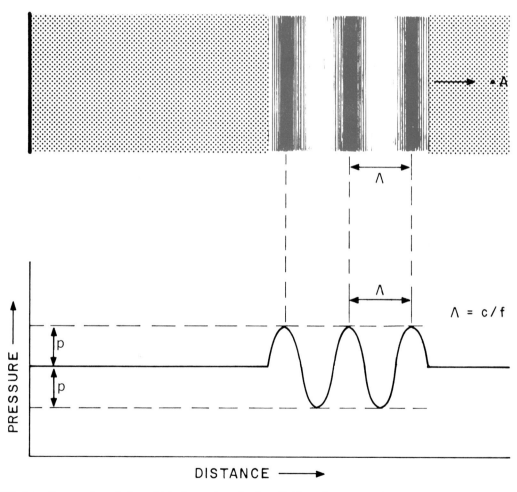

FIG. I-4. Propagation of sinusoidal ultrasonic pulse in a fluid medium at two instants of time. Lower plot shows ultrasonic pressure variation of peak amplitude p. Static pressure level is exhibited outside the region occupied by the pulse.

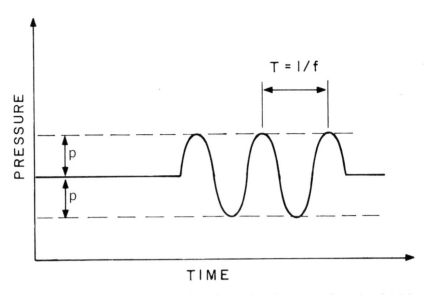

FIG. I-5. Pressure variations caused as ultrasonic pulse passes through point A in Figure I-4. The frequency of these variations is the same as that of the transducer vibrations.

This relation is obeyed since the transducer generates the same pressure level every 1/f seconds, and this pressure travels at a velocity equal to c. In water, 10-MHz operation produces a wavelength of 0.15 mm which is commensurate with retinal thickness; increasing the frequency to 20 MHz decreases the wavelength to 0.075 mm.

The concept of wavelength describes the spatial distribution of pressure at a single instant of time. It should be remembered, however, that ultrasonic pulses continually propagate through tissue structures at high velocities, causing rapid pressure oscillations as they travel through points within the eye. In fact, as shown in Figure I-5, the pressure at a point in the eye varies at the same high rate (e.g., 10 MHz) at which the transducer vibrates.

Thus far, longitudinal ultrasonic waves have been discussed. Several other types of ultrasonic waves can be generated in certain materials but are not important in ophthalmic examinations. Surface (Rayleigh) waves and shear (transverse) waves are examples of these. Shear waves are excited in solids when a transducer surface vibrates within one plane (Fig. I-6). This motion causes a shear in the adjacent region of the solid which is transmitted to progressively farther regions within the solid. Shear waves couple poorly into fluids and tissues and are dissipated by viscosity at very rapid rates so that they cannot be utilized in ophthalmic visualization systems.

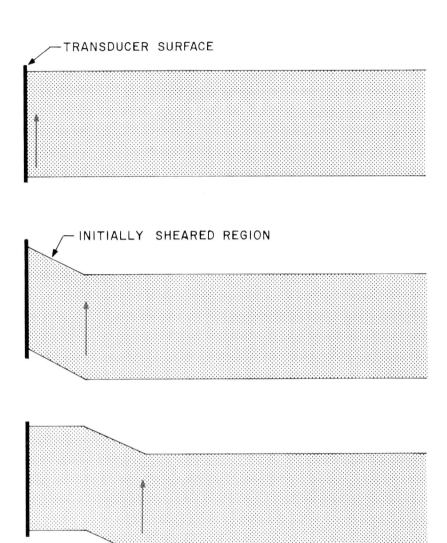

TRANSDUCER SURFACE

INITIALLY SHEARED REGION

SHEAR WAVE PROPAGATION

FIG. I-6. Generation and propagation of shear ultrasonic wave in a solid. The wave is generated by a shearing force at the transducer surface. Internal displacements are perpendicular to direction of propagation.

Reflection of Ultrasound

Ultrasonic pulses are reflected at boundaries between media that possess differing mechanical characteristics. Figure I-7 illustrates the extreme case of total reflection from a rigid wall bounding a fluid of depth L. When the incident compression reaches the wall, the expansive forces accompanying molecular collisions are redirected

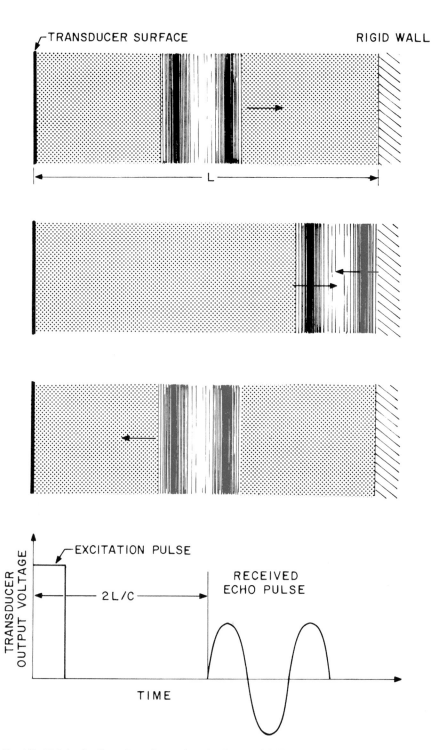

FIG. I-7. Total reflection of an ultrasonic pulse from a rigid boundary. The transducer output voltage displays both the excitation pulse and the echo pulse so that the total transit time can be measured.

back into the fluid and the same phenomena described above cause the pulse to travel through the fluid in the reverse direction. The reflected pulse arrives back at the transducer after a time interval equal to 2 L/c and generates an output transducer voltage as shown in the figure. Observation of this output voltage not only enables detection of the boundary but also specifies L if c is known. It should be noted that while the onset time of the echo voltage pulse depends only on L and c, the shape and time duration of the voltage pulse is dependent on characteristics of the ultrasonic pulse and transducer parameters as discussed subsequently.

In the eye a similar reflection arises whenever a pulse encounters a boundary between two ocular structures. However,

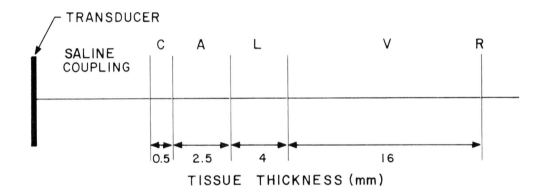

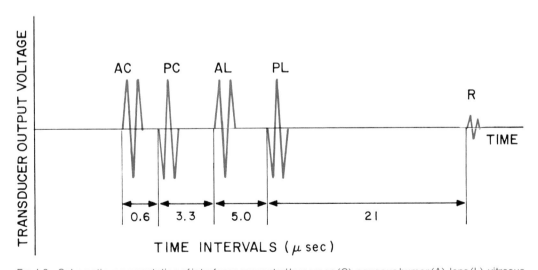

FIG. I-8. Schematic representation of interfaces presented by cornea (C), aqueous humor (A), lens (L), vitreous humor (V) and retina (R). Transducer voltage demonstrates echoes from anterior and posterior corneal surfaces (AC and PC), lens surfaces (AL and PL) and retina. Measured time intervals can be used with velocity data to determine the thickness of each ocular segment.

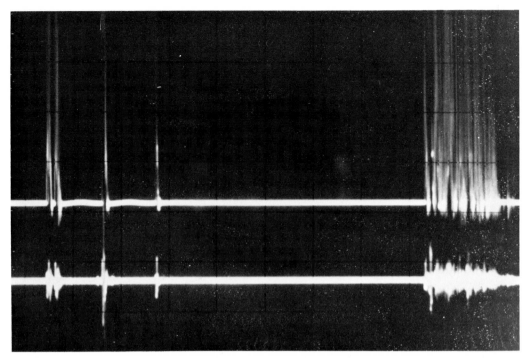

FIG. I-9. Echo voltages obtained from eye; lower series of echoes correspond to those illustrated in Figure I-8. Upper signals are processed video waveforms as described in Chapter II. Following ocular echoes, a complex echo pattern arises from scattering within orbital fat.

ocular tissues exhibit similar mechanical properties so that only a small fraction of the incident pulse is reflected. Most of the incident energy is transmitted through the boundary where it undergoes partial reflections at each successive interface.

The major reflective surfaces in the normal eye are those of the cornea, lens and rear wall layers. Figure I-8 shows a diagram of these surfaces with typical dimensions and also illustrates the transducer echo voltages which arise from each of them. Corresponding clinical results are shown in Figure I-9. The time interval between voltage pulses can be used to determine the thickness of the corresponding tissue segment since the pertinent propagation velocities are known. Specifically, the time interval between successive echoes is equal to $2 L/c$, where L is the corresponding tissue thickness. Thus, the lens echoes are separated by 5 μsec,* since L = 4 mm and c = 1,641 m/sec. Biometric systems using this approach are capable of measuring dimensions with accuracies near $\pm$250 microns and specially designed systems have achieved accuracies of $\pm$20 microns in axial length determinations.

* μsec denotes microsecond, which is 10^{-6} seconds; nanosec denotes 10^{-9} seconds.

The strength of ultrasonic reflections depends upon the characteristic acoustic impedances, Z, of adjacent tissues. The characteristic impedance of a tissue is defined as the product of its density, ρ, and propagation velocity:

$$Z = \rho c.$$

The ratio, R, of the pressure amplitude of the reflected pulse to that of the incident pulse is equal to:

$$R = \frac{Z_2 - Z_1}{Z_1 + Z_2}.$$

R is called the reflection coefficient and the subscripts refer to the first and second tissue structures, respectively (Fig. I-10).

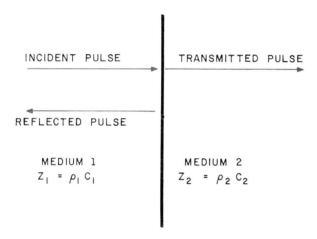

INCIDENT PULSE   TRANSMITTED PULSE

REFLECTED PULSE

MEDIUM 1   MEDIUM 2
$Z_1 = \rho_1 c_1$ $Z_2 = \rho_2 c_2$

FIG. I-10. Ray diagram showing paths of incident, reflected, and transmitted ultrasonic pulses at a tissue interface under normal incidence. The characteristic acoustic impedances of both tissues determine the relations between the amplitudes of these pulses.

The value of the reflection coefficient is an important identifying characteristic of a tissue boundary and in many cases can be ascertained from the magnitude of the corresponding echo voltage. Since R depends on $Z_2 - Z_1$, its value depends on the characteristic acoustic impedances of tissues on both sides of ocular boundaries. Thus, the reflection from, say, a foreign body (large Z) will be smaller if it is situated in a blood clot (moderate Z) than if it is situated in the vitreous humor (small Z). Within homogeneous structures such as

TABLE I-2. Ultrasonic Reflection Coefficients
(compiled from data in ref. 7)

Interface	Reflection Coefficients
Water—aluminum	0.85
Cornea—aqueous humor	−0.06
Aqueous humor—lens	0.07
Lens—vitreous humor	−0.07
Vitreous humor—retina	0.01
Retina—choroid	0.001

the normal vitreous, Z is a constant and no reflections arise. In heterogeneous structures (e.g., cataractous lens) Z can vary from point to point and, accordingly, echoes are generated from within these structures.

As shown in Table I-2, most normal and pathologic structures give rise to small reflections ranging from 7 per cent at the lens-aqueous humor interface to approximately 0.1 per cent at the chorio-retinal interface. Reflection coefficients exceeding 10 per cent are encountered with rigid foreign bodies. Negative values of R occur at interfaces such as the cornea-aqueous boundary, where Z_1 (cornea), is larger than Z_2 (aqueous). Physically, this implies that the compressive component of the incident wave is reflected as a rarefactive component and vice versa. The echo voltages generated from such surfaces are inverted because of this acoustic reversal.

Several factors modify the echo amplitudes observed in practice. If an ultrasonic beam impinges on a tissue boundary at an oblique angle, then the reflected pressure received at the transducer is less than that described above. The reflection coefficient in this case depends upon the angle of incidence, surface roughness and ultrasonic wavelength. The echo amplitudes from rough surfaces vary more slowly with angle of incidence than do those arising from smooth surfaces (Figs. I-11 and I-12). Echo strength can also change if the tissue boundary is sharply curved because of focusing and defocusing phenomena, as illustrated in Figure I-13. Finally, apparent reflectivities are modified because of attenuation arising from absorption and other factors which diminish the amplitudes of incident and reflected ultrasonic pulses.

Another important type of ultrasonic reflection is scattering which arises from small, closely spaced reflective surfaces such as those presented by internal tumor structures (small blood vessels, calcific deposits, cellular aggregates, etc.) and the connective tissue septae of orbital fat. Reflections from these distributed reflectors

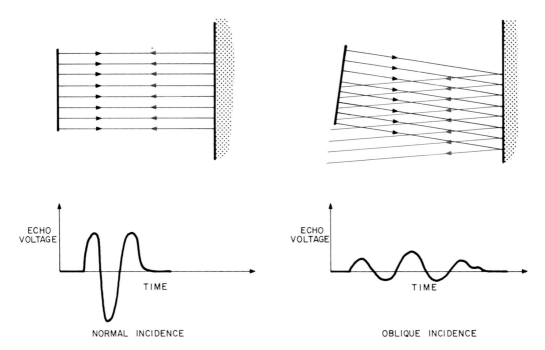

FIG. I-11. Reflection from planar interface at normal and oblique incidence. Oblique incidence results in lowered echo amplitude and increased duration due to the variation in transit times along different rays.

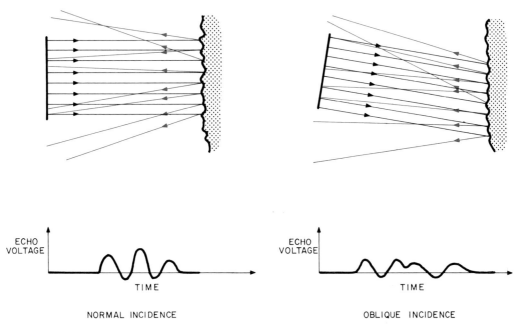

FIG. I-12. Reflection from rough interface. Surface roughness redirects energy in a variety of directions causing decreased echo amplitude and increased duration. Oblique incidence does not affect echo amplitude to the extent encountered with smooth surfaces.

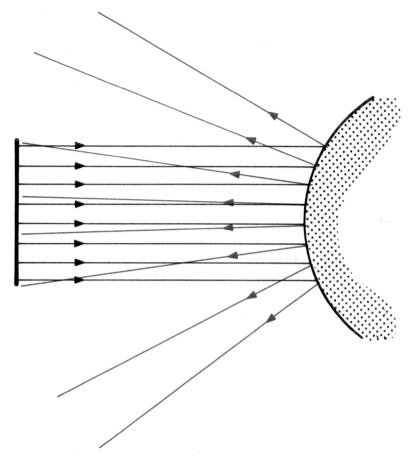

FIG. I-13. Reflection from curved surface. Beam spreading upon reflection reduces echo amplitudes.

cause complex echo voltages in which the contributions from many individual small scatterers are superimposed, as shown in Figures I-9 and I-14. The overall echo patterns are determined by numerous factors including geometric scatterer properties (size, shape, and orientation), the spatial distribution of scatterers, absorptivity and ultrasonic wavelength. Diagnostically useful information is often obtained by examining these echo patterns for features such as the rate at which their amplitudes diminish with increasing tissue depth. Frequency-dependent changes in these patterns could become an important factor in tissue identification. Scattering from biologic tissues is only poorly understood at present, and it is in this area that major advances must be achieved for greater accuracy in differential diagnosis.

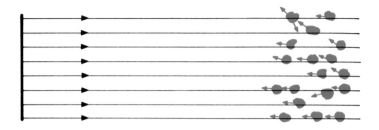

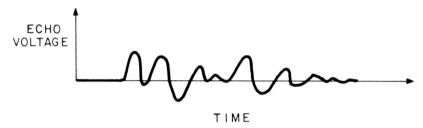

FIG. I-14. Scattering from distributed inhomogeneities. The echo voltage consists of the superposition of returns from many scatterers.

Absorption of Ultrasound

As an ultrasonic wave propagates through any medium it is progressively absorbed and ultimately appears as heat. Absorption arises from factors such as viscosity which prevent the density of a medium from responding instantaneously to ultrasonic pressure variations. In biologic media, absorption arises from many complex cellular and molecular phenomena that are, to a large extent, only poorly understood.

The heat produced through absorption is insignificant at the low ultrasonic power levels used in diagnostic systems. However, the absorptive diminution in ultrasonic wave amplitude is extremely important since it can drastically reduce echo amplitudes. Because absorption increases with increasing depth and frequency, it not only constrains the maximum tissue depth that can be examined but also limits the highest frequencies that can be employed.

Absorption increases exponentially with the distance traversed by an ultrasonic wave; as a wave travels a distance x, its pressure amplitude decreases by a factor $e^{-\alpha x}$, where α is the absorption coefficient of the medium. Absorptive losses are commonly denoted in terms of decibels (dB) as determined by computing $20 \log e^{-\alpha x}$. Since α usually increases linearly with frequency, it is common to specify absorptivity in terms of dB/cm-MHz. An absorptivity of 2 dB/cm-MHz means that at 10 MHz there will be an absorptive loss of 20 dB/cm, corresponding to a 90 per cent pressure reduction in 1 cm of tissue depth. Over a distance of 2 cm, absorption would lead to a 40-dB loss, corresponding to a pressure reduction of 99 per cent. These fractional reductions are experienced by both incident and reflected pulses.

TABLE I-3. Ultrasonic Absorption Coefficients

Substance	Absorptivity dB/cm-MHz	Reference
Aqueous humor	0.1	8
Lens	2	9
Vitreous humor	0.1	8
Fat	0.63	10

Materials vary widely in their absorption coefficients (Table I-3). Usually, materials with high propagation velocities (e.g., metals) exhibit low absorptivities, while materials with low velocities have high absorptivities. Air has such a large absorption coefficient that it cannot be used to transmit ultrasonic waves at frequencies in the MHz region. In the eye, reported absorptivities range from 0.1 dB/cm-MHz in the vitreous to 2 dB/cm-MHz in the lens. Some materials have absorption coefficients that increase with the square of ultrasonic frequency; however, most tissues exhibit values of α that are linearly proportional to frequency.[11]

Refraction of Ultrasound

An ultrasonic wave is redirected (refracted) whenever it obliquely traverses boundaries between media with different propagation velocities. Refraction is used to advantage in acoustic lenses. However, it also leads to defocusing and shifting of ultrasonic beams as they encounter curved tissue surfaces within the eye.

Figure I-15 illustrates the reflection and refraction that result when an ultrasonic pulse encounters a plane interface at an angle θ with respect to its normal. In this situation, a reflected pulse is generated at an angle θ while a transmitted pulse propagates into the second medium at an angle ϕ, which is determined from Snell's law

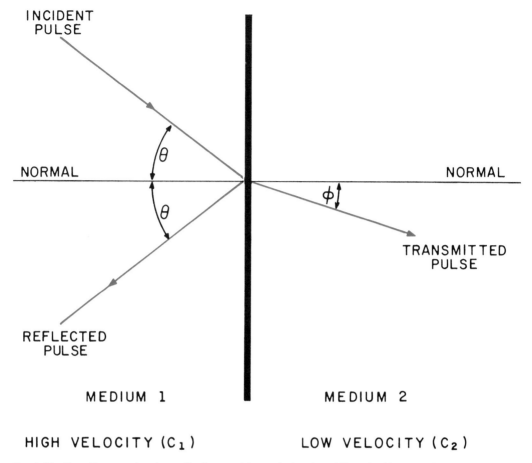

INCIDENT
PULSE

NORMAL   NORMAL

θ

θ

ϕ

TRANSMITTED
PULSE

REFLECTED
PULSE

MEDIUM 1   MEDIUM 2

HIGH VELOCITY (c_1) LOW VELOCITY (c_2)

FIG. I-15. Ray diagram showing reflection and transmission for oblique incidence at boundary between media with different propagation velocities.

$$\sin \phi = \frac{c_2}{c_1} \sin \theta$$

where c_1 and c_2 are the propagation velocities in the first and second media respectively. As evidenced by the above equation, refraction depends upon differences in propagation velocity, not upon variations in characteristic impedance. The physical basis for refraction is illustrated in Figure I-16, which shows sequential positions of an ultrasonic pulse at instants of time separated by a constant increment which for illustrative purposes is chosen to be 1 μsec. In this example, c_2 is less than c_1 so that as soon as part of the pulse enters the second medium it travels a smaller distance during the 1-μsec

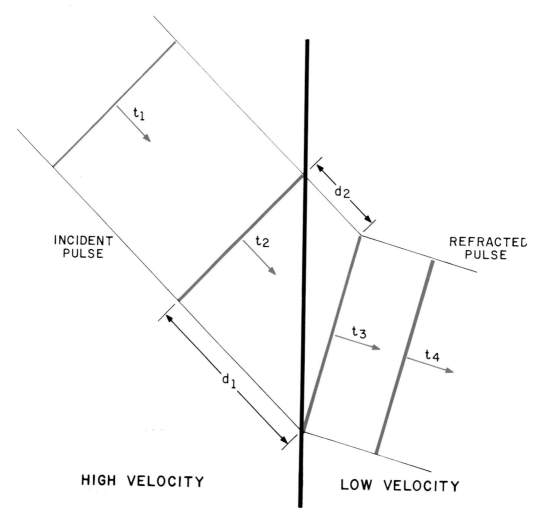

t_1

d_2

INCIDENT
PULSE

t_2

REFRACTED
PULSE

t_3

t_4

d_1

HIGH VELOCITY

LOW VELOCITY

FIG. I-16,   Sequential positions of incident and refracted ultrasonic pulses at planar boundary.

interval. At t_2, the top portion of the illustrated pulse just encounters the boundary; in the next microsecond, it will propagate over a relatively small distance, d_2, in the low-velocity medium. On the other hand, the bottom portion of the pulse is still propagating in the high-velocity medium during this period and travels a relatively large distance, d_1. The difference between d_1 and d_2 causes the transmitted pulse to be tilted to the degree noted in Snell's law.

The same type of refractive effects at curved surfaces can cause focusing or defocusing of transmitted pulses. Focusing may be accomplished by using high-velocity planoconcave lenses as illustrated in Figure I-17, which again shows the position of a propagating pulse at sequential time intervals. Focusing occurs at the con-

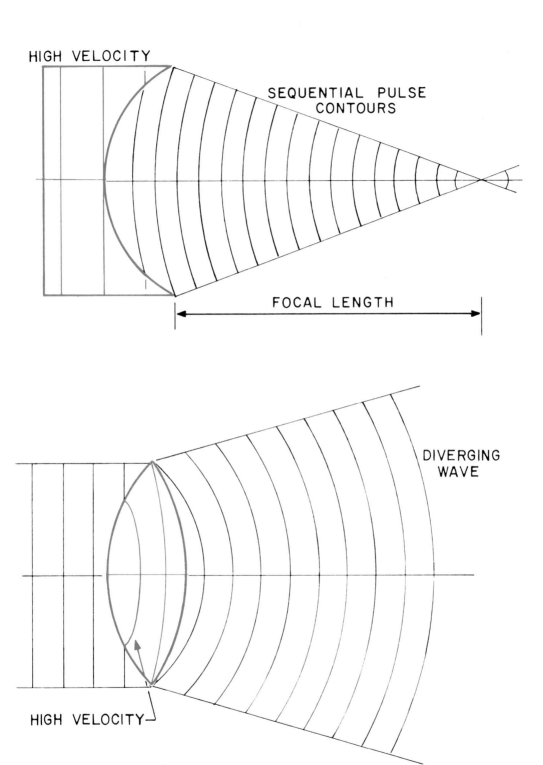

HIGH VELOCITY

SEQUENTIAL PULSE
CONTOURS

FOCAL LENGTH

DIVERGING
WAVE

HIGH VELOCITY

FIG. I-17. Refractive effects of curved high-velocity structures. *Top:* a high-velocity planoconcave lens focuses a plane ultrasonic wave. *Bottom:* the ocular lens causes defocusing.

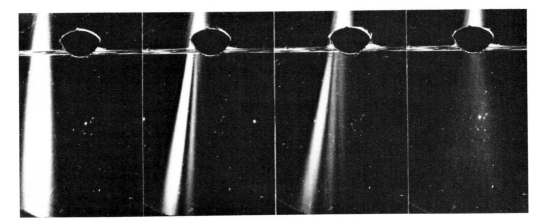

FIG. I-18. Schlieren photographs illustrating the effects of propagation through a porcine lens with a diameter of 1 cm. The beam was generated by a unfocused transducer (2.5 mm diameter, 3.5 MHz) which was scanned across the lens. The transducer is located above the lens. The horizontal line is a support membrane placed at the periphery of the lens.

cave surface because the portion of the pulse emerging from the lens travels more slowly than that portion still within the lens. The emerging pulse lies on concave contours that tend to converge at the focus of the lens. The focal length, F, is related to the lens radius of curvature, A, by the relation:

$$F = \frac{c_L}{c_L - c} A$$

where c_L and c refer to the lens and coupling medium propagation velocities. This relation is the same as that encountered in optics. (Converging optical lenses use convex surfaces because the propagation velocity of light is lower in lens materials than in air.) The

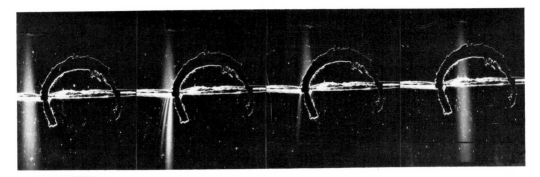

FIG. I-19. Schlieren photographs illustrating the effects of propagation through curved scleral section. The transducer is that used in Figure I-18.

actual focusing of transducer beams by acoustic lenses is modified by diffraction, which is treated in a subsequent section.

As also illustrated in Figure I-17, defocusing occurs when an ultrasonic pulse emerges from convex structures, such as the ocular lens, which exhibit high propagation velocities. In vitro experimental observation (Fig. I-18) of this effect has been obtained with a schlieren optical system which visually displays the geometry of ultrasonic beams. When a beam passes through the center of the lens, beam spreading and absorption losses are clearly demonstrated. If transmission occurs through peripheral lenticular segments, refraction leads to a shift in the direction of propagation. These effects impede examination of tissues posterior to the lens. However, propagation through the sclera does not alter beam characteristics unless the beam is almost tangent to the scleral surface[12,13,14] (Fig. I-19).

Axial Resolution

The degree to which tissue structure can be resolved with ultrasonic systems is limited in practice by factors such as absorption and diffraction. This section discusses how these phenomena affect axial (thickness) resolution. The next section discusses their impact on lateral (width) resolution.

The smallest tissue thickness that can be resolved by an ultrasonic system is termed its axial resolution and is determined by the time duration of the ultrasonic pulse. Short durations are needed to resolve thin tissue segments. This fact can be illustrated by considering the conditions needed to resolve the cornea which is typically 0.5 mm thick and gives rise to echoes separated by 0.6 μsec. Corneal echoes obtained with three different pulse durations are shown in Figure I-20. In the first two cases, the pulse duration is less than 0.6 μsec, so that the two corneal echoes can be distinguished. If the pulse duration exceeds 0.6 μsec, as in the third case, the echoes overlap and the corneal surfaces are not resolved.

In general, a pulse duration, T, yields an axial resolution equal to cT/2, where c represents the propagation velocity of the appropriate tissue structure. It is convenient to consider an average tissue velocity of 1.5 mm/μsec resulting in the relation:

$$\text{axial resolution} = 0.75\,T \quad (\text{mm})$$

where T is specified in μsec. This relation provides a convenient

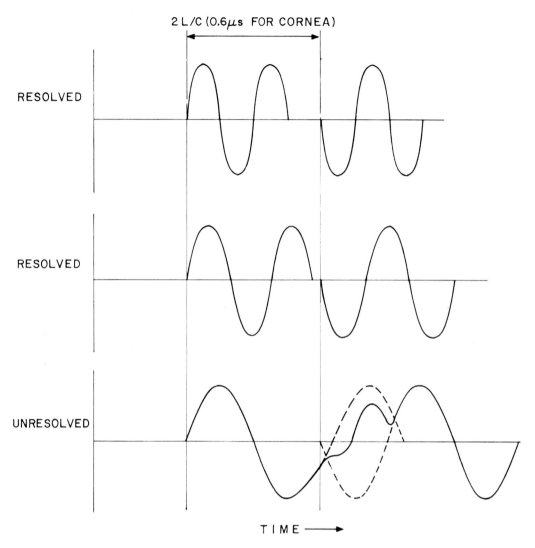

2 L/C (0.6µs FOR CORNEA)

RESOLVED

RESOLVED

UNRESOLVED

TIME ⟶

Fig. I-20. Effects of pulse duration on axial resolution. In the upper two examples, pulse duration is small enough to resolve both corneal surfaces. In the lower example, the pulse duration is too large for corneal resolution.

basis for determining axial resolution, since T can be determined by measuring the duration of an echo from a flat test object. For example, if a pulse duration of 0.15 µsec is observed, then tissue surfaces separated by 0.11 mm are resolvable. (This resolution represents the limit now attainable in clinical systems.)

Generation of ultrasonic pulses as short as 0.15 µsec necessitates careful transducer design and fabrication. Even with short excitation voltage pulses, ultrasonic pulse duration can be excessively large because of the "ringing" encountered in undamped transducers. As shown in Figure I-21, an excited transducer actually

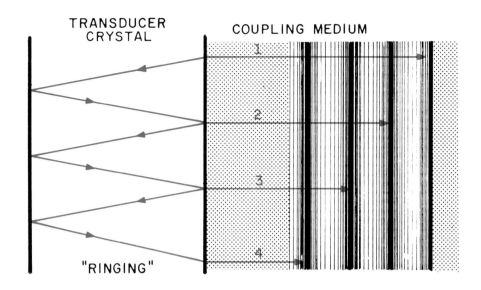

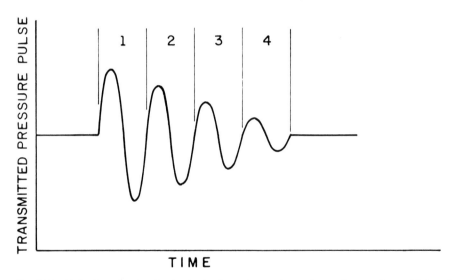

FIG. I-21. Pulse lengthening due to ringing in undamped transducer. Successive multiply reflected pulses are transmitted sequentially into the coupling medium.

generates two ultrasonic pulses at its front surface. One pulse propagates into the coupling medium while the other travels in the reverse direction through the transducer. This internal pulse repeatedly undergoes partial reflection and transmission at the two surfaces of the transducer crystal. Thus, many individual pulses, staggered in time, are transmitted into the fluid where they form a

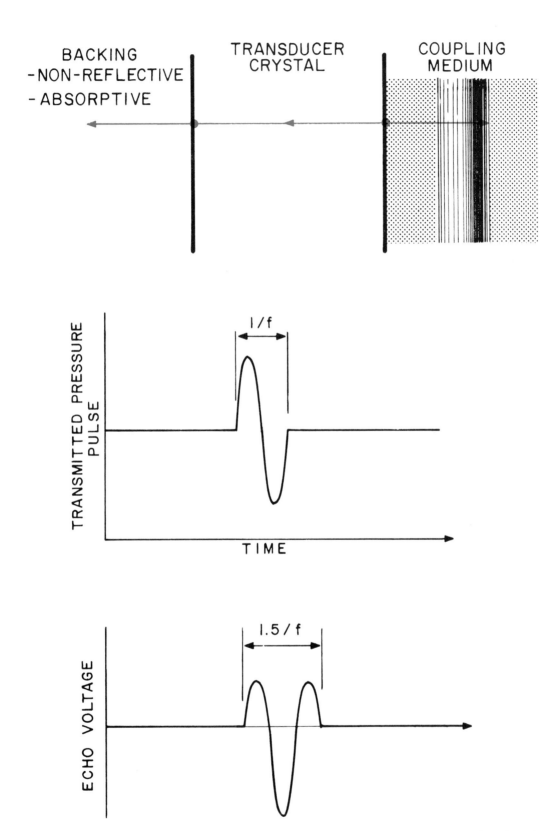

FIG. I-22. Ray diagram and waveforms for ideally backed transducer. During reception, the echo voltage is lengthened by one half cycle because of the small transit time through the transducer.

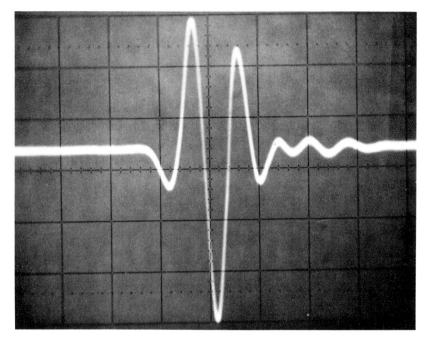

Fɪɢ. I-23. Echo voltage obtained for reflection from a flat glass plate using a damped 10 MHz transducer. Significant pulse amplitudes occur within a 0.15-μsec interval. Horizontal scale, 0.10 μsec/cm.

composite pulse of long duration. The same type of internal reflections occur during reception of ultrasonic echoes, further lengthening the effective pulse duration.

In a damped transducer internal reflections are suppressed by bonding a backing section to the rear crystal surface. The acoustic impedance of the backing material is matched to that of the crystal. Exact impedance matching reduces the reflection coefficient to zero, eliminating internal reflections. As shown in Figure I-22, echoes obtained with perfect matching have a total duration equal to 1.5/f, where f is the crystal's resonant frequency. Thus, pulse duration can be minimized by using transducers with high resonant frequencies. Although other electrical and mechanical considerations complicate this simple discussion,[15,16] damped transducers with responses close to the ideal case have been fabricated for diagnostic applications (Fig. I-23).

Short pulses commensurate with high-quality axial resolution can be achieved at high frequencies. However, absorption increases with frequency and the attendant diminution of echo amplitude impedes the use of resonant frequencies above 20 MHz for ocular examinations. At this center frequency, the minimum pulse duration is 0.075 μsec and an axial resolution of 0.056 mm is theoretically achievable; in practice, resolution on the order of 0.1 mm has been achieved. Orbital examinations require deeper tissue penetration and increased absorption losses hinder the use of frequencies above 10 MHz.

Lateral Resolution

Detailed examinations of the eye and orbit place stringent requirements not only on axial resolution but also on lateral resolution (sometimes specified in terms of angular or azimuthal resolution). Lateral resolution is equal to the width of the ultrasonic beam generated by the transducer. Small beamwidths are needed to measure lateral dimensions accurately, distinguish small objects, and delineate tissue contours.

The importance of lateral resolution is exemplified in the situation where a small reflecting object (e.g., an intraocular foreign body) is being examined. As shown in Figure I-24, the object will generate echoes as long as it is situated within the ultrasonic beam, so that its lateral position and size cannot be accurately assessed with a wide

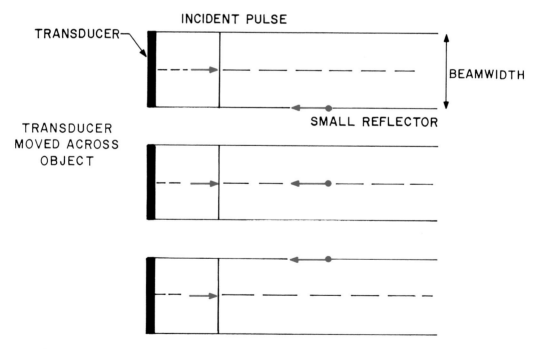

FIG. I-24. Diagrams illustrating lateral resolution which is equal to the width of an ultrasonic beam. A small reflector will generate echoes as long as it is located within the beamwidth; this is illustrated for three reflector postions.

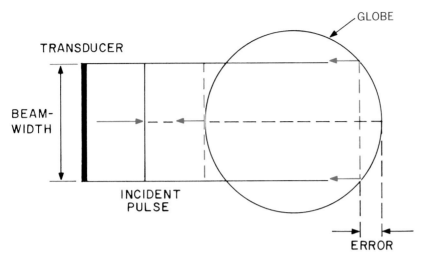

FIG. I-25. Biometric error due to large beamwidth. Initial portion of echo from posterior wall arises from off-axis points yielding an erroneously short measure of axial length.

beamwidth. In addition, if several such reflectors are located at the same tissue depth, they cannot be identified as separate entities unless their lateral spacing exceeds the beamwidth.

Lateral resolution is also a critical factor in examination of curved ocular surfaces. In axial length determinations, for example, a wide ultrasonic beam will give rise to retinal echoes originating from regions anterior to the point of interest (Fig. I-25). Accordingly, the vitreous chamber appears to have an erroneously shallow depth: a beamwidth of 1 cm can cause an error of 1 mm. Similar effects can obscure small surface irregularities that accompany initial tumor development and degenerative processes.

It might seem that ultrasonic beamwidths could be determined by the ray tracing techniques employed in geometric optics. However, this simple approach is inadequate since it does not account for diffraction which arises from the finite size of ultrasonic wavelengths. The following discussion shows how diffraction limits the lateral resolution attainable with, first, unfocused and, second, focused transducers.

Unfocused Transducers

Pulses produced by an unfocused transducer can be considered to arise from Huygens' point sources distributed over the flat circular surface of the transducer. Huygens' sources are used to describe the radiation of ultrasound waves in the same manner as that used

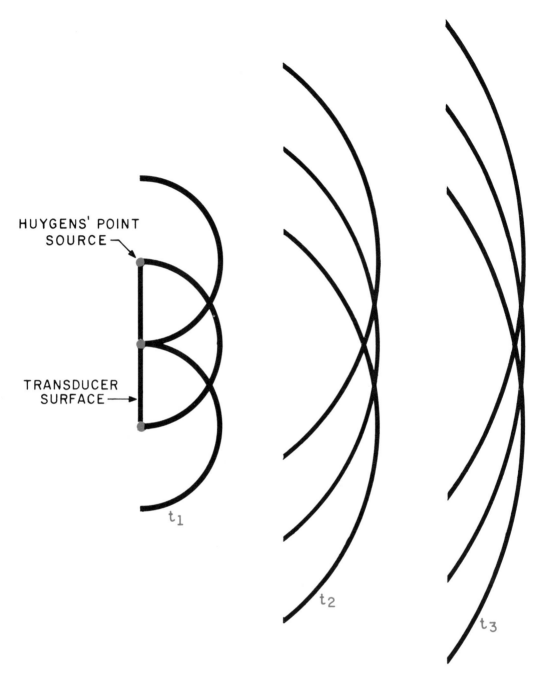

HUYGENS' POINT
SOURCE

TRANSDUCER
SURFACE

t_1

t_2

t_3

FIG. I-26. Ultrasonic wavefronts emanating from three Huygens' point sources. Resultant pulse components are shown at successive time intervals t_1, t_2, t_3.

when treating the radiation of light. Figure I-26 depicts the generation of an ultrasonic pulse from the superposition of spherical ultrasonic wavelets emanating from each point source. (For clarity, only three sources are diagrammed.) When a transducer is excited, each wavelet spreads through the transmission medium, causing large pressure amplitudes at points of constructive interference. On the other hand, no pressure variations occur at points of destructive interference where the component compressions from some point sources are exactly cancelled by the simultaneous rarefaction components from other sources. As the wavelets progressively spread through the medium, several distinctive effects are observed which have led to the concepts of near field (e.g., conditions at t_1) and far field (e.g., conditions at t_3).

Near-field (Fresnel region) conditions apply when the pulse is still near the transducer. The length of the near field is equal to a^2/Λ,

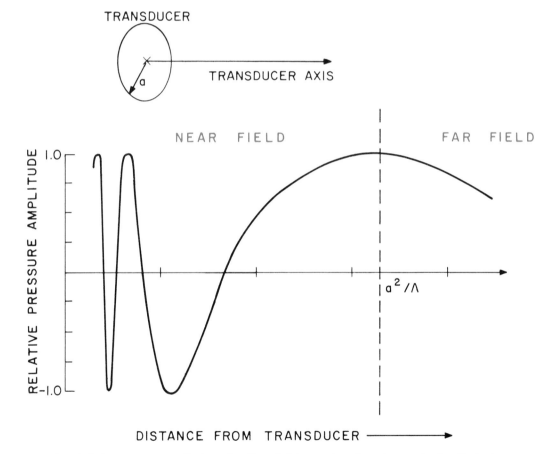

FIG. I-27. Relative pressure amplitude as function of distance along transducer axis. Amplitude decreases monotonically for distances larger than a^2/Λ.

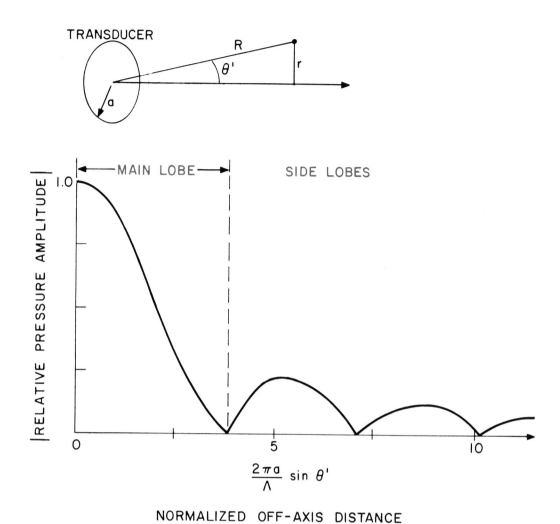

FIG. I-28. Dependence of far-field pressure amplitude upon angular position. Plot is drawn for points at a fixed distance, R, from transducer center and abscissa values are proportional to off-axis distance, r.

where a is the radius of the transducer rim. Here, little beam spreading occurs and the beamwidth is equal to the transducer diameter. Pulse amplitudes vary rapidly over small distances because of the complex interference patterns in this region. The sudden amplitude variations are strongly evident at points situated on the transducer axis (Fig. I-27). When the pulse passes from this region and enters the far field it experiences a gradual amplitude reduction due to far-field beam spreading.

In the far field (Fraunhofer region), the beamwidth progressively increases as the pulse travels a greater distance, R, from the transducer. If the beam cross section is examined, a distinctive lobed

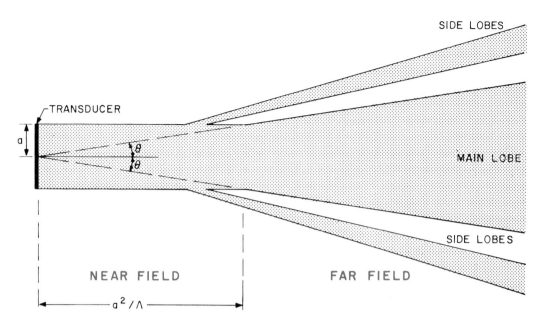

FIG. I-29. Beam pattern of an unfocused transducer showing near-field and far-field regions. The 3-dB angular width of the main lobe is 2 θ.

pattern is seen (Figs. I-28 and I-29). The central main lobe contains more than 80 per cent of the ultrasonic energy and exhibits a gradually tapered pressure amplitude. There are also several peripheral side lobes encircling the main lobe. Side lobes are characterized by small pressure amplitudes and are formed because of weak constructive interference; these low-amplitude regions result in corresponding weak tissue echoes which can assume importance if highly sensitive electronic amplifiers are used.

The effective beamwidth in the far field is usually measured between those points in the main lobe where the pressure amplitude falls by 3 dB to 70 per cent of its maximum value; this width is equal to 0.5 (Λ/a)R. Often it is more meaningful to specify the angle that describes the 3-dB periphery of the main lobe (Fig. I-29); this angle (in radians) is approximately equal to 0.5 Λ/a.

Ultrasonic wavelength and transducer dimensions determine both near-field and far-field characteristics. Figure I-30 summarizes the effects of Λ on beam characteristics. As Λ decreases (frequency increases) the length of the near field increases and the far-field beamwidth becomes narrower. Typically, a is 2.5 mm and Λ is 0.1 mm (15 MHz), yielding a near-field length of 62.5 mm and a far-field beam angle of 1.2 degrees.

Ocular examinations with unfocused transducers are usually

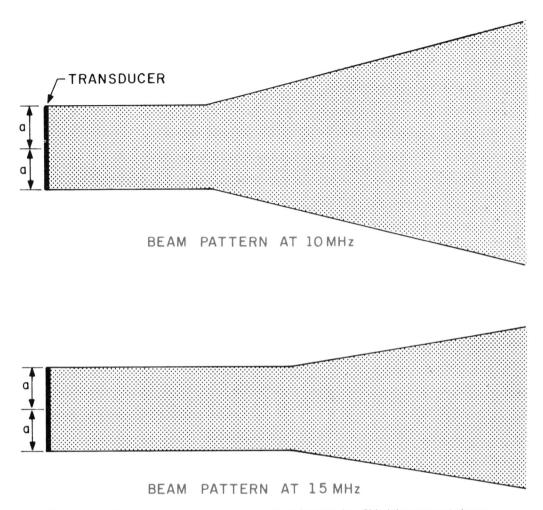

TRANSDUCER

a

a

BEAM PATTERN AT 10 MHz

a

a

BEAM PATTERN AT 15 MHz

FIG. I-30. Beam patterns of unfocused transducer at two frequencies. Side lobes are not shown.

performed within the near field where the beam is typically 5 mm wide. This degree of lateral resolution, too coarse for many ophthalmic examinations, can be improved by focusing as discussed below.

Focused Transducers

Transducers are focused by using acoustic lenses, as discussed in connection with refraction. However, the width of the resultant beam is not zero at the focal point as diagrammed in Figure I-17; rather, diffraction causes a small but finite beamwidth that depends on ultrasonic wavelength and transducer parameters.

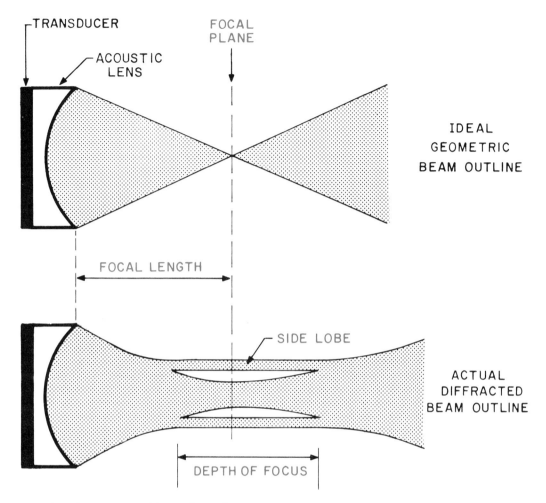

FIG. I-31. Beam pattern of focused transducer.

Analyses treating Huygens' point sources show that focused beams have profiles such as that shown in Figure I-31. In the focal plane, the beam exhibits a lobed structure of the same type encountered under unfocused far-field conditions. Here, the side lobes straddle the narrow focused region and the main lobe beamwidth is equal to $0.5(\Lambda/a) F$, where F is the focal length of the transducer and a again represents the radius of the transducer rim. Typically, Λ is 0.1 mm (15 MHz), a is 5 mm, and F is 30 mm, resulting in a beamwidth of 0.30 mm. The same transducer dimensions provide smaller beamwidths as frequency is increased.

In the design of clinical focused transducers, the desired beamwidth can be obtained by proper selection of wavelength and transducer parameters (a and F). However, several other factors must be considered when choosing a transducer which will permit adequate tissue examination.[17] Focal lengths must be chosen to provide focusing in the desired tissue region; focal lengths of 30 mm allow for intraocular focusing while larger focal lengths are needed for deeper orbital examinations. Furthermore, high frequencies cannot be used in the orbit because of absorption. These combined limitations on focal lengths and frequencies constrain lateral resolution in the orbit more severely than in the eye. In addition, clinical transducers must be weakly focused to generate narrow beams over relatively long tissue depths. Strong focusing, obtained with very large transducer diameters, is not usually desirable; although strong focusing produces very narrow beamwidths, it can do so only over unacceptably shallow tissue depths.

These discussions of unfocused and focused transducer beam patterns are applicable when the ultrasonic pulse contains several cycles of oscillation. They must be modified if the transducer generates a very short pulse such as the single cycle pulse illustrated in Figure I-22. Extremely short pulse durations do not allow enough time for standard interference patterns to develop. For a single-cycle pulse, the 3-dB main lobe width is equal to that quoted above but side lobe patterns and near-field characteristics differ in several respects from those discussed above.[18]

Composite Resolution

Composite (axial and lateral) resolution depends on frequency and transducer geometry. These factors in turn are influenced by the type of examination to be made. Ocular examinations present an environment where high-quality resolution can be achieved; orbital examinations must be carried out at lower resolution.

For an ideal transducer, both components of resolution improve as resonant frequency is increased; however, absorption also increases with frequency and limits the value that can be used in practice. In the eye, frequencies near 20 MHz have been used to attain an axial resolution of 0.1 mm; focal lengths of 30 mm (midvitreous focusing) together with a transducer radius of 5 mm allow lateral resolution of 0.2 mm. In orbital examinations, increased absorption limits frequencies to a maximum of 10 MHz. These low frequencies and necessarily long focal lengths (e.g., 60 mm) reduce axial resolution to approximately 0.3 mm and lateral resolution to 0.9 mm.

The discussions in the preceding sections have concerned the pulse-echo technique which is the most commonly used approach in medical ultrasonography. Other types of ultrasonic medical systems utilize Doppler, through-transmission, and holographic techniques.

Ultrasonic Doppler systems[19] measure the velocity of moving tissue elements such as red blood cells by sensing the frequency shift that occurs upon reflection from moving interfaces. Blood velocity in the ophthalmic artery, for example, can be established from the Doppler shift that occurs at a known angle of beam incidence. Flow rates can then be calculated if the vessel diameter is known; in some cases, this diameter can be ascertained from pulse-echo measurements.

Through-transmission systems use matched transmitting and receiving transducers placed across opposite surfaces of the body (e.g., across the breast). This technique can provide a measure of total ultrasonic attenuation along a chosen axis in the body. Through-transmission approaches have not been used in ophthalmology because of a lack of suitable transmission paths.

Ultrasonic holography[20,21] utilizes principles developed for optical holography. A continuous sinusoidal ultrasonic wave, after passing through the examined organ, is superimposed on a reference beam to form an acoustic hologram. Special optical techniques can be used to record the hologram on film which is placed in a coherent optical system to produce a three-dimensional representation of the imaged organ. These representations are distorted because of the large disparity between ultrasonic wavelengths and optical wavelengths used in image reconstruction. Because of this and other difficulties, much development will be required before useful holographic imaging of the eye and orbit can be achieved routinely.

Measurement of Ultrasonic Beam Parameters

Two basic factors in ultrasonic systems are the geometric features of ultrasonic beams (i.e., their shape, focal zone dimensions, etc.) and the ultrasonic intensity levels which are generated. These parameters must often be accurately determined for research applications. They can be studied by techniques which sense relatively minor perturbations associated with the physical attributes of ultrasonic radiation. Geometric beam structure can be assessed with small piezoelectric probes or scans of simple targets (e.g., wires) as described in Chapter II. Alternatively, this type of information can be obtained from schlieren optical systems as described below. Ultrasonic intensity levels are most commonly determined from radiation pressure measurements, also described below.

Schlieren Systems

Schlieren techniques use an optical system to produce a visible image of an ultrasonic beam. The light intensity at each point in a schlieren image is related to the average pressure amplitude within the imaged beam and provides a semiquantitative measure of beam strength.

In a schlieren system (Fig. I-32) a point source of light and a collimating lens combine to produce a plane wave of light which passes through a fluid-filled optical cell. The light exiting from the cell is focused by an integrating lens upon a small, opaque optical stop. If there are no ultrasonic waves propagating through the fluid in the optical cell, all light is blocked by the stop.

The transducer to be studied is placed in the optical cell and excited with a continuous-wave sinusoidal voltage. Ultrasonic waves perturb the index of refraction within the cell fluid so that the light emerging from the cell is nonplanar and, therefore, is no longer completely focused on the stop. That portion of light bypassing the stop contains spatial and amplitude information relating to beam structure. A reimaging lens converts this information into image form. (If the optical stop were not used, unaffected portions of the incident light would obscure the schlieren image.)

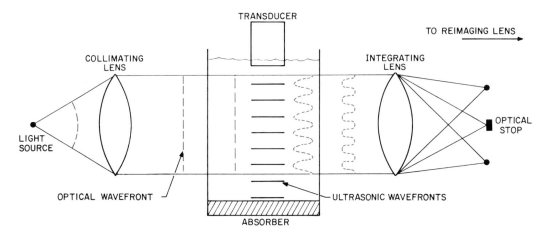

FIG. I-32. Diagram of schlieren system.

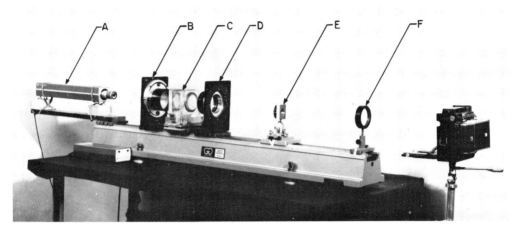

FIG.I-33. Schlieren system showing laser (A) used with spatial filter to simulate point source. Also shown are collimating lens (B), optical cell (C), integrating lens (D), optical stop mount (E) and reimaging lens (F). Noncoherent light sources can also be utilized in schlieren imaging.

Sensitive schlieren systems can be used to examine pulsed rather than continuous-wave beams, and similar optical systems (e.g., Bragg visualization systems) can be used to produce images of tissue structure.[22] The schlieren system shown in Figure I-33 has been extremely useful in studies of tissue propagation effects (Figs. I-18 and I-19).

Intensity Measurements

Ultrasonic intensity is defined as the amount of ultrasonic energy passing through a unit area in a unit time. In a plane ultrasonic wave the intensity, I, is simply related to the amplitude, p(t), of the ultrasonic pressure variations and the characteristic impedance of the transmission medium:

$$I = \frac{\overline{p^2(t)}}{Z}$$

where the superscript bar denotes an average over time. (I is usually specified in watts/cm^2.)

Determination of intensity usually involves a measurement of the power, P, (energy per unit time) radiated by a transducer through a cross-sectional area, W. Intensity is then calculated by dividing the measured power by this area, i.e.,

$$I = P/W.$$

The average ultrasonic power, P, emanating from a diagnostic transducer can be measured by calorimetry or by radiation pressure techniques. In calorimetry, a beam propagates through a thermally isolated fluid of known absorptivity. The temperature rise stemming from absorption of the incident ultrasonic beam is used to determine the incident ultrasonic power.

Radiation pressure can also be used to determine ultrasonic power. In the most common radiation pressure technique a beam is reflected at 45 degrees by a highly reflective plate suspended from an analytic balance. The balance serves to measure the small force on the plate which results from the redirection of wave momentum. This force is directly related to the incident ultrasonic power; a power level of one milliwatt produces a force of 0.067 milligram. Carefully designed measuring systems with sensitive balances are capable of measuring the low power levels encountered in diagnostic systems.[23]

In practice, there are several ways of specifying ultrasonic intensity. These depend upon the choice of cross-sectional area, W, and the selection of an appropriate temporal averaging interval. W can be selected to provide measures of average or peak spatial intensities. For example, average spatial intensity can be measured over the half-power (3-dB) points of a focused beam. Alternatively, the peak spatial intensity can be determined by defining W as a small, differential area centered at the focal point. Furthermore, diagnostic systems emit short ultrasonic pulses at regular intervals, and there are two meaningful ways of defining an appropriate period for temporal averaging. One approach specifies the average intensity during the "on time" of the ultrasonic pulse. Another approach quotes the average intensity existing between the initiation of one pulse and the onset of the next. Intensities arrived at using either of these averaging periods are related by the duty cycle of the system, which is the ratio of pulse duration to pulse repetition interval.

Biological Effects of High-intensity Ultrasound

In view of the widespread application of diagnostic ultrasound, it is important to note that the low intensities employed in current systems pose no known threat of tissue damage. Animal studies, the absence of reports of clinical damage, and extrapolation of laboratory data all point to the safety afforded by present diagnostic

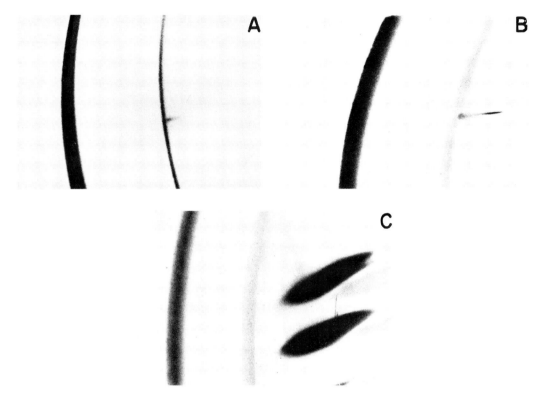

FIG. I-34. Slit-lamp photographs of experimental cataracts in the rabbit lens. *A*: Incipient haze cataract. *B*: Anterior haze cataract with incipient, thread-like opaque cataract. *C*: Large opaque cataracts produced by identical exposures at adjacent lenticular sites.

systems.[24,25] At high intensities, however, animal studies reveal that physical alterations can be produced in ocular tissues.

The cataractogenic effects of high-intensity ultrasound have been examined by several investigators starting with Zeiss[26] in 1938. Further work by Lavine et al.[27] and Torchia, Purnell and Sokollu[28] served to define threshold values of intensity and exposure time needed to produce cataracts in the rabbit eye. Work in our laboratories has been devoted to studying cataract production at higher frequencies and intensities.[29,30] In these in vivo studies, focused continuous-wave ultrasound (0.4 mm beamwidth) was applied to a large series of rabbit eyes. The smallest lesions observed were haze cataracts discernible only with slit lamp techniques as shown in Figure I-34. At progressively higher exposures, haze cataracts become larger and eventually develop a thread-like region of total opacity. At still higher exposures, the totally opaque region grows rapidly and can extend throughout the entire lens thickness. All of these cataracts are formed immediately and are irreversible.

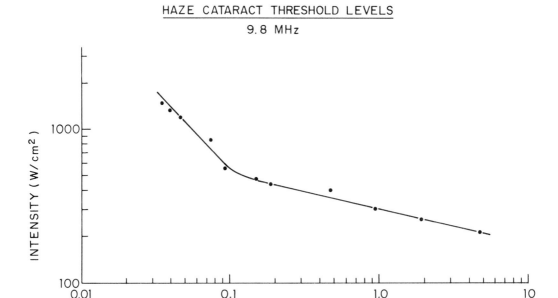

HAZE CATARACT THRESHOLD LEVELS
9.8 MHz

FIG. I-35. Intensity levels and exposure durations needed to produce haze cataracts at 9.8 MHz. Average intensity within the 3-dB beamwidth is specified.

The intensity exposure-time conjugates required to produce minimal haze cataracts are shown in Figure I-35. The requisite intensity levels far exceed the time-averaged intensities used in diagnosis, which are less than 0.1 watt/cm^2 (100 milliwatts/cm^2). The "threshold" curve exhibits two distinct regions. For times shorter than 100 msec, the threshold intensity is inversely proportional to exposure time, implying that a constant energy level is needed for cataract production. For lower intensities, and correspondingly longer exposure times (longer than 100 msec), disproportionately high intensities are required. These data and other observations suggest that a thermal mechanism is responsible for cataract production. At high intensities, cataracts are produced after the absorption of a constant amount of energy has established a "critical" temperature within the lens. At lower intensities, the required exposure times are long enough to permit significant amounts of heat to be conducted from the insonified volume; this conduction necessitates relatively high energy levels to establish the critical temperature within the lens.[31]

Other types of ocular damage that have been examined experimentally include chorioretinal lesions, vitreous liquefaction and corneal opacification. Baum[32] and Moore et al.[33] studied effects at frequencies near 1 MHz, intensities on the order of 1 watt/cm^2, and

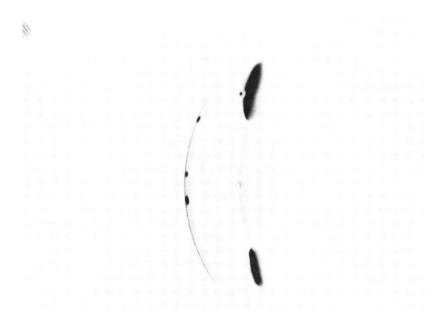

FIG. I-36. Slit-lamp photograph demonstrating small corneal opacities produced by insonification at adjacent sites.

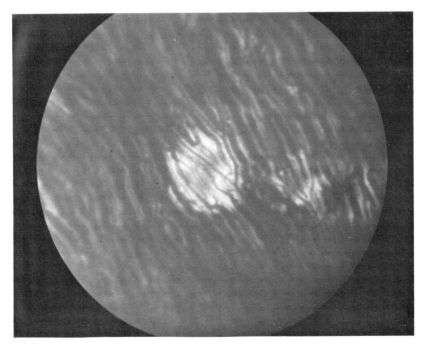

FIG. I-37. Funduscopic photograph showing effects of high-intensity ultrasound on choroidal vasculature.

time durations of a few minutes. They observed both reversible and irreversible effects including corneal opacification, conjunctival injection, and edema of the ciliary body. Baum concluded that the "safe" range for ultrasonic irradiation was 0.25 watts/cm² for 5 min to 1.0 watt/cm² for 3 min. Donn[34] reported that liquefaction of the vitreous body could not be accomplished at 900 watts/cm² but occurred at lower levels if an air bubble had been previously injected into the vitreous. Rosenberg and Purnell[35] have reported the production of gross visible lesions of the ciliary body. Purnell, Sokollu, Torchia, and Taner[36] have studied the production of chorioretinal lesions by ultrasound at 7 MHz. At the onset of insonification, they noted a blanching of choroidal circulation which might tend to increase the efficacy of thermal damage mechanisms.

Figures I-36 and I-37 show experimental in vivo results[37] obtained in our laboratories using the same beam characteristics employed in the cataract studies described above. Figure I-36 shows the localized corneal opacities which can be produced at intensities that exceed cataractogenic levels. These lesions first appear in the central zone of the corneal stroma and are irreversible. Choroidal damage, produced in albino rabbits under similar experimental conditions, is illustrated in Figure I-37. This type of lesion can be

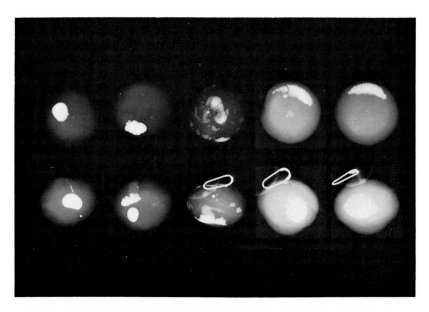

FIG. I-38. X-rays of intact bovine eyes after injection of Ethiodol, a radiopaque oil-based dye. *Far left:* Typical control eye, injected with dye but not irradiated. *Second:* An eye after 20 min of continuous-wave irradiation; *third:* after 10 min of pulsed irradiation (pulse repetition frequency 10 Hz); *fourth:* after 2 min of pulsed irradiation (6 Hz); *fifth:* after 20 min of pulsed irradiation (6 Hz). Upper and lower rows show X-rays taken in orthogonal planes.

seen to develop during insonification and involves a diminution of circulation within a well-defined area of the choroidal vascular bed. In some cases, the effect is transitory and normal circulation resumes within a few seconds after insonification ceases. Permanent damage as shown here can lead to subsequent disruptive and degenerative changes, including scleral ectasia.

Several phenomena might be involved in producing tissue alterations that have been observed experimentally. Heat production, mediated through absorption, would seem to be the direct cause of many types of damage. Other damage mechanisms might involve mechanical stressing, cavitation, streaming, and radiation pressure. Cavitation involves the sudden collapse of gas bubbles that can form if sufficiently large pressure excursions are established within an ultrasonic beam. Cavitation is accompanied by extremely large pressures and other phenomena that can cause gross tissue disruption. Streaming results from average pressure gradients set up by small nonlinear effects in the acoustic properties of fluids. On a large scale, streaming can cause flow within ocular fluids; on a small scale, streaming forces can cause cellular damage. Radiation pressure is a steady force exerted at reflective tissue boundaries. In animal experiments, radiation pressure has been observed to cause movements of detached retinas[36] and vitreous opacities.[38] The last phenomenon shows potential application in clinical dispersion of vitreous hemorrhage (Fig. I-38).

Much research remains to be performed before ultrasonically induced tissue alterations are understood in detail. This research will be important in guiding the development of future diagnostic systems and is essential if promising therapeutic applications of ultrasound in ophthalmology are to be evaluated. In terms of present clinical safety, it is important to note that the above examples of tissue alterations were achieved at intensity levels far exceeding those used in diagnostic systems. There has not been any confirmed report of ocular damage encountered at diagnostic levels. In fact, animal experiments using 1- to 4-hr exposures to a diagnostic system failed to produce detectable structural changes in the eye.[25]

References Cited

1. Mundt, G. H., and Hughes, W. F.: Ultrasonics in ocular diagnosis. Am. J. Ophthalmol., 41:488–498, 1956.
2. Willard, G.: Temperature coefficients of ultrasonic velocity in solutions. J. Acoust. Soc. Am., 19:235–241, 1947.
3. Jansson, F., and Kock, E.: Determination of the velocity of ultrasound in the human lens and vitreous. Acta Ophthalmol., 40:420–433, 1962.

4. Frucht, A. H.: Die Schallgeschwindigkeit in Menoschlichen und Tierischen Geweben. Z. Ges. Exp. Med., 120:526–557, 1953.
5. Coleman, D. J., Lizzi, F. L., Franzen, L. A., and Abramson, D. H.: A determination of the velocity of ultrasound in cataractous lenses. In: Ultrasonography in Ophthalmology. Edited by J. Francois and F. Goes. Basel, S. Karger, 1975, pp. 246–251.
6. Oksala, A., and Lehtinen, A.: Measurement of the velocity of sound in some parts of the eye. Acta Ophthalmol., 36:633–639, 1958.
7. Baum, G., and Greenwood, I.: The application of ultrasonic locating techniques to ophthalmology; part I. Am. J. Ophthalmol., 46:319–329, 1958.
8. Begui, Z. E.: Acoustic properties of the refractive media of the eye. J. Acoust. Soc. Am., 26:365–368, 1954.
9. Filipczynski, L., et al.: Visualizing internal structures of the eye by means of ultrasonics. Proc. Vibr. Probl., 4:357–368, 1967.
10. Wells, P. N. T.: Physical Principles of Ultrasonic Diagnosis. New York, Academic Press, 1969, p. 25.
11. Dunn, F.: Ultrasonic absorption by biological materials. In: Ultrasonic Energy. Edited by Elizabeth Kelly. Urbana, University of Illinois Press, 1965, pp. 51–65.
12. Lizzi, F., Burt, W., and Coleman, D. J.: Effects of ocular structures on the propagation of ultrasound in the eye. Arch. Ophthalmol., 84:635–640, 1970.
13. Oksala, A., and Hakkinen, L.: Experimental studies of the behavior of ultrasound in the sclera and cornea. In: Ophthalmic Ultrasound. Edited by K. Gitter, A. Keeney, L. Sarin and D. Meyer. St. Louis, C. V. Mosby Co., 1969, pp. 59–63.
14. Oksala, A., and Varonen, E.: The effect of the lens on the ultrasonic field in diagnosis of the eye by ultrasound. Acta Ophthalmol., 43:260–267, 1965.
15. Kossoff, G.: The effects of backing and matching on the performance of piezoelectric ceramic transducers. IEEE Trans. Sonics Ultrason., 13:20–30, 1966.
16. Redwood, M.: Transient performance of a piezoelectric transducer. J. Acoust. Soc. Am., 33:527–535, 1961.
17. Kossoff, G.: Design of narrow beamwidth transducers. J. Acoust. Soc. Am., 35:905–912, 1963.
18. Lizzi, F.: Transient radiation patterns in ophthalmic ultrasonography. Doctoral thesis, Columbia University, School of Engineering and Applied Sciences, New York, 1971.
19. Baker, D. W.: Pulsed doppler blood-flow sensing. IEEE Trans. Sonics Ultrason., 17:170–185, 1970.
20. Metherell, A. F., El-Sum. H. M. A., Dreher, J. J., and Larmore, L.: Introduction to acoustical holography. J. Acoust. Soc. Am., 42:733–742, 1967.
21. Greguss, P., and Bertenyi, A.: Ultrasonic holography in ophthalmology. In: Ophthalmic Ultrasound. Edited by K. A. Gitter, A. H. Keeney, L. K. Sarin, and D. Meyer. St. Louis, C. V. Mosby Co., 1969, pp. 81–87.
22. Smith, R. A., Wade, G., Powers, J., and Landry, J.: Studies of resolution in a Bragg imaging system. J. Acoust. Soc. Am., 49:1062–1068, 1971.
23. Rooney, J. A.: Determination of acoustic power outputs in the microwatt-milliwatt range. Ultrasound Med. Biol., 1:13–16, 1973.
24. Dunn, F. and Fry, F.: Ultrasonic threshold dosages for the mammalian central nervous system. IEEE Trans. Biomed. Eng. 18:253–256, 1971.
25. Ziskin, M., Romayandanda, N., and Harris, K.: Ophthalmologic effect of ultrasound at diagnostic intensities. J. Clin. Ultrasound, 2:119–122, 1974.
26. Zeiss, E.: Effects of ultrasound on excised bovine lenses. Graefe. Arch. Ophthalmol., 139:301–322, 1938.
27. Lavine, O., et al.: Effects of ultrasonic waves on the refractive media of the eye. Arch. Ophthalmol., 47:204–219, 1952.
28. Torchia, R. T., Purnell, E. W., and Sokollu, A.: Cataract production by ultrasound. Am. J. Ophthalmol., 64:305–309, 1967.
29. Coleman, D. J., Lizzi, F., Burt, W., and Wen, H.: Some properties of ultrasonically induced cataracts. Am. J. Ophthalmol., 71:1284–1288, 1971.

30. Lizzi, F. L., Packer, A. J., and Coleman, D. J.: Experimental cataract production by high frequency ultrasound. Submitted for publication.
31. Carstensen, E. L., Miller, M. W., and Linke, C. A.: Biological effects of ultrasound. J. Biol. Phys. 2:173–192, 1974.
32. Baum, G.: The effect of ultrasonic radiation upon the eye and ocular adnexa. Am. J. Ophthalmol., 42:696–706, 1956.
33. Moore, C. H., et al.: Some effects of ultrasonic energy on the rabbit eye, Arch. Ophthalmol., 54:922–930, 1955.
34. Donn, A.: Ultrasonic wave liquefaction of vitreous humor in living rabbits. Arch. Ophthalmol., 53:215–223, 1955.
35. Rosenberg, R. S., and Purnell, E. W.: Effects of ultrasonic radiation to the ciliary body. Am. J. Ophthalmol., 63:403–409, 1967.
36. Purnell, E. W., Sokollu, A., Torchia, R., and Taner, N.: Focal chorioretinitis produced by ultrasound. Invest. Ophthalmol., 3:657–664, 1964.
37. Lizzi, F. L., Packer, A. J., and Coleman, D. J.: Experimental ocular lesions produced by high-frequency ultrasound. Presented at the 1976 Annual Meeting of the Acoustical Society of America, Washington, 1976.
38. Coleman, D. J., Lizzi, F., Weininger, R., and Burt, W.: Vitreous dispersion by ultrasound. Ann. Ophthalmol., 2:389–396, 1970.

Additional References

Hueter, T., and Bolt, R.: Sonics. Techniques for the Use of Sound and Ultrasound in Engineering and Science. New York, John Wiley and Sons, Inc., 1955.
Kinsler, L., and Frey, A.: Fundamentals of Acoustics, 2nd ed. New York, John Wiley and Sons, Inc., 1962.

II

Ultrasonic
Systems

THREE types of ultrasonic systems find application in ophthalmology; these have been termed A-, B- and M-mode systems. Each of these presents morphologic information in a distinctive display format. A-mode systems graphically display tissue boundaries as a function of distance along any selected axis (Fig. II-1). These systems, the first to be used in ophthalmology, are important for quantifying echo characteristics and for biometric applications. B-mode systems,[1] introduced in the late 1950s, produce cross-sectional representations of ocular and orbital anatomy (Fig. II-2) which are readily interpreted; these images have proven extremely useful in the diagnosis of a broad spectrum of disease states. M-mode systems present graphical displays showing time histories of tissue motion along a selected axis of the eye (Fig. II-3).

While the basic physical principles discussed in Chapter I underlie the operation of all ultrasonic systems, it is electronic technology which translates these principles into practical clinical systems. Electronic devices are used in generating ultrasonic pulses, processing echoes and displaying ultrasonograms. This chapter describes how electronic units are used in A-, B- and M-mode systems and how they influence the quality of clinical results. It also discusses the means of recognizing and eliminating misleading results stemming from improper system adjustments.

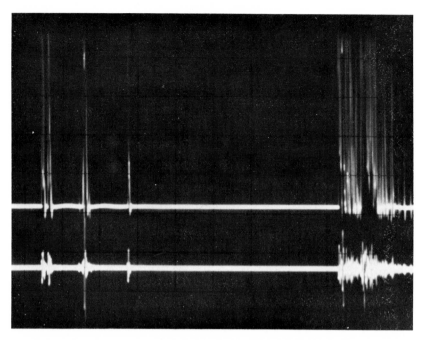

FIG. II-1. A-mode results showing effective tissue reflectivity (vertical axis) versus time or, equivalently, distance. Video signals (*top*) and R.F. signals (*bottom*) arise from boundaries shown in Figure I-8.

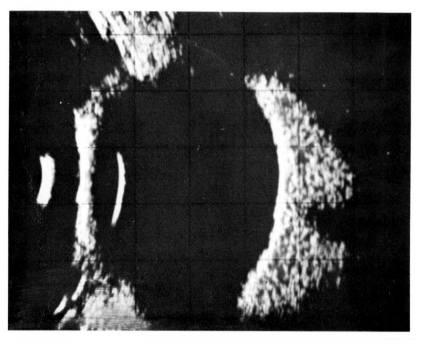

FIG. II-2. B-mode image of normal eye, depicting major ocular structures and retrobulbar fat. The nonreflective optic nerve appears as a dark region within the speckled fat pattern.

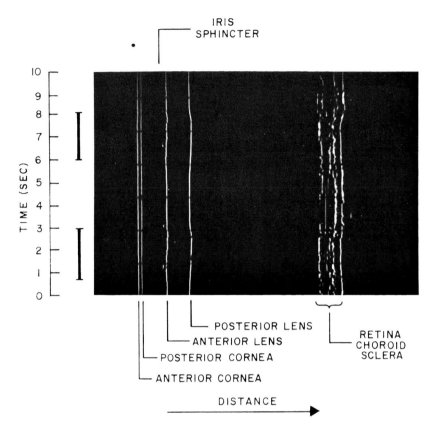

IRIS
SPHINCTER

POSTERIOR LENS
ANTERIOR LENS
POSTERIOR CORNEA
ANTERIOR CORNEA

RETINA
CHOROID
SCLERA

DISTANCE

Fig. II-3. M-mode time history showing positions of tissue interfaces as functions of time. (Vertical bars indicate periods of accommodation.)

Throughout this chapter emphasis is given to the overall quality of an ultrasonogram in terms of three parameters: resolution, sensitivity and dynamic range. Resolution has already been defined in Chapter I. Sensitivity refers to the weakest reflector which can be detected in a displayed ultrasonogram. Dynamic range describes the spread of echo amplitudes which is accurately portrayed in an ultrasonogram.

A-mode Systems

A-mode systems are the most fundamental ultrasonic systems and form the basis for more complex modes of operation. The standard A-mode configuration, shown in Figure II-4, consists of an electronic pulser which excites the transducer, a receiver which processes echo voltage pulses, and a display unit which presents

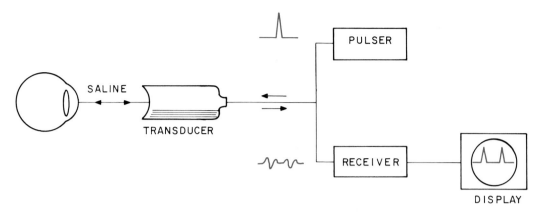

FIG. II-4. Schematic diagram of A-mode system and typical voltage waveforms.

the echo signals. Electronic pulser, receiver and display units are found in all ultrasonic systems. They are often contained within a single chassis connected to the transducer by an electrically shielded cable. The operation of each of these units is discussed in the following sections. Most attention is given to the receiver since it provides a large degree of operator interaction which can be of great value in clinical examinations.

Electronic Pulser

The electronic pulser repeatedly "shock excites" the transducer with short voltage pulses applied across the electrodes of its piezo-electric element. Each excitation results in the generation of an ultrasonic pulse. The pulse repetition rate must be low enough to allow all returning echoes to be received by the transducer before the next ultrasonic pulse is generated. Typically, a 1-KHz rate is used so that a pulse is generated at 1-msec periods while only 67 μsec are needed to allow reception of echoes from the deepest portions of the orbit.

The duration of the excitation pulse is an important factor in determining the resolution of an ultrasonic system. Long excitation pulses result in correspondingly long ultrasonic pulses and concomitant poor axial resolution. The amplitude of the excitation pulse is important in achieving adequate sensitivity. Typically, 200- to 400-volt amplitudes result in ultrasonic pulses large enough to produce detectable echoes from weakly reflecting interfaces such as the vitreoretinal interface.

In many systems, a "damping" or "energy" control allows the

excitation pulse to be varied between the extremes of a short, low-amplitude pulse (providing high resolution but low sensitivity) and a long, high-amplitude pulse (providing low resolution but high sensitivity). The clinician must decide the combination of resolution and sensitivity most advantageous in a given situation.

Electronic Receiver

Following transducer excitation, echoes from ocular and orbital interfaces impinge upon the transducer. The voltage pulses generated in response to these ultrasonic echoes must be modified before they can be displayed in a useful format. The required modifications are carried out by an electronic receiver. First, echo voltage pulses are envelope detected to simplify their waveforms. Second, they are amplified to augment their initially low levels. A receiver can also incorporate additional processing techniques such as time-varied gain to compensate for tissue absorption. Each of these operations is discussed in the following sections.

ENVELOPE DETECTION. An echo voltage pulse generated by a transducer is illustrated in Figure II-5. This "radio-frequency" (R.F.) pulse exhibits several cycles of oscillation with maxima and minima which define the signal's envelope. Detection networks are used to obtain this envelope or "video" signal for A-mode display. Video signals are usually sufficient for locating and identifying reflective structures. They are more readily processed and interpreted than the more complex R.F. signals.

Rectification, the first process in isolating the video signal, converts the bipolar R.F. signal to a unipolar voltage. In half wave rectification, this is accomplished by eliminating all signal components of one polarity. In full wave rectification, all R.F. cycles are converted to a single polarity. This total conversion permits better estimates of the signal envelope. Full wave rectification is especially desirable in biometry since it preserves the initial portion of every echo pulse regardless of its polarity, and thus maintains an accurate representation of the timing between all echoes. The video signal is then obtained by using a filter to smooth the rapid oscillations in the rectified waveform. The filter time constant must be adjusted to provide sufficient smoothing without introducing excessive pulse lengthening.

R.F. and video signals obtained from the anterior segment of the eye are illustrated in Figure II-6. While the video signals of the eye are readily interpreted, they do not convey all of the information inherent in the R.F. signals. Specifically, the relative polarity of the

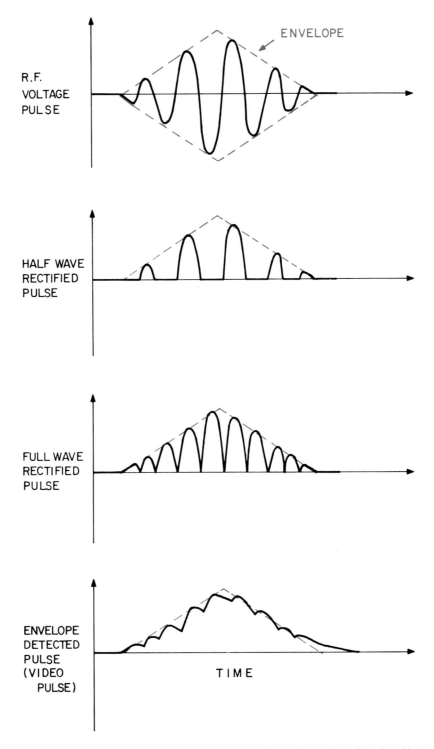

R.F.
VOLTAGE
PULSE

ENVELOPE

HALF WAVE
RECTIFIED
PULSE

FULL WAVE
RECTIFIED
PULSE

ENVELOPE
DETECTED
PULSE
(VIDEO
PULSE)

TIME

FIG. II-5. Echo voltage waveforms illustrating procedures in envelope detection. Note elimination of initial half cycle in half wave rectification.

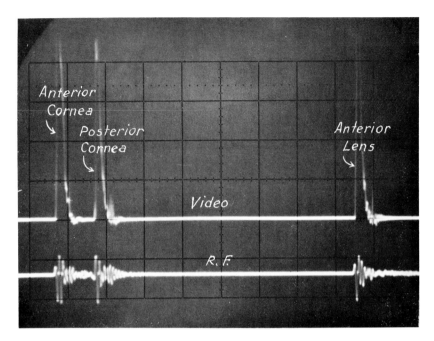

Fig. II-6. Anterior segment of eye, demonstrating resolution at 20 MHz and polarity change in radio frequency waveform between anterior and posterior corneal echoes.

reflection coefficient is shown by the polarity of the initial cycle in each R.F. signal but cannot be discerned from the video signal. Research is now being directed to other, more subtle features of R.F. signals using techniques such as spectrum analysis (discussed in a subsequent section).

AMPLIFICATION. Prior to their display in ultrasonograms, video signals pass through electronic amplifiers. Here their voltage levels are multiplied by a gain factor that effectively provides a controllable vertical scale in A-mode displays. Gains on the order of 100 (40 dB)* are needed to raise the amplitudes of these signals from their initially low levels (e.g., 1 millivolt) to levels that are compatible with display requirements. Amplifiers must be carefully designed and operated to provide accurate representations of input echo signals. The most important factors in amplification are bandwidth, saturation, noise and dynamic range.

The short-duration video pulses undergoing amplification contain a broad spectrum or "bandwidth" of frequency components which must be accommodated by an amplifier. The bandwidth of a pulse is approximately equal to the reciprocal of its duration. If this bandwidth is reduced by a smaller amplifier bandwidth, the amplified pulses will be stretched in time and axial resolution will suffer.

*A voltage ratio, K, is expressed in decibels by computing 20 log K.

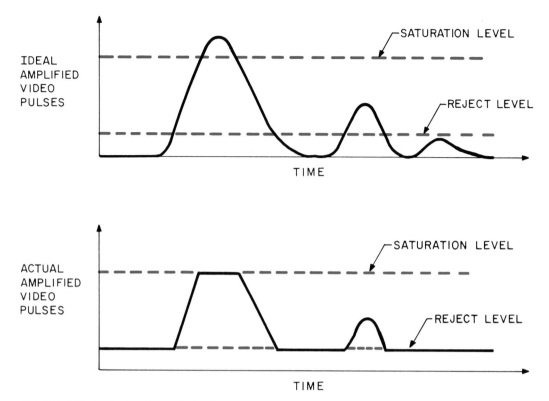

FIG. II-7. Effects of saturation and rejection on video signals. Both saturation and rejection can cause loss of important signal features, as shown in lower waveforms.

Amplification of 0.15-μsec pulses, therefore, necessitates an amplifier bandwidth of at least 7 MHz.

A factor of prime importance when adjusting amplifier gain is saturation which occurs whenever the amplified pulse reaches the maximum level (e.g., 5 volts) that the amplifier can supply. If an input signal is too large (or if the gain is too high), saturation occurs and can eliminate clinically significant information about echo strength (Fig. II-7). Saturation is always encountered at the very beginning of an A-mode display when a part of the large excitation pulse is picked up by the amplifier. This so-called main bang causes a dead space directly in front of the transducer and obliterates echoes from very close objects. It is of no consequence as long as an adequate standoff distance is provided by the coupling medium.

Electronic noise limits the detection of small echoes and can present especially severe problems with large bandwidth amplifiers. Noise consists of small, random voltage variations that arise because of statistical fluctuations, such as thermal motion, of electrons in resistors, transistors, and other components. At high gains, the

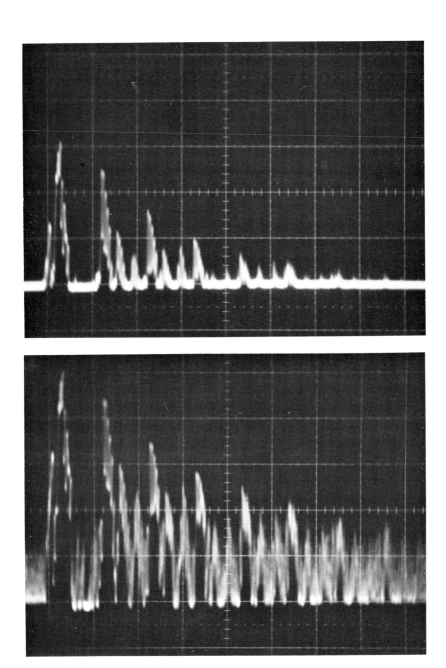

FIG. II-8. A-mode signals obtained at low gain (*top*) and high gain (*bottom*). Random noise signals ("grass") are apparent at high gain.

resultant noise signals appear as "grass" in an ultrasonogram and obscure small echoes (Fig. II-8). (Noise causes the all-too-familiar "snow" in television monitors.) Most ultrasonic units possess reject controls which establish a threshold level that can be set to prevent the grass from being displayed in A-mode ultrasonograms. Reject controls, if improperly adjusted, can suppress the display of small or modest echoes which may be diagnostically significant (Fig. II-7).

Saturation and noise combine to determine the dynamic range of an amplifier. Dynamic range is defined as the spread of input signal amplitudes which result in meaningful output signals. The largest useful input signal is that which just causes saturation; the smallest useful input signal is that which yields an output just above the amplifier noise level. Typical video amplifiers have dynamic ranges of 40 dB; i.e., the maximum input signal is 100 times larger than the minimum input signal. This range is usually sufficient for accurate displays of tissue echoes.

TIME VARIED GAIN. Time varied gain (TVG) can partly compensate for the effects of tissue absorption on echo amplitudes. As noted in Chapter I, absorption causes a progressive loss in the strength of a propagating ultrasonic pulse. Absorptive attenuation of echo strength increases exponentially with distance (Fig. II-9). Compensation for this effect involves increasing amplifier gain with time, t, in a manner which is the inverse of absorptive decay. The appropriate gain is of the form of $e^{\alpha ct}$, where α is the absorption coefficient and c is the velocity of ultrasonic propagation. While TVG is useful, it cannot compensate exactly for absorption in the eye and orbit because absorption coefficients differ greatly in specific ocular and orbital tissues. (Time varied gain is sometimes termed STC or sensitivity time control.)

LOGARITHMIC AMPLIFICATION. Logarithmic amplification is often employed to extend the effective dynamic range of an amplifier. In a standard (linear) amplifier, the gain, G, is independent of the input signal level and an output voltage is equal to G times the corresponding input pulse. In a logarithmic amplifier, the output voltage is proportional to the logarithm of the input voltage. As shown in Figure II-10, this type of amplification yields a large gain for small signals and a small gain for large signals. Thus a logarithmic characteristic reduces differences in echo levels and permits a wider range of input signals to fall between the noise and saturation levels of an amplifier. Logarithmic amplification can be used effectively in B-mode systems where it compresses the large range of input echo signals to the small range of brightness levels that can be displayed on oscilloscopes.

Other nonlinear characteristics have also been used to advantage in ultrasonography. An S-shaped function, for example, provides largest gain at intermediate signal levels and has proven useful in A-mode examinations.[2] However, such nonlinear amplification

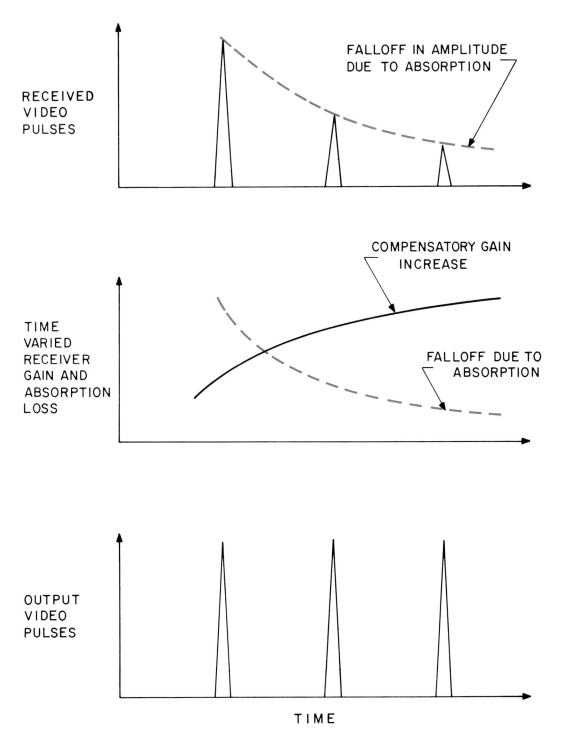

FIG. II-9. Time varied gain (TVG). *Top:* Echoes from equally strong reflectors are progressively reduced by absorption in intervening tissue. *Center:* TVG gain and absorption characteristics. *Bottom:* Processed voltages after application of TVG.

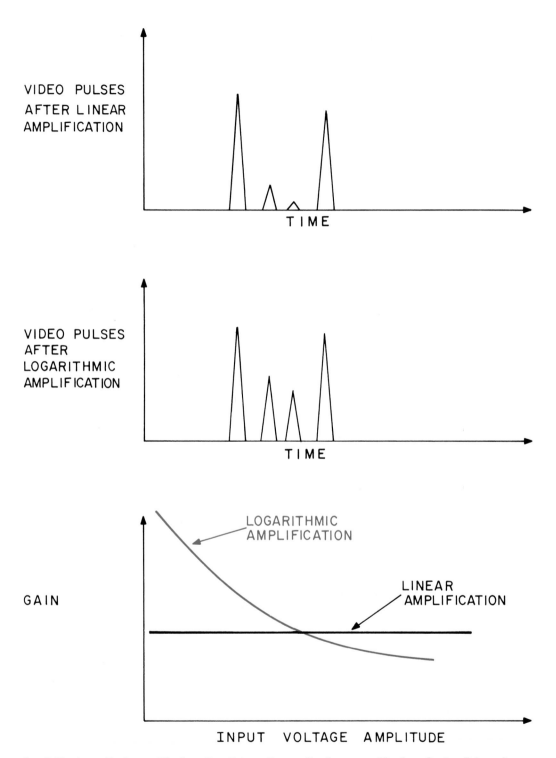

FIG. II-10. Logarithmic amplification. *Top:* Echo voltages after linear amplification. *Center:* Echo voltages after logarithmic amplification. *Bottom:* Comparison of linear and logarithmic gain characteristics.

makes it difficult to recognize relative echo amplitudes and to compare clinical echo patterns with those obtained in standard systems. Characteristic A-mode patterns can be easily distorted unless great care is exercised in adjusting all system parameters.

Oscilloscope Display

After being processed by the receiver, echo voltages are displayed on an oscilloscope. In A-mode operation, the oscilloscope displays a graph of the video signals as a function of time. It is appropriate at this point to describe briefly the operation of oscilloscopes, which are similar to television monitors. An oscilloscope contains a display tube with a phosphorescent screen which glows when struck by an electron beam emitted from a "gun" at the base of the tube. Horizontal and vertical movements of the electron beam are controlled by voltages applied to deflection plates (Fig. II-11). Even the brightness produced by the beam can be controlled for intensity-modulated (Z-axis) display. Different display screen phosphors are available to provide a given color and image persistence.

In A-mode presentations, the horizontal deflection plates are supplied with a voltage that increases linearly with time after transducer excitation. Thus, horizontal position across the screen represents elapsed time, which in turn is proportional to distance from the transducer. At the same time, the vertical plates are supplied with the processed video signals. These simultaneous operations sweep the electron beam over the oscilloscope screen in a manner that corresponds to a plot of signal amplitude versus distance, yielding the desired graphical display. This process is repeated each time the transducer is excited; excitation rates (e.g., 1 KHz) are high enough to produce flicker-free A-mode displays.

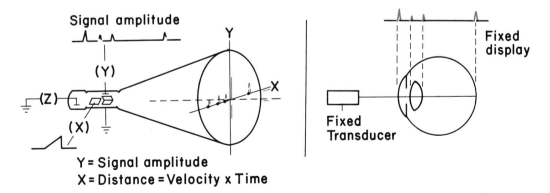

FIG. II-11. Oscilloscope presentation of A-mode signals. Vertical display axis (Y) represents signal amplitude while horizontal axis (X) represents transit time (distance). Brightness (Z) is constant.

The vertical scale in these displays can be varied through amplifier gain adjustments. The time axis can be magnified by increasing the slope of the horizontal deflection voltage so that less time is required to sweep the light spot across the entire screen. To interpret clinical results and determine tissue dimensions, it is necessary to note the oscilloscope sweep setting which specifies this time magnification or, equivalently, to display standard voltage pulses (markers) separated by known time intervals. When these time scales are known, the horizontal axis can be interpreted in terms of tissue depth.

Summary of A-mode Controls

It is useful at this point to summarize the controls that are available with typical A-mode systems and to outline the effects which these controls exert on system performance. Subsequent chapters will present clinical results illustrating optimum adjustments for specific diagnostic situations.

Table II-1 lists the most important controls associated with the pulser, receiver, and display units. The pulser damping control affects system sensitivity and resolution. Since these factors cannot be optimized simultaneously, the clinician must decide upon an appropriate compromise. In ocular examinations, resolution is usually more important than sensitivity; in orbital examination the reverse usually holds true.

The receiver provides a great deal of operational flexibility. Gain control permits direct adjustment of sensitivity and should be set at

TABLE II-1. Basic A-mode Controls

Electronic Unit	Control	Function Controlled	System Parameters Affected
Pulser	Damping	Transducer excitation	Sensitivity Resolution
Receiver	Time constant	Envelope detection	Resolution
	Gain (sensitivity)	Amplification	Sensitivity Saturation Dynamic range
	Reject	Noise display suppression	Dynamic range
Oscilloscope	Time base	Magnification	Depth scale

a level which allows clear display of weak echoes. Gain and reject controls must be adjusted jointly to provide an adequate dynamic range in the ultrasonogram. High gain settings must be used carefully to avoid receiver saturation, while reject levels must be set only slightly above the noise level so that the display of "grass" is suppressed without the unnecessary elimination of weak echoes. If time varied gain is used, its rate of increase must be set to compensate for absorptivity losses without causing excessive saturation.

The most important display control relates to the horizontal time axis in the ultrasonogram which represents tissue depth. The time sweep of the oscilloscope should be chosen to provide a useful magnification of the tissue being studied. The time interval represented by each division on the oscilloscope screen must be specified either by recording the oscilloscope time scale or displaying calibrated time markers.

The electronic units utilized in A-mode systems are also employed in B- and M-mode systems. In these more complex modes of operation, the considerations which have been described here are fully applicable. It is expeditious to adjust for proper A-mode operation before using these other modes.

B-mode Systems

B-mode systems combine transducer scanning and electronic processing to produce cross-sectional images of the eye and orbit. The quality of these images depends upon the factors already discussed for A-mode systems. However, there are additional electronic, mechanical and acoustic considerations which should be understood for optimal clinical utilization and proper diagnostic interpretation. Furthermore, B-mode images are susceptible to several types of artifacts which are readily recognized and which can often be eliminated. In addition to treating these topics, the following sections discuss useful image enhancement techniques and describe color-coded and isometric B-mode systems which convey quantitative reflectivity information.

B-mode Image Generation

The simplest B-mode systems utilize a linear transducer scan motion, as shown in Figure II-12. Although the scan is continuous, it is convenient to first consider a fixed transducer location. Echo signals are processed as in A-mode operation. However, the resulting B-mode video signals are not used to control the vertical deflec-

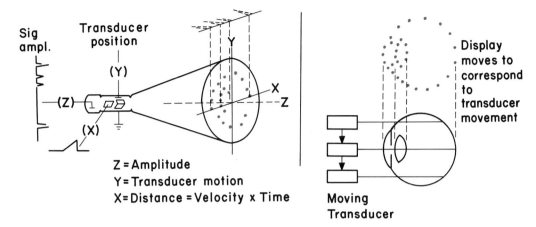

FIG. II-12. B-mode imaging with linear scan pattern. X and Y display axes correspond to spatial coordinates as ascertained from transit time and transducer position, respectively. Brightness corresponds to signal amplitude and is indicative of tissue reflectivity.

tion plates of an oscilloscope. Instead, these signals are used to regulate the intensity of the oscilloscope's electron beam as it is swept horizontally across the screen. In this intensity (or Z-axis) modulation, if no echo is present, the beam is completely suppressed so that the screen remains dark. When an echo occurs, the beam is energized and its intensity is modulated to produce a spot with brightness proportionate to the amplitude of the echo voltage. Thus, the display presents tissue reflectivity in terms of brightness as a function of time or, equivalently, distance from the transducer.

In B-mode systems, the transducer is scanned progressively across the eye and the intensity modulated display axis is scanned down the oscilloscope screen in a corresponding fashion. The correspondence is achieved by applying the voltage from a position-sensing device (potentiometer) mounted on the transducer to the vertical deflection plates of the oscilloscope. Thus, the points which appear on the oscilloscope screen indicate the two-dimensional position of reflective surfaces in the scanned tissue.

In these images, sharply demarcated boundaries (e.g., the anterior lens surface) which generate well-defined A-mode echoes are displayed as distinct surfaces; acoustically homogeneous regions (e.g., the normal vitreous) are displayed as dark areas; acoustically heterogeneous areas (e.g., the orbital fat) which generate many closely spaced A-mode echoes are displayed as correspondingly speckled brightness patterns. The images presented by conventional oscilloscopes do not persist during the entire scan operation, which usually takes a few seconds. Therefore, they are viewed after time exposure photography or by presentation on storage oscilloscopes which store and repeatedly display B-mode images. (Storage oscil-loscopes are useful for monitoring examinations but possess poor resolution and gray scale characteristics.)

Scan Patterns

B-mode systems can employ various scan patterns, as shown in Figure II-13. The most useful patterns are those in which the ultra-sonic beam is perpendicularly aligned with reflective tissue surfaces.

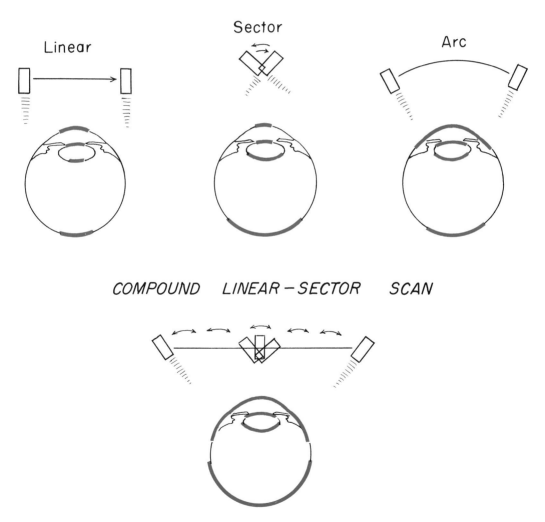

SIMPLE SCAN PATTERNS

Linear

Sector

Arc

COMPOUND LINEAR – SECTOR SCAN

FIG. II-13. Transducer scan patterns. Simple linear, sector and arc patterns allow partial imaging of ocular surfaces. The most complete coverage results from compound scanning.

With perpendicular alignment, echoes travel directly back to the transducer rather than being redirected along a misaligned path that bypasses the transducer. Linear scan patterns can achieve perpendicularity only over small segments of curved ocular surfaces such as those of the retina; therefore, they provide images of limited portions of the eye. Sector scan patterns are more compatible with these curved surfaces and allow echoes from large segments of posterior surfaces to be captured for B-mode presentations. Arc scan patterns also permit perpendicular alignment over large ocular regions.

Compound scanning combines several scan motions to achieve the most complete coverage of the eye and orbit. The compound scan pattern utilized in our laboratory combines a repetitive sector scan superimposed on a slower linear scan. With this combination each tissue element is viewed from several directions, assuring normal illumination of most boundaries at some instant during the scan. Another useful compound scan pattern combines sector and arc scans.

Compound scanning requires carefully designed electronic circuitry. Control signals from both linear and sine-cosine potentiometers must be combined so that the oscilloscope display axis can accurately follow the appropriate translation and sector motions of the transducer. Scan inaccuracies in compound scan systems are especially serious because they can prevent proper superposition of tissue elements as they are viewed from different transducer angles. Inadequate superposition can cause a single tissue element to appear at a different image location each time it is viewed from a different transducer position.

Transducer scan units can be motorized or manually controlled. A manually controlled system has been employed in these laboratories. This approach provides a great degree of flexibility and allows detailed examination of selected tissue areas.[3] However, irregularities in hand motions can cause the transducer to dwell for relatively long periods over some tissue elements. Because these elements are illuminated with more ultrasonic pulses than other areas, their brightness is exaggerated in the B-mode image. This artifact does not interfere with the geometric definition of tissue structure but it does preclude quantitative assessments of reflectivity from image brightness. When quantitative reflectivity levels are of interest, a sector scan is used together with an optical encoder to provide uniform illumination rates in spite of irregular manual control. The encoder senses transducer orientation and triggers a single excitation pulse each time the transducer is sectored through a preset angular increment (e.g., 0.3 degree).

Rapid scanning can also be achieved with manual or motorized systems.[4,5] Motor-driven sector scans can generate several images per second for continuous viewing on oscilloscopes or television monitors. These displays allow rapid surveying of the eye and orbit and permit tissue evaluation during eye rotation. Rapid imaging can also be accomplished with a set of adjacent transducers that are excited in rapid succession to simulate high-speed transducer scanning.[6] A more sophisticated technique employs arrays containing many independent piezoelectric elements.[7,8] In effect, these elements approximate Huygens' sources and, by properly sequencing their excitation, the beam they form can be focused and steered within the examined tissue. This electronic scanning can be performed at very high rates and offers great promise for diagnostic systems.

Direct contact B-mode systems are not well suited for ophthalmic examinations but are widely used in obstetrics and gynecology. A transducer is manually scanned across the body surface which has been coated with a thin layer of coupling oil or gel. The resulting complex scan pattern is followed via potentiometers mounted on a series of shafts connected to the transducer.

B-mode Image Quality

Under ideal conditions, the light intensities in B-mode images correspond precisely to the acoustic reflectivity at each tissue point. In linear and sector scans, image intensity should represent reflectivity at a specific angle of beam incidence. In compound scans each tissue element is viewed from several aspects and image intensity ideally represents an average reflectivity (averaged over the appropriate range of angular beam incidence). In practice, these representations are constrained by the limited intensity ranges of oscilloscopes and the small dynamic ranges of films. A display dynamic range of about 15 dB can be obtained by carefully controlling all system parameters. This dynamic range can also be achieved in photography by careful choice of film exposure and development to assure the desired film "gamma" or transfer characteristic. Effective dynamic range can be increased by prior logarithmic amplification; however, it is often most expedient to use B-mode images for assessments of general anatomy and to obtain A-mode results along specifically chosen directions for quantitative reflectivity information.

The resolution inherent in B-mode images can be limited by large oscilloscope spot sizes or inadequate Z-axis bandwidth. However, these are usually not the limiting factors and resolution is most often governed by the same considerations that determine A-mode resolution. Axial resolution is determined by the duration of the ultrasonic pulse; thus, excessively long pulses will cause thickening of line segments in the image and prevent detection of closely spaced surfaces.

Lateral resolution is determined by the ultrasonic beamwidth. Wide beams exaggerate the apparent width of reflective structures in a manner that depends upon the scan pattern being used. To

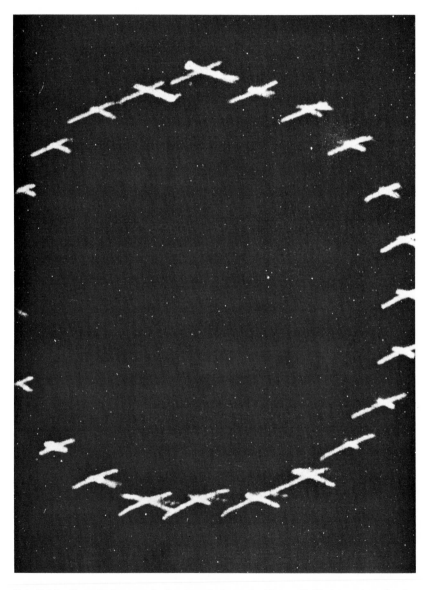

FIG. II-14. B-mode image of wire target shown in Figure II-15. Arcs at each wire location arise from finite beamwidth. Sector scans from two transducer locations were used to generate this image.

examine this effect, consider transverse scans across a long thin wire. In a linear scan, the wire appears as a line segment with a width equal to the effective beamwidth. Similarly, in a sector scan the image of the wire appears as an arc. In a compound scan, the image of the wire contains a number of intersecting arcs corresponding to the constituent sector scans. For example, Figure II-14 shows a B-mode image of a cylindrical array of thin wires (Fig. II-15) that were

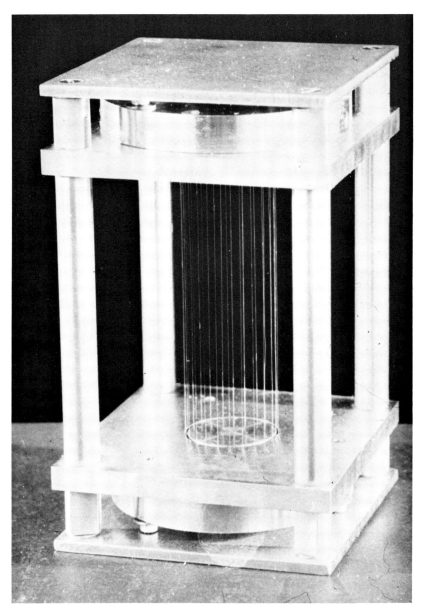

FIG. II-15. Calibration target consisting of cylindrical array of thin wires.

sector scanned from two locations to simulate a compound scan. Note that the arcs intersect at points which locate the positions of the wires; if optimal gain settings could be used in clinical applications it would be possible to display only these points of intersection and thereby realize better angular resolution than that available with a single sector scan. However, such optimization is difficult in practical situations.

Just as in A-mode operation, absorption limits the resolution attainable with B-mode systems. High-resolution images of the eye can be obtained at 20 MHz but only a thin layer of the orbit can be penetrated at this high frequency. Deeper orbital penetration requires lower frequencies (on the order of 5 to 10 MHz).

B-mode Artifacts

B-mode images are susceptible to artifacts resulting from ultrasonic and electronic sources. The most commonly encountered artifacts are listed in Table II-2 and are described below.

B-mode artifacts can arise because of differences in the propagation velocities of various tissues. For example, Figure II-16 illustrates distortions stemming from the relatively high velocity within the ocular lens. Along a central path (OA) through the lens, the rear wall appears to be displaced anteriorly because the high lenticular velocity decreases the transit time from the transducer to point A.

TABLE II-2. Types of B-mode Artifacts

Source	Effects
ACOUSTIC ARTIFACTS	
Velocity differences	Displacement artifact Contour distortion
Absorption	Shadowing
Multiple reflections	Surface duplication
ELECTRONIC ARTIFACTS	
Noise	"Snow"
Saturation	Obliteration of texture
Saturation (occurring with texture enhancement)	"Swiss cheese" artifact
Inadequate superposition	Blurring and duplication

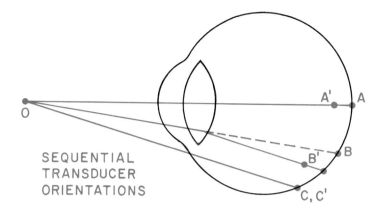

SEQUENTIAL
TRANSDUCER
ORIENTATIONS

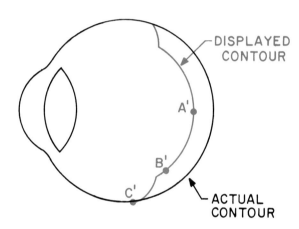

FIG. II-16. Artifacts due to high lenticular propagation velocity. *Top:* Transducer orientation and propagation paths for sector scan centered at 0. *Bottom:* Comparison of actual and displayed contours. Distortions arise from decreased transit time (A') and refraction (B').

(This shortening is also present on an A-scan.) In addition, scan paths passing obliquely through the lens (for example, OB) subject the ultrasonic pulse to refraction so that the point actually being imaged does not lie along the transducer axis. On the other hand, paths bypassing the lens result in undistorted imaging. The overall effect of these phenomena is to distort the contours of tissues located behind the lens. These distortions can be aggravated in compound scans since each posterior tissue element is viewed along several paths through the lens.

Another type of artifact, acoustic shadowing, decreases the image light intensity in tissue regions posterior to highly absorptive structures such as the lens and certain types of tumors. Shadowing often facilitates differential diagnosis by allowing the clinician to categorize tumors according to their absorptivity. Because of these effects, the most accurate results are obtained only when the transducer scan paths do not traverse the lens. Carefully oriented scans through the sclera result in only minimal degradations from velocity and absorption effects.

Multiple acoustic reflections constitute another source of artifacts, introducing duplication of tissue contours as shown in Figure II-17. Here, ultrasonic echoes from the cornea and lens return to the transducer where they are partially reflected back toward the eye. These echoes are then reflected by the cornea and arrive for a second time at the transducer after the transit time determined by the transducer-cornea separation. The multiply reflected echoes appear in both A-mode signals and B-mode images, where they usually appear as phantom surfaces within the vitreous or in posterior regions. Recognition of multiple reflections is straightforward: changing the transducer-cornea standoff distance alters the location of the artifacts with relation to the eye. These artifacts can be eliminated by making this standoff distance equal to the maximum tissue depth to be examined.

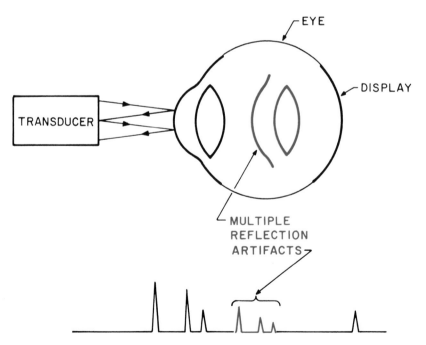

FIG. II-17. Artifacts from multiple reflections. Echoes from the cornea and lens are reflected at the transducer and, again, at the cornea. Both A- and B-mode results present these multiply reflected pulses at locations corresponding to total multiple-path transit times.

Electronic artifacts can assume several forms. "Snow" can appear on B-mode images if electronic noise is not rejected prior to display. Saturation can cause heterogeneous structures such as orbital fat to appear as uniformly bright areas. (With the texture enhancement processing described below, saturation causes "Swiss cheese" artifacts.) Improperly adjusted compound scan systems can cause tissue details to be severely blurred or duplicated because of faulty superposition. Recognition of these artifacts is aided by careful monitoring of A-mode signals.

Electronic Image Processing

Diagnostically useful tissue characteristics may be enhanced with electronic processing techniques prior to image display.[9] Image enhancement techniques are most useful for viewing heterogeneous structures such as tumors that exhibit densely packed reflecting elements. Often these internal features cause only minor perturbations in A-mode signals and appear as indistinct areas in standard B-mode images. More distinctive and informative displays of these structures can be formed by using techniques which (1) clearly delineate major contours or (2) emphasize internal structural patterns or texture. The second approach is especially useful and has been employed in the majority of B-mode images that are presented in subsequent chapters.

The first type of image processing, contour enhancement, displays only those interfaces which are distinctly resolved. In this technique, illustrated in Figure II-18, video signals do not directly modulate the intensity on the oscilloscope screen. Instead, whenever the video signal rises above a preset threshold, it triggers a standardized voltage pulse of fixed amplitude and duration. These standard "display" pulses are presented in B-mode format. Thus, all reflecting surfaces that are clearly resolved are displayed with equal brightness. Closely spaced internal surfaces that cause only minor signal variations are not displayed. A B-mode image obtained using this technique is shown in Figure II-19.

The second, more useful, form of processing emphasizes internal texture. Here, video signals are first differentiated: this yields a voltage signal proportional to the slope of the original video signal. After differentiation the originally rapid, small signal variations due to poorly resolved internal structures appear as relatively large voltages. This differentiated signal could be displayed directly in B-mode format. However, it has been found more advantageous to use the differentiated signal to trigger standard display pulses so that all textural features are represented with equal brightness (Fig. II-19).

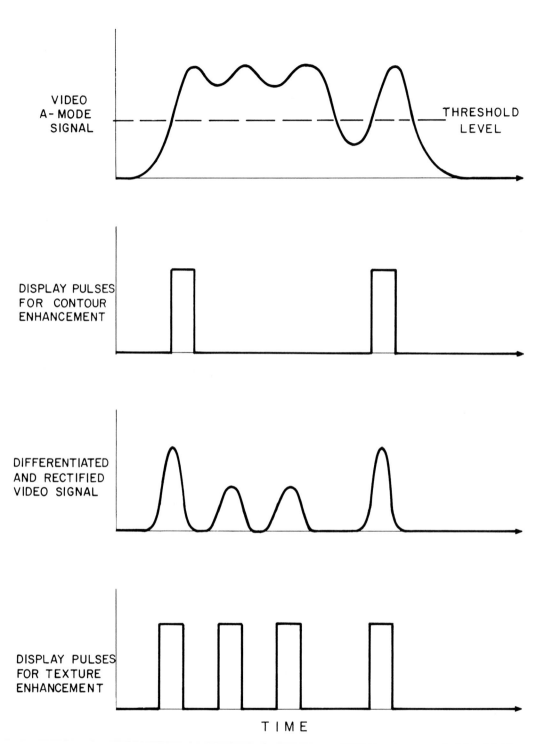

FIG. II-18. Voltage waveforms encountered in image processing techniques. In contour enhancement, video signals trigger standard display pulses. In texture enhancement, differentiated video signals trigger display pulses.

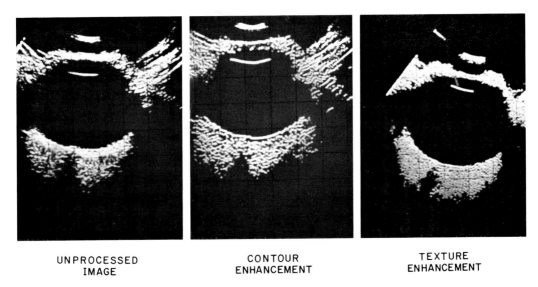

| UNPROCESSED IMAGE | CONTOUR ENHANCEMENT | TEXTURE ENHANCEMENT |

FIG. II-19. B-mode images illustrating contour and texture enhancement. Contour enhancement emphasizes well-resolved interfaces and sharply delineates surfaces such as the anterior retina. Texture enhancement presents internal structural details with equal brightness. This is apparent in the display of orbital fat.

(Differentiated signals are also rectified so that only positive slopes in A-mode signals are displayed; this prevents each signal ripple from triggering display pulses at both its rising and falling segments.)

Images obtained with these pulsed enhancement techniques exhibit no gray scale. Enhancement is realized at the expense of amplitude information which can be obtained from supplementary A-mode observations along paths that can be superimposed on the B-mode image.

Other enhancement techniques (e.g., double differentiation) are sometimes encountered.[10] When employing any of these techniques, it is important to understand the underlying electronic processing for proper diagnosis and recognition of artifacts. Saturation, for example, can result in different artifacts depending upon the type of processing involved. In standard B-mode images, areas of saturation appear as uniformly bright areas. On the other hand, saturation followed by the differentiation used in texture enhancement will produce very small signals since the slope of the saturated signal is nearly zero. Thus, each area of saturation will appear as a dark patch in the enhanced B-mode image, sometimes creating a "Swiss cheese" pattern of artifactual vacuoles (color plates A and B).

Color B-mode Images

The ability of conventional B-mode images to convey amplitude information is constrained by the minimal brightness range (under

20 dB) that can be generated by an oscilloscope and recorded on film. A promising approach to overcoming this limitation depicts echo amplitude by color, rather than brightness, in B-mode images. For example, low amplitudes might be presented in blue, moderate amplitudes in green, and high amplitudes in red.

Several approaches to color-encoded images are possible. Digital techniques utilize analog-to-digital converters, memory arrays and encoding logic.[11] Photographic techniques color code carefully photographed B-mode images which are scanned by an isodensi-tometer.[12]

The color system employed in these laboratories[13] utilizes a standard B-mode system but incorporates an electronic scan converter in place of an oscilloscope. The scan converter captures signals from the receiver and stores them in B-mode format. The signals are stored as a charge distribution that is retained within an electronic storage tube. When transducer scanning is completed, the storage tube is repeatedly read out by its scanning electron beam. Just as in a television camera, the image is read out in a raster format, so that it is compatible with display on TV monitors. The signals being read out pass through logic networks which compare their amplitudes to a series of reference levels. These networks then excite the combination of monitor display guns which produce the color indicative of echo amplitude.

The scan converter allows an image to be viewed for more than 30 minutes after data acquistion. During this observation time, the physician can vary the amplitude ranges represented by each of eight colors and thus obtain a finer partitioning of echo amplitudes. He can also adjust the read-out scan to "zoom in" on an ocular or orbital region of particular interest (color plates C and D).

Isometric B-mode Displays

Isometric display[14] constitutes another approach to presenting echo amplitude data in B-mode images. (This technique is an extended version of deflection modulation presentations.[15]) In isometric displays, B-mode data are treated as three-dimensional entities; two dimensions (X, Y) specify spatial tissue coordinates; the third dimension (S) represents echo amplitude and is displayed in relief. Analog circuitry is used to display isometric presentations of these three-dimensional structures on an oscilloscope (color plates E–H). Operator controls are available to vary the simulated tilt and rotation of the displayed projection. This interactive feature greatly enhances the subjective appreciation of B-mode data.

The isometric system again utilizes a scan converter to provide

B-mode signals corresponding to X, Y, and S. During a scan, these signals are captured and subsequently undergo repetitive readout, processing and display. The processing can best be understood by considering the tilting of stored B-scan signals which represent a top (plan) view of tissue reflectivity.

The simulation of tilting, illustrated in Figure II-20, involves separate processing of X, Y, and S signals. X signals are applied unaltered to the horizontal deflection plates of the oscilloscope. The Y signals are first multiplied by the cosine of the tilt angle β, before application to the vertical deflection plates. This multiplication introduces the appropriate isometric spatial foreshortening. (In the extreme case where $\beta = 90$ degrees, an edge view is produced.) Simultaneously, echo amplitudes, S, are superimposed as vertical displacements on the spatial X, Y format; S signals are first multiplied by sine β before being applied to the vertical deflection plates. (In the case of an edge view $\beta = 90$ degrees and maximal projections of S signals are displayed.)

Simultaneous rotation and tilting can be simulated through similar signal manipulations prior to display. Signal weighting factors are introduced by sine-cosine potentiometers and amplifiers which can be adjusted by simple operator controls to vary the viewing aspect simulated in the display.

M-mode Systems

M-mode systems, sometimes termed TM (time-motion) systems, have been developed to examine temporal variations in tissue dimensions and have found widespread diagnostic application in cardiology. Although M-mode operation has not been widely employed in ophthalmology, it has provided high-resolution data concerning accommodation and vascular pulsations within tumors and the choroid.[16]

In M-mode operation, a transducer is aligned along a selected axis within the eye. Then, as shown in Figure II-21, the transducer remains fixed while processed echo voltages intensity modulate an oscilloscope beam, delineating the position of each tissue interface. As time progresses, the horizontal display axis is slowly swept down the oscilloscope screen. If all tissue structures remain stationary, a series of parallel lines is displayed. If tissue positions fluctuate with time, corresponding variations occur in the distances between these lines so that a complete time history of tissue position is portrayed.

The M-mode results shown in Figure II-3 detail dimensional variations along the visual axis during accommodation. It should be noted that dimensional changes in high-velocity structures (the lens

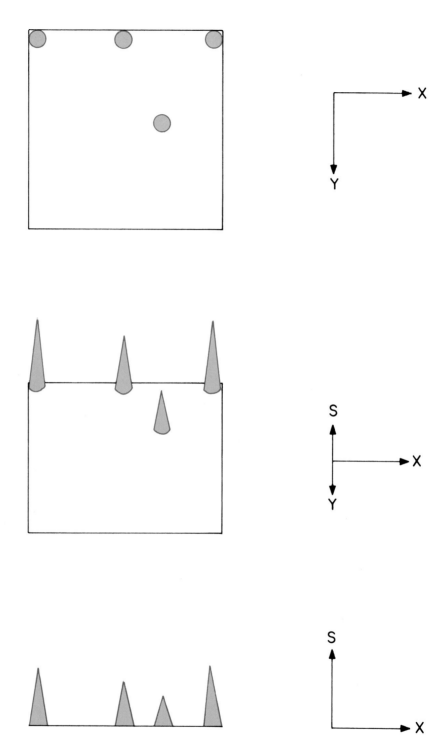

Fig. II-20. Schematic B-mode images illustrating isometric display format. *Top:* Conventional image (equivalent to plan view). *Center:* Tilted presentation showing reflectivity (S) in relief. *Bottom:* Simulated edge view.

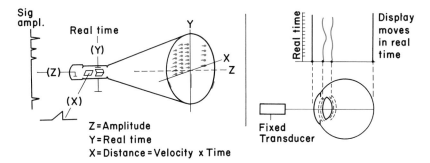

Sig
ampl.

Real time
(Y)

Y

X
Z

(Z)

(X)

Z = Amplitude
Y = Real time
X = Distance = Velocity x Time

Real time

Fixed
Transducer

Display
moves
in real
time

F𝗂𝗀. II-21. M-mode system operation. Horizontal display axis corresponds to distance (transit time). Brightness is used to locate tissue surfaces. Vertical axis corresponds to real time.

in this case) can cause apparent shifts in positions of posterior structures such as the retina. A thickening of the lens, for example, increases the high-velocity path length traversed by the ultrasonic pulse; this occurrence shortens the total transit time to and from the retina and causes an apparent anterior displacement in retinal position. Such effects are easily recognized and actual tissue dimensions can be calculated using available velocity data.

System Calibration

An ultrasonic system must be calibrated periodically if reproducible clinical results are to be obtained. Periodic calibration assures proper system adjustment; it also identifies malfunctions in electronic equipment and variations in transducer characteristics.

Several calibration techniques have been described in the literature.[17,18] In the most accurate and complete calibration approaches, electronic test equipment is used to monitor system responses to a series of voltage waveforms. Simpler calibration procedures are usually sufficient for current diagnostic systems. These procedures employ echoes from test objects to determine the resolution, sensitivity, and geometric fidelity of ultrasonic systems. These measurements are briefly outlined in the following sections for, first, A-mode systems and, second, B-mode systems.

A-mode Calibration

Straightforward procedures can be used to assess the resolution and sensitivity of an A-mode system. Axial resolution can be determined by measuring the duration of an echo returned from the front surface of a flat glass plate. Pulse duration is defined by the 3-dB width of the video signal where the voltage has dropped to 70 per cent of its maximum value. In this measurement, care must be taken to achieve normal beam incidence by adjusting the transducer orientation to maximize echo amplitude. In addition, saturation must be avoided in this and all other calibration procedures.

Lateral resolution can be estimated from a linear, transverse scan across a thin wire the diameter of which is less than the expected beamwidth. The wire should be located at a distance equal to the penetration depth used in tissue examinations. Lateral resolution is equal to the scan displacement which causes the wire echo to decrease by 3 dB from its maximum value.

Sensitivity can be specified in several ways. A useful approach is to calibrate the system so that echo amplitudes are referred to those obtained from a flat glass plate. The plate is located at a representative standoff distance and viewed with normal beam incidence. The gain control is set at its clinical level and a calibrated attenuator, included in many receivers, is used to reduce the plate echo signal by a known amount, usually specified in dB. The resulting echo height establishes a level on the oscilloscope display which bears a known relationship to the plate echo. By using several attenuator settings, the entire display graticule can be calibrated. For complete clinical examinations, it should be possible to view echoes that are 40 to 80 dB below the plate echo.

B-mode Calibration

The geometric fidelity of a B-mode system should be evaluated to ensure accurate spatial representation of tissue morphology. Measurements must be made to ascertain spatial magnification and to ensure proper superposition for compound scanning.

These measurements[19] utilize test targets of known geometry such as the circular array of wires shown in Figure II-15. The dimensions of this target's B-mode image can be used to determine image magnification. The image also permits the oscilloscope deflection amplifiers to be adjusted for equal vertical and horizontal magnification. Unequal magnifications cause the displayed image to assume an elliptical shape rather than the correct circular configuration.

The same target also permits the superposition of a compound scan system to be evaluated and adjusted. As previously described, the B-mode image of each wire exhibits a number of intersecting arc segments arising from component sector scans executed at different transducer positions. These arcs should intersect within a small region corresponding to the actual wire location. Potentiometer circuitry should be adjusted to obtain this superposition so that proper echo registration is achieved in tissue examinations.

Axial and lateral resolution can be measured by noting the apparent thickness and width of each wire. Alternatively, pairs of wires with varied spacing can be scanned to determine the minimum detectable separations. As in all B-mode imaging, the oscilloscope intensity should be set at moderate levels to prevent the blooming and resultant image blurring which occur at high electron-beam intensities.

Ultrasonic Spectrum Analysis

A recently developed technique employs spectrum analysis of echoes returned from ocular and orbital structures. Ultrasonic spectrum analysis is still in its research stages but has already provided clinical data not available with conventional ultrasonography. The technique is analogous to optical spectroscopy where white light is decomposed into its constituent colors to ascertain optical reflectivity and absorptivity as functions of wavelength. Ultrasonic spectrum analysis decomposes short echo pulses into their constituent sinusoidal components to determine acoustic reflectivity and attenuation as functions of frequency.

Spectrum analysis of tissue echoes is motivated by several considerations. First, spectral data can be used for quantitative studies of reflection and attenuation. Second, spectral data can provide statistically reliable descriptions of scattering from random tissue structures such as intraocular tumors. Third, it is more convenient to compensate for extraneous transducer and system parameters in the frequency domain than in the time domain: this compensation provides data which are primarily sensitive to tissue properties alone.

Several types of systems can be used in spectrum analysis. Lele[20] has used an electronic spectrum analyzer to study attenuation in cardiac tissues. Waag[21] has employed swept-frequency excitation with a bistatic transducer configuration. Purnell and Sokollu[22] have used electrical filters to generate frequency coded, color B-mode images. The clinical system developed in these laboratories[23,24] employs a gated spectrum analyzer to provide on-line results which are digitized for subsequent computer processing and entry into a computer library. The following sections briefly describe this system and present typical clinical results.

Figure II-22 presents a simplified block diagram of the spectrum analysis system which has been interfaced with the A- and B-mode system described in previous sections. In clinical operation, B-mode results serve to locate ocular and orbital abnormalities. Then, R.F. echo signals from these structures are gated for spectral processing; proper tissue selection is facilitated by superimposing the gate location on A- and B-mode displays.

Usually, echoes are gated from a 1.5 mm tissue depth. Gated echo signals are applied to a spectrum analyzer with an output

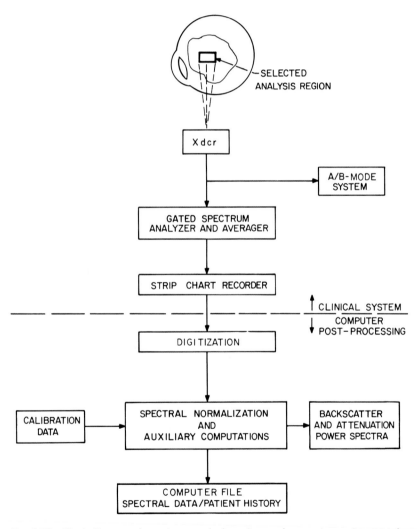

FIG. II-22. Block diagram of spectrum analysis system and computer post-processing techniques.

voltage proportional to the signal energy contained within a narrow frequency band. The center frequency of this band is automatically swept from 5 to 15 MHz to produce a complete spectrum for display on a strip chart recorder.

The system also incorporates a spectral averaging mode to accommodate analysis of random tissues such as intraocular tumors, vitreous hemorrhages, and orbital fat. In this mode the transducer is scanned across the area of interest and spectra from adjacent transducer orientations are determined by the spectrum analyzer. These individual spectra are applied to an on-line digital averager which computes the mean backscatter power spectra of the scanned tissue. Typically, 14 independent spectra are used to form this average.

After clinical data acquisition, calibration spectra are obtained from an optically flat glass plate located at the same range as the examined tissue. Calibration spectra are used to normalize tissue spectra and thereby minimize the effects of frequency-dependent system and transducer characteristics. Normalization is carried out in a computer after tissue and calibration data have been digitized. Other computer processing includes estimation of spectral slopes and ratios for attenuation determinations. Processed spectra are entered into a computer file indexed according to disease.

Clinical Results

Catalogued tissue spectra are examined to identify characteristic tissue "signatures" in terms of absolute reflectance, spectral configuration (resonances, frequency slopes, etc.) and attenuation spectra. While data interpretation is still in its formative stages, several features of potential diagnostic utility have been observed. These are discussed with reference to Figure II-23, which illustrates typical backscatter spectra for ocular structures.

Detached retinas and retinas overlying choroidal tumors produce scalloped backscatter spectra with resonant peaks resulting from constructive interference between anterior and posterior surface echoes. This resonance can cause reflectivity variations of 10 dB over frequency intervals as small as 1.5 MHz. The frequency separation between resonant peaks can be used to estimate retinal thickness. In addition, extrapolation of the resonant pattern to zero frequency can be used to determine the relative polarities of the reflection coefficients at each surface.

Diffuse vitreous hemorrhages yield Rayleigh spectra that increase as f^4 over the 5 to 15 MHz frequency band. This spectral

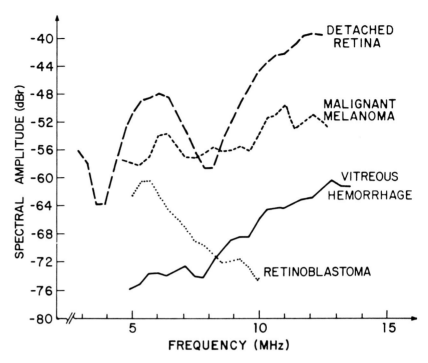

FIG. II-23. Backscatter spectra for ocular pathology. Spectral amplitude is specified in dBr to denote dB levels referenced to the reflectivity of a water-glass interface.

shape is consistent with scattering from a uniformly random distribution of particles the radii of which are much smaller than the incident ultrasonic wavelengths. In contrast to this shape, ocular tumors often yield spectra which are relatively flat (e.g., malignant melanoma) or negatively sloped.

Orbital structures have also been examined with the spectral system. Thyroid ophthalmopathy has been found to cause statistically significant alterations in the spectra of orbital fat. Spectral resonances indicative of structural periodicities have been observed in isolated areas of orbital fat.

Attenuation characteristics have been studied with the spectral system. The effects of acoustic attenuation are clearly evidenced in Figure II-24, which presents backscatter spectra obtained at various depths in orbital fat. At deep sites, the spectra assume a large negative slope because of cumulative attenuation losses which increase with frequency. Ratios of these spectra at sequential depths can be used to estimate attenuation rates.[25] These "attenuation spectra" are used to compensate backscatter spectra of orbital structures for losses in intervening fat. Attenuation spectra of pathologic tissues are now being measured for potential application in differential diagnosis.

NORMAL ORBITAL FAT SPECTRA

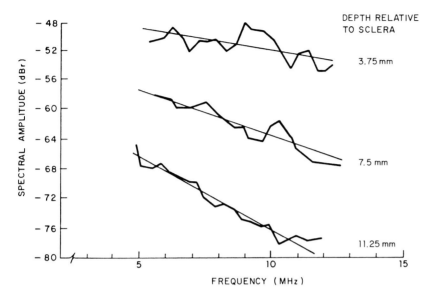

FIG. II-24. Backscatter spectra of orbital fat at three penetration depths.

References Cited

1. Baum, G., and Greenwood, I.: The application of ultrasonic locating techniques to ophthalmology—part 2. Ultrasonic visualization of soft tissues. Arch. Ophthalmol., 60:263–279, 1958.
2. Ossoinig, K. C.: Quantitative echography—the basis of tissue differentiation. J. Clin. Ultrasound, 2:33–46, 1974.
3. Coleman, D. J., Konig, W. F., and Katz, L.: A hand-operated ultrasound scan system for ophthalmic evaluation. Am. J. Ophthalmol., 68:256–363, 1969.
4. Bronson, N.: Development of a simple B-scan ultrasonoscope. Trans. Am. Ophthalmol. Soc., 70:365–408, 1972.
5. Filipczynski, L.: Compound and rapid scan ultrasonic imaging of eye structures. In: Ophthalmic Ultrasound. Edited by K. A. Gitter, A. H. Keeney, L. K. Sarin, and D. Meyer. St. Louis, C. V. Mosby Co., 1969, pp. 207–212.
6. King, D. L.: Real-time cross-sectional ultrasonic imaging of the heart using a linear array multi-element transducer. J. Clin. Ultrasound, 1:196–200, 1973.
7. Maginness, M. G., et al.: A cardiac dynamics visualization system. Proceedings IEEE Ultrasonics Symposium, 1973, pp. 4–6.
8. Somer, J. C., Oosterbaan, W. A., and Freund, E. J.: Ultrasonic tomographic imaging of the brain with an electronic sector scanning system. Proceedings IEEE Ultrasonics Symposium, 1973, pp. 43–48.
9. Lizzi, F. L., and Katz, L. L.: Signal processing for ultrasonic characterization of ocular tissue. Proceedings Electro-Optical Systems Design Conference, 1973, pp. 231–236.
10. Kossoff, G.: Improved techniques in ultrasonic cross-sectional echography. Ultrasonics, 10:221–229, 1972.

11. Liebesny, J. P., and Lele, P. P.: Enhancement of ultrasonic B-scans by chromatic encoding. Proceedings IEEE Ultrasonics Symposium, 1973, pp. 37–38.
12. Baum, G.: Quantized ultrasonography. Ultrasonics, 10:14–15, 1972.
13. Coleman, D. J., and Katz, L.: Color coding of B-scan ultrasonograms. Arch. Ophthalmol. 91:429–431, 1974.
14. Coleman, D. J., Katz, L., and Lizzi, F. L.: Isometric, three-dimensional viewing of ultrasonograms. Arch. Ophthalmol., 93:1362–1365, 1975.
15. Baum, G.: Problems in ultrasonographic localization and attempts at their solution. *In*: Ophthalmic Ultrasound. Edited by K. A. Gitter, A. H. Keeney, L. K. Sarin, and D. Meyer. St. Louis, C. V. Mosby Co., 1969, pp. 231–237.
16. Coleman, D. J., and Weininger, R.: Ultrasonic M-mode technique in ophthalmology. Arch. Ophthalmol., 82:475, 1969.
17. Bronson, N. R.: Quantitative ultrasonography. Arch. Ophthalmol., 81:460–472, 1969.
18. Buschmann, W. H.: Reproducible calibrations: the basis of ultrasonic differential diagnosis in A-mode and B-mode examination of eye and orbit. *In*: Ultrasonography in Ophthalmology. Edited by M. Wainstock. Boston, Little, Brown and Co., 1969, pp. 761–792.
19. Erikson, K. R., Carson, P. L., and Stewart, H. F.: Field evaluation of the AIUM standard 100 mm test object. *In*: Ultrasound in Medicine, Vol. II. Edited by D. White and R. Barnes. New York, Plenum Press, 1976, pp. 445–451.
20. Lele, P., and Namery, J.: A computer-based ultrasonic system for the detection and mapping of myocardial infarcts. Proc. San Diego Biomed. Symp., 13:121–132, 1974.
21. Waag, R. C., and Lerner, R. M.: Tissue macrostructure determination with swept-frequency ultrasound. IEEE Ultrasonics Symposium, 1973, pp. 63–66.
22. Purnell, E. W., Sokollu, A., Holasek, E., and Cappaert, W.: Clinical spectra-color ultrasonography. J. Clin. Ultrasound, 3:187–189, 1975.
23. Lizzi, F. L., and Laviola, M. A.: Power spectra measurements of ultrasonic backscatter from ocular tissue. IEEE Ultrasonics Symposium, 1975, pp. 29–32.
24. Lizzi, F. L., and Laviola, M. A.: Ultrasonic spectral investigations for tissue characterization. *In*: Ultrasound in Medicine, Vol. II. Edited by D. White and R. Barnes. New York, Plenum Press, 1976, pp. 427–440.
25. Lizzi, F. L., St. Louis, L., and Coleman, D. J.: Applications of spectral analysis in medical ultrasonography. Ultrasonics, 14:77–80, 1976.

Additional References

Frederick, J. R.: Ultrasonic Engineering. New York, John Wiley and Sons, Inc., 1965.
Wells, P. N. T.: Physical Principles of Ultrasonic Diagnosis. New York, Academic Press, 1969.

CHAPTER III

Ultrasonic Biometry

Ultrasonic Biometry

SINCE the first use of ultrasonography in the eye,[1] investigators have applied this method to the measurement of ocular dimensions. Successful results enabled ultrasonic biometry of the eye to supplant more traditional optical and radiographic methods. The present widespread application of ultrasound in ocular measurement stems from its capacity to provide rapid, objective and accurate results. The clinical procedure is convenient to both subject and examiner. Low-intensity pulsed ultrasonic methods (as opposed to radiographic methods) produce no known harmful effects on ocular tissue.[2] With ultrasonic methods, ocular dimensions are obtained independently for each segment along the visual axis. With standard optical methods, these measurements are not independent; each measurement requires correction for effects produced in more anterior ocular segments.

The two main clinical uses of ultrasonic biometry have been: (1) axial measurement—for anatomic or physiologic correlative studies such as intraocular lens determination, studies of anterior chamber depth/lens thickness ratios in glaucoma or axial length/lens thickness variations, and (2) morphologic assessment—for comparative studies such as size and growth of intraocular tumors or thickness of extraocular muscles.

In both of these areas, accurate and precise measurements are required that may be obtained by special examining techniques and by attention to the principles of physics and ultrasound.

There are four principal areas of concern in making accurate ultrasonic measurements. These are:

1. Proper alignment of the transducer

   The transducer beam must be assiduously aligned along the desired axis of measurement, whether it be optical axis, visual axis, or maximum height of a tumor. Special techniques are required for axial globe measurements since significant error is produced by a shift of a few degrees of transducer orientation.

2. Distortion-free measurement

   The transducer or standoff must not compress or distort the globe or the tissue being examined. Obviously, even minimal compression of the cornea by the transducer can induce a major error in axial length.

3. High-frequency, narrow beamwidth transducer

   The measuring beam must be narrow in order to avoid errors in measurement of curved surfaces. The error in using a wide beam transducer is analogous to trying to measure the depth of a rounded cup bottom with a wide ruler; the true depth of the cup cannot be reached.

   The highest frequency transducer able to produce the desired depth of penetration should be used in order to obtain greatest accuracy. This is analogous to using a ruler with finer division points for greater accuracy. The importance of this principle in ultrasonic measurement is underlined by the fact that an error of 0.3 mm in axial length determination corresponds to approximately 1 diopter of refractive error.

4. Measurement system standardization

   The time distance between echoes must be accurately determined and, if conversion to millimeters is desired, tissue velocity correction factors must be properly applied. Measurements can be made from a photograph using standard time/distance reference marks, or more accurately can be made electronically with an interval counter.

In selecting the equipment and techniques to be followed for ultrasonic biometry, each of these four principles requires careful consideration. Obviously, certain desired goals will require more accuracy than others. Compromises in techniques can be permitted only when gross approximations are required.

Numerous studies have been performed using ultrasound to provide measurements of the eye and orbit which have not previously been obtainable in vivo.[3-23] The most obvious such measurement is that of globe length. While radiographic techniques have been devised to measure the globe length, e.g., those of Stenstrom[24] and Sorsby,[25] these are not widely applicable, because of the inherent danger of radiation damage to the lens and retina, and because of the subjective end-point used for estimation of the posterior pole position. Leary[15] and Sorsby[21] provided an extensive review of globe length measurement using ultrasound. In one notable series of experiments, they compared optical, ultrasonic and radiographic measurements. Even with a relatively low transducer frequency (4 MHz), using a membrane-covered standoff on the transducer and optic axis alignment, they found that the ultrasonic technique was the preferred method. Their series of measurements of axial lengths of developing children's eyes is a classic study. Other investigators[26-38] have demonstrated improved techniques for increased accuracy of ultrasonic measurement, alignment and electronic aids to measurement. These will be discussed in the section on techniques in this chapter.

Gernet[39-42] used ultrasonic biometry in determining the role of the lens in producing emmetropization of the eye. He also demonstrated that measuring the axial length was necessary in diagnosing the disease he labeled "gigantophthalmia," which is enlargement of the entire globe.[43] This entity cannot be diagnosed when only the corneal diameter and curvature can be measured.

The lens position changes during accommodation have been studied by Coleman[44] using a high-frequency (20-MHz) transducer. The demonstrated mass movement of the lens during accommodation led to a revised hypothesis of the accommodative mechanism.[5]

Other valuable clinical uses of ultrasonic biometry include studies of anterior chamber depth and lens thickness in patients with glaucoma.[46-63] Abramson[64-66] and others[67-69] have studied the effects of pilocarpine on both the anterior chamber depth and lens thickness.

Axial length changes in progressive myopia have been evaluated by several investigators.[70-90] Schwartz[91] made a study of monozygotic twins to determine the effectiveness of mydriatics and cycloplegics in retarding progressive myopia. Another clinical use of ultrasonic biometry is in the determination of axial length to specify accurately dioptric power of keratoprostheses[92-94] and intraocular lenses[95-98] during presurgical preparation. Obtaining the position of

TABLE III-1.   Selected Clinical Applications of Biometry

Investigator	Year	Application
1. Yamamoto[23]	1960	Axial length
2. Araki[26]	1961	Axial length
3. Jansson[13]	1963	Axial length
4. Leary[15]	1963	Refraction
5. Rivara[20]	1963	Axial length
6. Sorsby[21]	1963	Axial length
7. Franceschetti[6]	1965	Axial length
8. Gernet[10]	1965	Axial length
9. Rivara and Zingerian[134]	1965	Volume
10. Buschmann[108]	1967	Exophthalmometry
11. Coleman[27]	1967	Axial length
12. Giglio[11]	1967	Axial length
13. Bronson[100]	1968	Foreign body localization
14. Gernet[43]	1968	Gigantophthalmia
15. Lowe[53]	1968	Anterior chamber, lens (glaucoma)
16. Oksala[35]	1968	Lens thickness
17. Coleman[4]	1969	Axial length
18. Delmarcelle[47]	1969	Anterior chamber, lens (glaucoma)
19. Francois and Goes[75]	1969	Myopia
20. Gernet[50]	1969	Anterior chamber, lens (glaucoma)
21. Weekers[63]	1969	Anterior chamber, lens (glaucoma)
22. Coleman[5]	1970	Accommodation, lens
23. Luyckx-Bacus[59]	1971	Anterior chamber, lens (glaucoma)
24. Abramson[64]	1972	Anterior chamber, lens (glaucoma)
25. Coleman[93]	1972	Keratoprosthesis
26. Gernet and Worst[95]	1973	Lens implants
27. Trier[22]	1973	Axial length
28. Gernet[124]	1973	Aniseikonia

an intraocular foreign body[99-104] and documenting chronologic change in ocular tumor size[105] are other frequent uses of ocular ultrasonic biometry.

Table III-1 provides representative references on the many clinical applications of biometry. While this summary is not an exhaustive survey of the many uses of biometry, it does serve to indicate the importance and wide application of this method. Other bibliographies of ultrasonic biometry have been compiled by Hamard et al,[105a] Vanysek et al.,[106] Giglio,[12] and Gitter et al.[107]

Ultrasonic measurements provide a way of exploring new facets of ocular anatomy and physiology. While the value of ultrasound in visual axis measurements and diagnosis of ocular disease has become well documented,[108-123] there are many biometric applications which remain unexplored. While the rigorous observance of specific physical principles is essential for accurate ultrasonic biometry, attention to these same principles is also necessary for purely clinical evaluations as well, for, in essence, the more accurately ultrasound can display surfaces and tissues, the more precise and reliable will be the clinical judgments based on these displays.

The accuracy and precision presently attainable in ultrasonic systems must now be considered, as well as the means by which they can be improved with specific reference to the requirements of both diagnosis and physiologic research.

Accuracy refers to the ability of a system to provide a measurement which is close to the true value; *precision* refers to the reproducibility of the measurement. System design and implementation have resulted in significant improvements in both these parameters. We will now discuss some of the considerations in selecting the optimal biometric system for the goals desired.

Ultrasonic Biometric Systems

The carefully aligned and directed A-mode system is the most commonly used and most accurate ultrasound modality for biometry of the eye. All systems for ultrasonic biometry include a transducer, a receiver and a display system. The physical considerations for each of these components have already been discussed in Chapters I and II. The role, the accuracy, and the significance of the components in a biometric system will be discussed in turn.

Transducer

The nature of the examining beam is of critical importance for both axial and lateral resolution. First, it should be stressed that the higher the frequency of the transmitted (and returned) echoes the shorter the wavelength, and, hence, the more accurate the resolving power of the system for separating discrete echoes. Secondly, a narrowly focused beam will have greater lateral resolution than will a wide beam. This is particularly important in examination of concave ophthalmic structures, since echoes from the edges of the wide beam return from positions on the concave surfaces that are not truly the most posterior aspect of the structure (Fig. III-1).

In addition to the concept of axial resolution of two closely spaced surfaces, we should also consider the related but separate problem of measurement of distantly separated surfaces. Frequency is the most important parameter in determining accuracy in measurements of large distances. The time of arrival of an echo cannot be

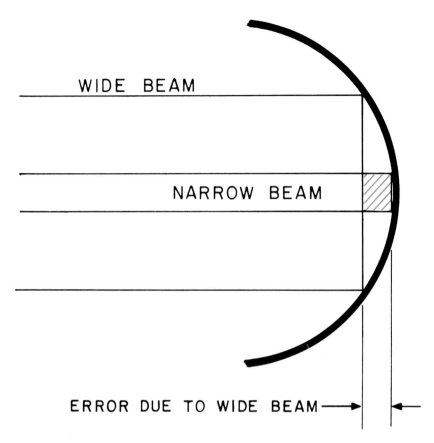

WIDE BEAM

NARROW BEAM

ERROR DUE TO WIDE BEAM ⟶

FIG. III-1. Schematic representation comparing measurements to the posterior pole of an eye using wide and narrow beam transducers. The wider beam produces a greater axial measurement error, since the first returned echoes come from the first surface seen, not from the back of the eye.

measured more exactly than a fraction of its first quarter cycle, i.e., to within a fraction of the time during which the voltage pulse rises to its first maximum. As the frequency of the examining transducer is increased (independently of the damping) the time duration of the first quarter cycle decreases, shortening the uncertainty in the time measurement so that better accuracy is attainable. At 10 MHz, a quarter cycle is only 25 nanosec long (corresponding to a tissue depth of 0.02 mm, assuming a velocity of 1,532 m/sec as in vitreous); at 20 MHz, these values become 12.5 nanosec and 0.01 mm of tissue depth (Fig. III-2). Thus at 20 MHz, a tissue measurement to equivalent first quarter cycles should not err by more than 10 microns, as compared to an error of twice this value at 10 MHz.

In considering the accuracy of measurements, it must be borne in mind that the points of measurement on both the "start" and "end" are important. First quarter cycles, e.g., the first quarter cycle

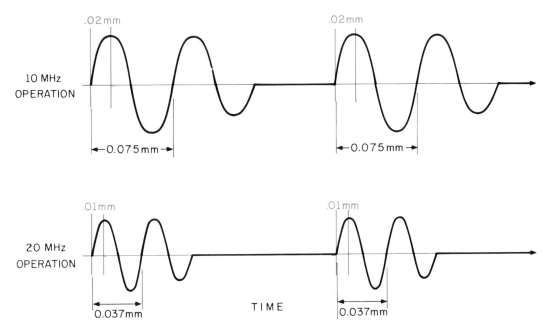

FIG. III-2. Schematic representation comparing the wavelength of ultrasound in the eye at 10 and 20 MHz. The 20-MHz wavelength is one-half the 10-MHz wavelength, thus providing twice the potential accuracy of measurement.

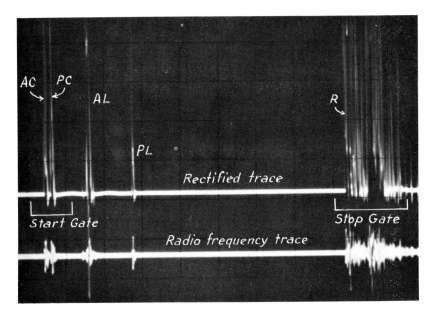

FIG. III-3. A-scan along the optic axis at 20 MHz showing the separation of corneal echoes and the resolution of dimensions typical at this frequency. The positions of "gates," which can be manually positioned for electronic measurement of tissue dimensions, are drawn in to indicate measurement of the cornea-to-vitreoretinal interface distance. (AC = anterior cornea, PC = posterior cornea, AL = anterior lens, PL = posterior lens, R = retina.)

of the corneal echo to the first quarter cycle of the lens echo, should be measured at corresponding voltage levels.

Increasing the frequency and focusing of the transducer results in improvements in both axial resolution and accuracy. However, tissue absorption also increases with frequency so that sensitivity is degraded. It has been found that a frequency of 20 MHz provides both high resolution and accuracy while providing sensitivity sufficient to detect echoes from the posterior ocular wall surfaces (Fig. III-3). Even higher-frequency transducers with resultant higher accuracy may be used for purely anterior segment biometry.

In addition to the all-important transducer frequency and the width of the ultrasound beam, the receiver which processes the information received from the transducer must be carefully considered.

Receiver

The receiver serves to process the output voltage pulses from the transducer into a form suitable for the display system employed. Receivers were discussed in Chapter II. The receiver adds no information to the returned echoes and in fact can distort waveshapes and thereby cause a loss of the information contained in the transducer output. The receiver can also critically influence attempts to achieve high overall accuracy. In particular, the process of rectification and rejection can result in loss of a part of the initial portion of the echoes unless these circuits are carefully designed. (Rectification, as noted in Chapter II, means converting bipolar signals to positive signals to produce a unipolar "envelope" of the reflected waves.) Since half wave rectification is less expensive to implement than full wave rectification, half wave rectification is employed in many ultrasonic systems. In this process either the positive or negative half of the alternating (R.F.) echo waveform is eliminated, rather than being converted to its opposite. Thus the first half cycle of an echo may be discarded and lost depending on its polarity (Fig. III-4). This process could delay the measured arrival time of some echoes by the time duration of a half cycle and result in correspondingly less accuracy. These systems are thus not recommended for biometry.

Ocular reflection patterns vary in polarity depending on the acoustic impedance of the various media, so that the initial half cycles of echoes will vary in polarity depending on whether the waves are going from a high impedance tissue to a lower impedance tissue or vice versa. Thus, half wave rectification will affect many time intervals such as the aqueous-lens and lens-vitreous intervals, and, again, the accuracy of measurements will be significantly degraded. This error can be avoided by employing full wave rectification which transforms the waveforms into unipolar signals without eliminating any portion of them. This full wave process is essential to allow maximum utilization of the accuracy inherent in the transducer output.

Another common feature employed in receivers is the electronic rejection of signals under a certain threshold level so that noise and small extraneous signals are not displayed. Since the echo voltages do not rise instantaneously, the rejection of noise may result in the elimination of the initial portion of the echo below the threshold level. If the peak amplitude of the first half cycle is not greater than the threshold level, a significant time lag will occur between the actual onset of an echo and its displayed waveform. This time error is a function of echo amplitude, a feature which varies through the eye. This is more of a problem, for example, with the vitreoretinal interface echo (low amplitude) than with the anterior corneal echo (high amplitude). Automatic gain control can remedy this situation by setting all peak echo amplitudes at the same voltage level so that rejection will alter all echoes by the same time interval.

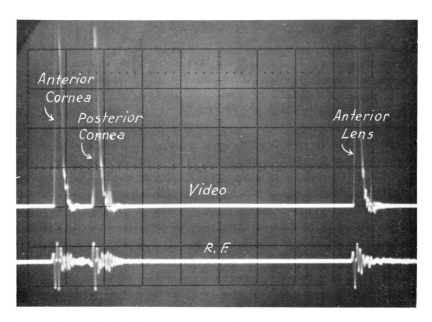

Fig. III-4. Electronically expanded view of the anterior segment of the eye shown in Figure III-3, again demonstrating the resolution available at 20 MHz and also demonstrating the polarity change in the radio-frequency waveform between anterior and posterior corneal echoes.

Finally, almost all systems display not the R.F. echo waveform but a video signal which is the envelope of this waveform. The time duration of the R.F. signal is smaller than that of its envelope-detected waveform, so that resolution is degraded in video signals. Thus to preserve all the resolution possible for accurate measurements it is desirable to employ radio frequency signals in all biometry methods where accurate measurements are desired and carried out on photographs of the oscilloscope screen.

Clinical Procedure

Visual Axis Ophthalmometry

In ophthalmometry, the dimensions of interest are usually those along the visual axis. Errors will result if the transducer is not aligned so that the path of the ultrasonic beam is along this axis. Jansson[125] has calculated that an error of 5 degrees in transducer orientation can result in an error of 0.1 mm in the measurement of the length of the visual axis. An error of this magnitude can be expected if the transducer is aimed along the path which provides maximum lens

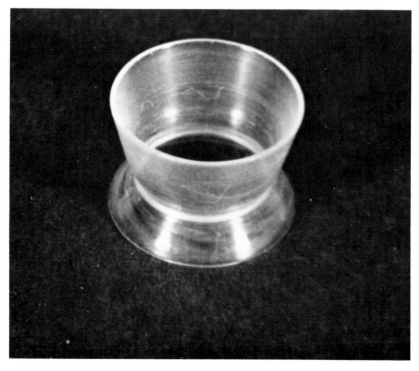

FIG. III-5A. A contact eye cup for axial measurement.

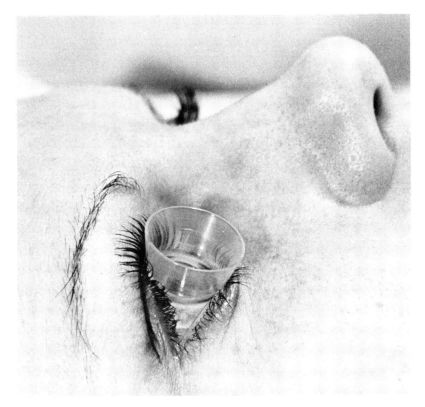

FIG. III-5B. Contact eye cup help in position by lids. The "cup" is filled with saline and the transducer can be aimed along the desired axis, while monitoring the A-mode display.

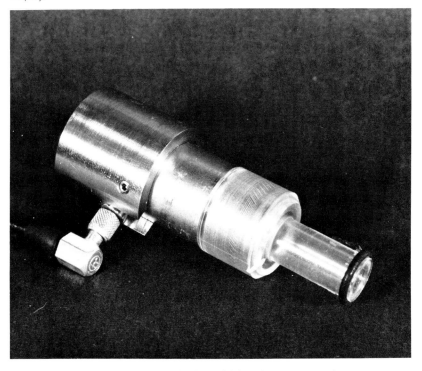

FIG. III-6. Water-filled standoff probe for axial length measurement.

echoes, i.e., the optic axis. Since the accuracy of the remainder of the system can be better than 0.1 mm, overall accuracy will be degraded by this procedure.

Alignment of the transducer with the visual axis has been used by many different observers. It was determined at an early stage that actual compression of the front of the globe by the transducer led to two major inaccuracies: flattening of the cornea and misalignment of the transducer beam.[126] Rivara devised a technique (which was adapted by Gernet)[127] that used a cup held between the lids. The cup was shaped to fit the sclera and was open at the bottom. With the patient supine, saline was used to fill the cup. The transducer was dipped into the front of the cup, away from the cornea, allowing measurement without touching the eye itself (Fig. III-5).

Leary[15] made use of what has been called a "water standoff probe." With this technique, a water-filled plastic cylinder is placed over the front of the transducer with the water column contained by the transducer face at one end and by a thin membrane (e.g., plastic wrap) over the open end of the tube. The membrane touches the cornea lightly, but, because of its flexibility, little deformation of the cornea occurs. The transducer's main bang thus does not interfere with the corneal echo (Fig. III-6).

Visual and Optical Axis Alignment

Yamamoto[128] provided an early solution to the problem of axis alignment. He devised a transducer crystal with a central area scraped to translucency so that a light shining through the transducer could be visualized by the examined subject.

Since then, other systems for visual alignment of the transducer have been devised. One of these is our own,[4] which uses a plastic cylinder around the transducer as in Leary's system, but uses the cornea of the eye to replace the membrane. The probe standoff is positioned slightly away or barely touching the limbus of the eye so that a meniscus of saline provides the only contact between the eye and the transducer. The patient aligns his own eye by looking through the center of the transducer at an alignment device or a light (Figs. III-7 through -11). This technique, with a variation in the transducer-eye coupling, has also been advocated by Giglio.[129] In Giglio's technique, a standoff cylinder is tapered to a small opening. The cylinder is filled before touching the eye so that a meniscus of fluid within the cylinder occludes the opening. Giglio has also developed a device which can move this cylinder to the patient's eye and away in only a few milliseconds between blinks, so that an anesthetic is not required for the measurement.

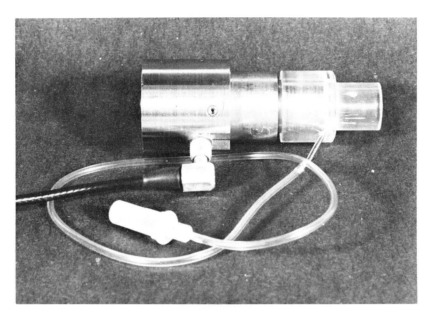

FIG. III-7. Open-end, limbus-supported probe with a focused 20-MHz transducer.

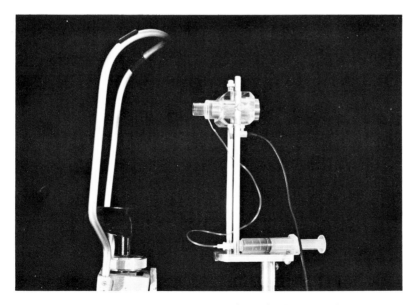

FIG. III-8. The transducer with limbus-supported standoff is mounted on a base that can be brought to the eye while the chin and forehead are stabilized.

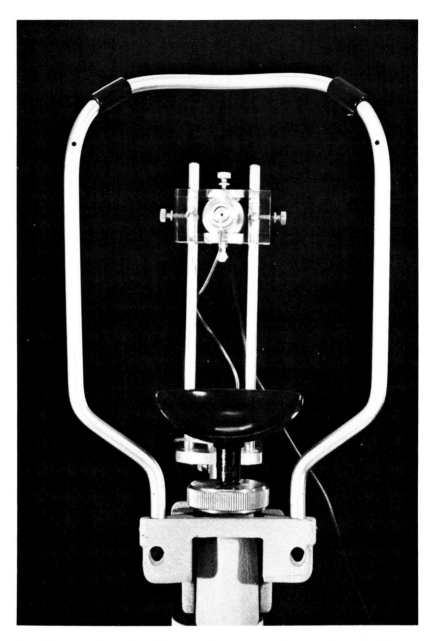

Fɪɢ. III-9. An end-on view of the transducer showing the central opening through which a fixation light can be viewed.

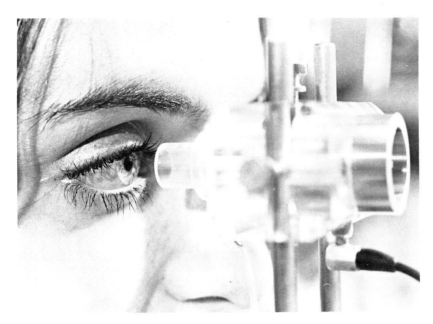

FIG. III-10A. The standoff is positioned on the limbus of the eye after a local anesthetic is instilled. Saline provides a meniscus of fluid contact between the rim and the limbus so that no pressure is exerted on the eye.

We have found many other standoff arrangements to be of value for specific projects, depending on horizontal or vertical approach and the transducer frequency and focal characteristics (Figs. III-12, -13).

The most accurate system which we have devised allows the patient to align the visual axis of his own eye (again with a standoff at the limbus) on a series of optotypes by means of a front surface mirror. The transducer is aimed at the eye through a hole in this mirror, so that as the patient fixates the optotype through this hole measurement along the visual axis is assured (Figs. III-14, -15).

In general, the less cumbersome method of aligning the patient's eye with a light source (i.e., using the visual axis) is easily reproducible and is the most useful for required measurements.

In making measurements along the optical axis, transducer alignment can be checked by observing three features of the display. First, the anterior and posterior lens echoes should be maximally separated. Second, the posterior lens echo amplitude should be maximal and nearly as high as that of the anterior lens echo. Third, the vitreous compartment dimension from the posterior lens to vitreoretinal interface should be maximized, while simultaneously the posterior lens echo amplitude is maximized. Accuracy can be further enhanced by averaging measurements.

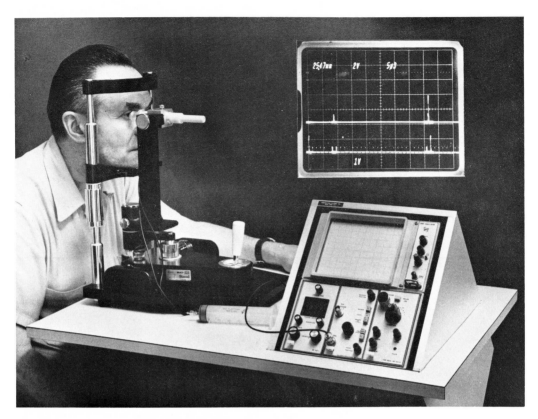

Fig. III-10B. Biometric ruler devised by Sonometrics Systems, Inc., for the determination of axial length, based upon equipment developed in our laboratory. A very thin (.02-mm) silicone membrane covers the front end of the transducer collar, preventing leakage and maintaining a constant fluid level. When the transducer is optimally aligned along the optical axis, the echoes produced by the cornea, the anterior and posterior lens capsules and the retina are used to determine the dimensions of the anterior chamber, the lens and the vitreous compartment. The acoustic velocity values for each ocular tissue are manually adjusted on a dial below the oscilloscope face. The tissue thickness measurements of the structure are automatically computed and portrayed on the oscilloscope screen as depicted in the inset.

A-mode Measurement

As noted above and in Chapter II, the accuracy of measurement depends on recognition of, and measurement at, the first quarter cycle of each echo. This means that A-mode techniques are more accurate than intensity modulated techniques. Also the A-mode technique must have sufficient full wave video rectification and sufficient receiver bandwidth so that the first quarter cycle is recognized. When full wave rectification is used, sufficient gain must be present in both measured echoes so that the first quarter cycle can be seen. Also, either an electronic counter or sufficient magnification of the oscilloscope screen must be possible so that the physical

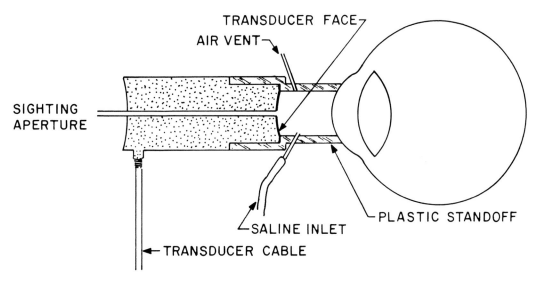

FIG. III-11. Schematic view of probe shown in previous figures. Saline is injected into the chamber from below. An air vent is provided on the top of the chamber. The patient fixates on a light source through the transducer to give visual axis alignment.

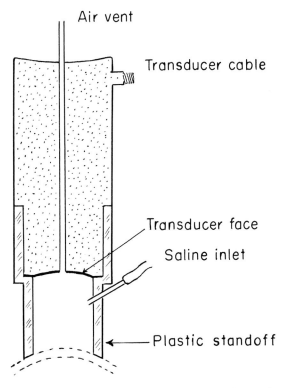

FIG. III-12. The same transducer as shown in the previous figures positioned vertically, using the sighting aperture as an air vent.

width of the oscilloscope trace (or photograph of it) does not become a problem in measurement.

Anatomic and Physical Problems of Measurement

We have already mentioned that distortion or flattening of the cornea may be a physical problem in A-mode measurement. A second problem is that the iris tends to interrupt the transducer beam so that a distinct differentiation between iris and anterior lens surfaces is not possible. With high enough resolution, 15 to 20 MHz, the peak of the second or anterior lens echo can be reliably discerned from the iris echo. Dilation of the pupil, if the experimental procedure will allow, will entirely avoid the problem of the iris interference with the anterior lens echo.

A third problem often encountered is that the patient, by squeezing the lids, will distort the eye. A drop of local anesthetic, such as proparacaine hydrochloride, in the patient's eye will usually permit comfortable examination for 15 to 30 minutes. Most patients have a tendency to squeeze their eyes when an anesthetic is not used, and this can greatly alter the dimensions of the globe.

A fourth problem in axial measurement that we have often observed is the presence of low-amplitude echoes preceding the definite vitreoretinal interface echo. This problem is often noted

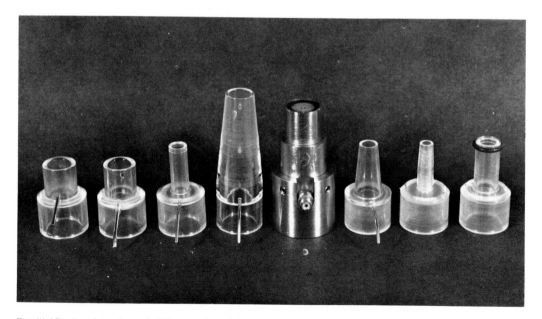

Fig. III-13. A variety of standoff tips found useful in specific measurement applications. These are shown with the 20-MHz focused transducer used in most of our biometric determinations.

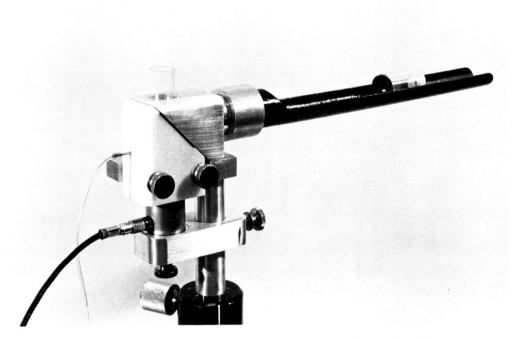

FIG. III-14. A device for visual axis alignment using an optotype and a front surface mirror.

when the vitreoretinal interface returns a relatively low echo, indicating that the transducer alignment is slightly off axis. Careful transducer alignment usually negates this difficulty. Occasionally an artifactual "multiple" of the corneal echo or the posterior vitreous hyaloid face causes spurious echoes to appear anterior to the retina.

Computation of Axial Measurement

Once the elapsed time between various echoes on the A-scan trace has been obtained, it is necessary to multiply these measurements by appropriate tissue velocities to determine a true axial measurement. Jansson's[125] velocities of 1,532 m/sec for aqueous and vitreous and 1,640.5 m/sec for lens are used as standards by most ophthalmic investigators. Other data in the literature have been reported and are summarized in Table III-2. These velocity constants are obviously of critical importance since they are multiplied by the time measurements obtained by biometry to arrive at distance measurements. Any inaccuracy in the velocity constant will thus cause inaccuracy in the final result. Nevertheless, for most experiments which determine a *change* in axial measurement under various

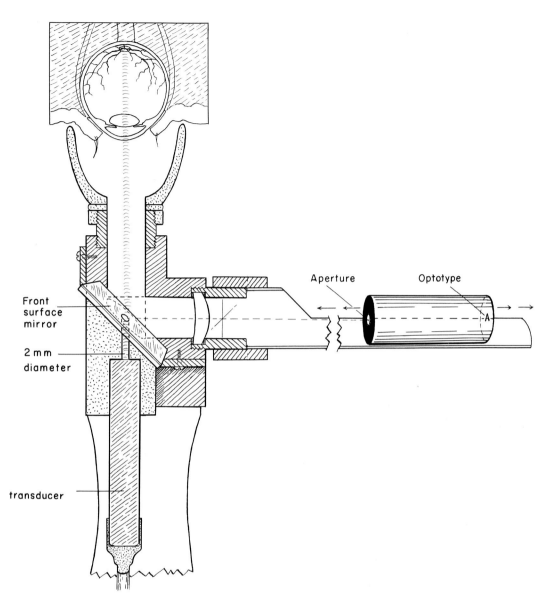

Front
surface
mirror

2 mm
diameter

transducer

Aperture

Optotype

A

FIG. III-15. Schematic representation of the visual axis aligner shown in Figure III-14.

physiologic or pharmacologic states, the constants do not provide a major source of error. They can, however, produce substantial errors in absolute measurements. Present data for aqueous and vitreous velocity constants are probably highly accurate, but the accepted lens velocity requires reexamination. However, since the anterior-to-posterior thickness of the lens is a small fraction of the total anterior-to-posterior length of the globe, the effect of a small error in the lens velocity is not as serious as the same percentage of error would be in the vitreous propagation velocity.

TISSUE THICKNESS = VELOCITY OF SOUND IN TISSUE X TIME

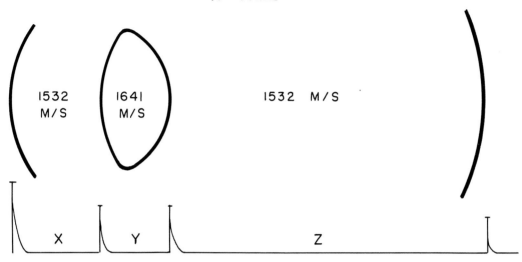

1532 M/S

1641 M/S

1532 M/S

X   Y   Z

FIG. III-16. The axial length of the eye is determined by measuring the sound transmission time between each major interface of anterior chamber (X), lens (Y), and vitreous compartment (Z), and multiplying the appropriate transmission time by the velocity of sound in that tissue. These three values added together provide the axial length of the eye.

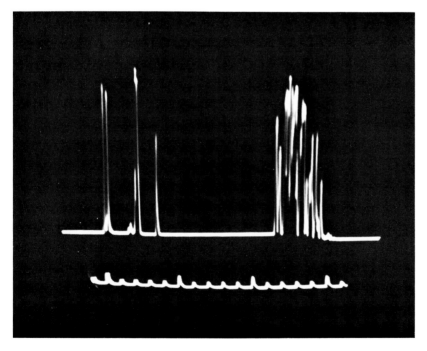

FIG. III-17. A-scan along the optic axis shown above a time marker scale used to indicate tissue depth. Each large marker corresponds to approximately 1 cm, and each small marker corresponds to approximately 2 mm, of tissue thickness.

Table III-2. Velocity of Sound (m/sec) in Human and Animal Tissues

Investigator and Year	Animal	Temperature and Frequency	Cornea	Aqueous	Lens	Cataractous Lens	Vitreous	Sclera	Other
Willard, G. 1947		10 MHz							Water $V_t = 1557 - .0245(74\text{-}T)^2$ V_t is velocity in meters per second
Ludwig, G. 1950	Human	24–25°C at 2.5 & 1.5 MHz							Muscle—1540 (range: 1490–1610) Spleen—1515 Liver—1553 Kidney—1558 Brain—1506
	Hog								Brain—1515
	Dog								Muscle—1575–1585
	Cow								Water—1490
Frucht, A. H. 1952	Human	24°C at 1.8 MHz							Pectoral muscle— 1530–1600 Fat—1445–1485
Frucht, A. H. 1953	Calf	24°C at 1.8 MHz							Muscle—1574 Fat—1465
	Pig								Muscle—1577 Fat—1444
	Horse								Muscle—1579 Fat—1443
Rudiger, W. (from Buschmann) 1953		24°C		1497	1616		1516		Fat—1443
Begui, Z. E. 1954	Calf	26–31°C							Fat—1476

Reference	Animal	Conditions							Notes
Goldman, D. E. and Richards, J. R. 1954	Dog	26°C at 4 & 12 MHz							Thigh (perpendicular)—1576; parallel—1592 Liver—1581 Kidney—1559 Heart—1572 Spleen—1570
	Rabbit								Thigh (perpendicular)—1587; (parallel)—1603 Liver—1575
Goldman, D. E. and Heuter, T. F.	Human	24°C at 1.8 MHz 37°C at 2.26 MHz 37°C at .8 MHz							Fat—1476 Meningioma—1540 Skull bone—3360
Oksala, A. and Lehtinen, A. 1958	Cow	22°C at 4 MHz	1550	1495	1650		1495	1630	
Oksala, A. and Lehtinen, A. 1959	Human	22°C at 4 MHz							
Barone, A. and Scafati, A. 1960	Rabbit Cavia Horse	25.05°C 27.80°C 27.07°C	1580	1470	1530	1570	1470	1660	Citrated blood 1530–1540
Yamamoto, Y., et al. 1961	Cow Pig Human	5 MHz							Skin—1581 Skin—1588 Skin—1601
Araki, M. 1961	Pig Human	5 MHz	1609	1546	1627 1638		1498 1514	1609 1613	

TABLE III-2 (Continued)

Investigator and Year	Animal	Temperature and Frequency	Cornea	Aqueous	Lens	Cataractous Lens	Vitreous	Sclera	Other
Jansson, F. and Sundmark, E. 1961	Pig Human	22°C 34.1°C & 35.2°C at 4 MHz			1665 1641		1510 1530		
Rivara, A. and Sanna, G. 1962	Pig Human	37°C at 4 MHz	1587.92 1586.38	1529.63	1672.75 1647.11		1531.53 1523.20	1655.76 1646.75	
Jansson, F. and Kock, E. 1962	Human Physiologic solution	37°C at 4 MHz		1532	1640.5	1543–1665	1532.4		
Nover, A. and Glanschneider, D. 1965	Human	37°C at 12 MHz	1610	1540	1645	1655–1691	1540	1650	Malignant melanoma 1660 Lid carcinoma—1585
Kossoff, G., Robinson, Garrett 1965		24°C							Muscle—1590 Fat—1440 Nerve, brain—1510
Tschewnenko, A. 1965	Human	37°C	1639	1534	1647		1534	1650	
Vanysek, J., Preisova, J., Obraz, J. 1969	Human	37°C	1639	1534	1647		1534	1650	

Reference	Species	Conditions			Measurements
Buschmann, W., Voss, M. and Kemmering, S. 1970	Human	37°C 6–14 MHz			External eye muscles 1631; Orbital fat—1462; Optic nerve—1615
Christmann, C., Ehler, E. 1971	Human				Humerus bone—2632; Radius—3073; Ulna—2787
VanVenrooij, G. 1971	Human	22°C at 2 MHz			Blood—1550–1570; CSF—1499; Meningioma—1524; Glioma—1529
Bradley, E. and Sacerio, J. 1972	Human	37°C			Blood—1560–1580
Craven, J., et al. 1973	Human	37°C at 5 MHz			Proximal radius—3406 (range 3210–3540) decreased with age
Sterns, G. K., Coleman, D. J., Ellsworth, R. M. 1974	Human	37°C at 22 MHz	1659 (child)	1629	Retinoblastoma—1535–1600; Clotted blood—1604
Coleman, D. J. et al. 1975	Human	37°C at 15 MHz			

The formula that we use for computing axial length is based on three transit time measurements of the eye: (1) anterior cornea to anterior lens, (2) anterior lens to posterior lens, and (3) posterior lens to vitreoretinal interface. In our method, using an interval counter, we use the cornea as a prime reference point and avoid moving the initial counter gate. Thus, to make the three measurements enumerated above, simple subtraction (examples will be discussed in detail below) provides us with the transit time of the anterior chamber, the lens and the vitreous compartment.

Each of these time measurements is then multiplied by the appropriate velocity constant to arrive at tissue measurements. The time from anterior cornea to anterior lens is multiplied by 1,532 m/sec to calculate the corresponding thickness. The time from anterior to posterior lens is multiplied by 1,640.5 m/sec to provide the thickness of the lens. The time from the posterior lens to the vitreoretinal interface is multiplied by 1,532 m/sec to provide the thickness of the vitreous compartment. These three values added together provide the total axial length of the eye (Fig. III-16).

Two small potential errors are inherent in this method. First, the cornea has an axial thickness of 0.5 to 0.6 mm and is not measured separately and corrected for by a velocity constant. Since this thickness is small the potential error from any difference in velocity constant is exceedingly small.

Second, the axial length is determined to the *vitreoretinal interface* and not to Bruch's membrane or to the posterior scleral wall. These features should be remembered when comparing axial measurements using ultrasound to those found by measuring histologic sections or to subjective visual data.

Measurements from Photographs

The display system presents the echo-generated voltage pulses from the eye in a form suitable for obtaining measurements. The most commonly employed method consists of a visual display of the echo waveforms on an oscilloscope screen. In biometry, this display can be photographed and time intervals measured by means of a vernier caliper. Since random errors can occur from effects such as small movements of the transducer or the subject's eye, it is important to obtain and average several readings. This process entails taking a large number of photographs in succession and repeating the measurements. This is time consuming but reduces measurement error.

The accuracy and precision attainable in measuring a linear distance over the relatively short dimension of a photograph are inherently poor. Difficulties arise, first, in determination of the time of origin of each echo, and, second, in accurate placement of the caliper points. Increasing the oscilloscope time base alleviates these problems but precludes viewing the entire ocular region simultaneously. These difficulties can introduce significant observer variation.

An alternative approach consists of dividing the echoes into several groups and displaying them simultaneously on separate traces on an oscilloscope. This procedure increases the accuracy and precision attainable but still makes averaging inconvenient. This solution sacrifices much of the flexibility possessed by the ultrasonic approach. It becomes inconvenient in applications such as foreign body localization where relative positions are important. These are more readily carried out when the entire eye is visualized on one trace.

Measurement of elapsed time between echoes can be made photographically or electronically. In the photographic technique a time reference scale must be used. It can be obtained by using a time marker built into the apparatus, which produces spikes on a horizontal baseline, or it can be obtained by using a "standard" block to provide spikes on the display that correspond to a "constant" tissue thickness.

The time marker system uses an oscillator as a clock to provide spikes at specified time intervals either on the trace baseline or on a separate trace immediately adjacent to the scan trace. The spikes are designed to correspond to a tissue thickness at a constant predetermined velocity, i.e., a 2-mm spacing corresponds to 2 mm of tissue at the calibration velocity. This selected velocity is usually that of water (1,500 m/sec) or of saline (1,530 m/sec). This technique provides only an approximation of tissue thickness and without careful equipment design is not particularly accurate (Fig. III-17).

The equipment instruction manual should be read carefully to determine the calibration velocity used, as it varies with different manufacturers. Crude biometry techniques do not correct for the difference in velocity of the lens and vitreous. At the very least, a correction factor of 1.07 should be used to account for the average lens difference. The correction factor is derived by dividing the lens velocity (1641 m/sec) by the aqueous and vitreous velocity (1532 m/sec), i.e.:

$$\frac{1641}{1532} = 1.07$$

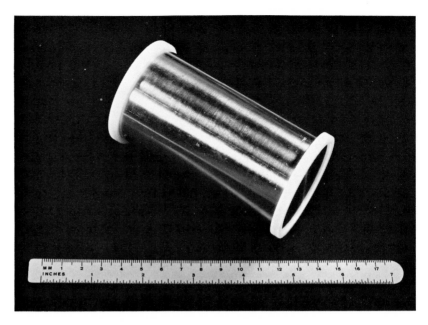

FIG. III-18. A metal standard block used for calibrating the photograph of the A-scan. The block, physically 10 cm long, produces echoes from end to end that correspond to a tissue thickness of 2.5 cm, due to the great difference in sound velocities in this metal and the eye. The block is initially calibrated by using an electronic interval counter.

With this technique, a lens thickness (e.g., 3.7 mm) computed by a time marker would be multiplied by 1.07 to give a corrected lens thickness of 3.96 mm. Thus, the derived axial length would be corrected by .26 mm to account for the faster velocity of sound through the lens. This method may be adequate for many observers, but when an electronic interval counter is not available we recommend the use of a standard calibration block. It requires only slightly more time and effort and is far more accurate.

Use of a standard, as Gernet has recommended,[124] provides a more accurate way of scaling photographs. In this method, a piece of metal (or plastic) with a propagation velocity many times that of tissue is used. Gernet used an aluminum block with a velocity approximately four times that of the eye. Since the velocity is great, a block approximately 10 cm long (4 times longer than the eye) will give echoes on the oscilloscope that correspond to approximately the length of the eye (Fig. III-18). The photograph of ocular echoes, when compared to a photograph of the echoes from a calibrated block, will thus allow appropriate scaling of the eye in terms of time (microseconds) or of comparable tissue thickness (millimeters).

The advantage of using a metal block with four times the velocity of the eye is that any inaccuracy in calibrating its length will cause only one-fourth as large an error in ocular measurements. For greatest accuracy with this method, the temperature of the bar as well as its composition must be accurately controlled (Fig. III-19).

The time for sound to traverse the standard block is measured with an interval counter and remains as its calibrated time transmission value. Thus, when the echoes from the block are photographed, the time between the echoes is always the same known value, even though the distance between the echo spikes may vary according to the settings on the equipment dials. Comparison of an eye with a standard thus allows calibration of the eye tissue transmission times.

With the standard block technique, a photograph of the echoes from the block is taken immediately after the photograph of the subject eye, while all the equipment dials are unchanged. Each of the eye distances is then measured and the distance between the block ends is measured from the photograph. The ratio of the total eye distance to the standard block distance on the photographs is

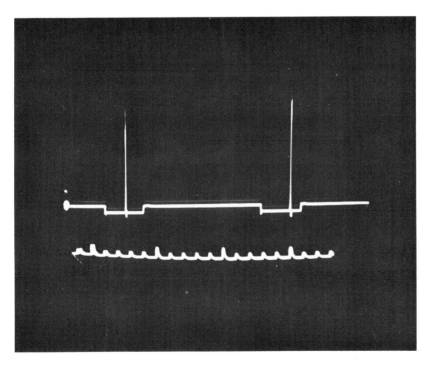

FIG. III-19. Photograph of the echoes returned from the standard block shown in Figure III-18. This photograph is then compared to the A-scan of the examined eye taken with all equipment settings unchanged.

then multiplied by the time interval constant for the standard block to give the total time for sound to traverse the eye. The lens, aqueous and vitreous compartments are then scaled.

As an example, consider the following eye lengths measured from a photograph:

Cornea to lens	13.4 mm
Anterior lens to posterior lens	15.9 mm
Posterior lens to retina	69.0 mm
Total	98.3 mm
Known standard measure	100.0 mm

The transmission time for the known standard is known to be 32.0 μsec. Therefore, each millimeter on the oscilloscope is 0.32 μsec. This factor multiplied by the measured lengths and the appropriate velocities provides the value for the total length of the eye:

Cornea to lens
$$13.4 \text{ mm} \times 1.532 \text{ mm}/\mu\text{sec} \times 0.32 \times 0.5 = 3.28 \text{ mm}$$
Anterior lens to posterior lens
$$15.9 \text{ mm} \times 1.641 \text{ mm}/\mu\text{sec} \times 0.32 \times 0.5 = 4.17 \text{ mm}$$
Posterior lens to retina
$$69.0 \text{ mm} \times 1.532 \text{ mm}/\mu\text{sec} \times 0.32 \times 0.5 = 16.91 \text{ mm}$$
Total length of the eye $= 24.36$ mm

Velocities have been expressed in mm/μsec by multiplying by 10^{-3}. The factor 0.5 accounts for the two-way travel.

The standard must be measured each time the equipment is used for biometry to provide a comparison scale, as even a slight variation in dial settings would produce a major error.

Using frequencies of 20 MHz, and with care, this method is probably accurate to within 0.1 mm of tissue thickness.

Measurements with an Electronic Interval Counter

Many of the difficulties of photographic recording and measurements can be circumvented by the use of an electronic interval counter.[27] This device measures the interval between echoes by electronically counting the number of pulses from an accurate oscillator which occur during the measured interval. The measurements become very accurate as the oscillator frequency is increased, since there are more pulses within a given time interval. This is analogous to using a ruler with finer divisions. At 50 MHz approximately 1,500 pulses are generated in the time interval between the corneal and rear wall echoes, and the smallest interval which can be measured is on the order of 0.02 mm (20 microns). Averaging a series of counter readings can decrease this already small interval significantly, thus providing even greater measurement precision.

The interval counter allows measurements to be made between any two echoes by means of adjustable voltage "gates" or "windows" which are monitored on an oscilloscope simultaneously with an A-scan presentation of the ocular echoes (Fig. III-20). The counter will present a digital readout of the interval between the first echoes occurring within each gate position. Thus, the first (start) gate can be positioned around the first corneal echo and the second (stop) gate positioned to detect a specified subsequent echo such as the retina. Averaging can be simply and rapidly accomplished by taking several readings for each echo. The counter can display readouts extremely rapidly (for example, five displays per second) or can itself average over a specified time period, thus providing a large average sample in a relatively short time period.

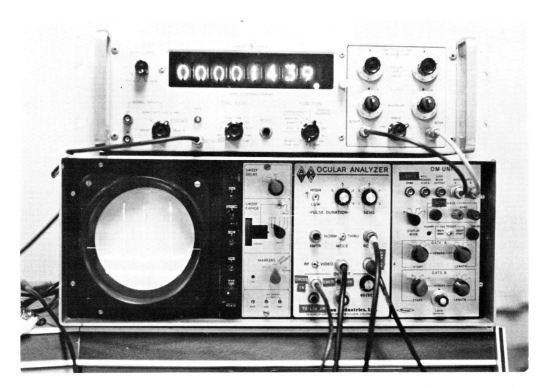

Fig. III-20. An electronic interval counter measurement system for providing exceptionally accurate time measurements between echoes. Gates or windows are positioned on the baseline around selected echoes. The time between the first echo in the "start" gate and the first echo in the "stop" gate is shown automatically and continuously on the interval counter.

This method, which we originated and prefer for our biometric applications, provides objective measurements of extremely high accuracy while preserving the flexibility of the A-scan system in studying many biometric problems. This approach can be conveniently employed to study many conditions since only an A-scan normal or perpendicular to the pertinent anatomy, together with a simple, manual adjustment of the voltage gate to select the desired echoes, is necessary. Continuous, real time monitoring of ocular dimensions and their variations under influences such as drugs or accommodation is thus available. The accuracy attainable with this system is independent of the dimensions studied. No alterations are required to measure large distances.

Measurements with the interval counter proceed exactly as in the example given for the standard block, except that the counter automatically provides the time for each of the eye components. After dividing by two to obtain one-way transit time, the computations are as follows:

Cornea to lens	2.09 μsec × 1532 m/sec = 3.20 mm
Anterior lens to posterior lens	2.48 μsec × 1641 m/sec = 4.07 mm
Posterior lens to retina	10.78 μsec × 1532 m/sec
	= 16.51 mm
Total length	23.78 mm

These time intervals can be measured repeatedly to improve accuracy. For example, ten readings for each interval can be made at the rate of three or more readings per second, so that in ten seconds ten separate total measurements can be made and averaged. Averaging can provide an additional decimal place in accuracy. This system provides the greatest accuracy for ultrasonic biometry. If high frequencies (i.e., 20 MHz) are used, the measurements can be accurate to approximately 0.02 mm or 20 microns.

Axial Length Measurement for Intraocular Lens Implant or Keratoprosthesis

Since most patients selected for intraocular lens implantation or keratoprosthesis do not have good central vision with the eye being considered for surgery, visual axis determination is not possible and the optic axis measurement must be utilized. The special problems encountered in obtaining these measurements should again be emphasized.

First, the selection of suitable echoes requires practice and skill. The transducer must be aligned so that the amplitude of the anterior and posterior lens echoes are maximized as to amplitude while the distance from the cornea to the vitreoretinal interface spike is simultaneously maximized. Globe compression must also be avoided during this procedure.

Second, since the lens thickness is critical, a spurious apparent anterior lens surface echo produced by the iris should be avoided by dilating the pupil and the true anterior lens echo should be carefully identified on the oscilloscope screen or photograph.

In calculating the axial length in cataract patients, we use the lens velocity of 1629 m/sec[130] as most cataractous lenses in our studies have a lower density than normal lenses. If a thin lens is found on measurement, i.e., a lens which measures less than 3.5 mm, this may indicate the more unusual clinical situation of a "dense" or sclerotic lens in which the velocity of sound lies in a higher range of 1660 m/sec.[130] In this instance, we suggest supplying two separate axial length measurements labeled "normal cataract" for the velocity computation using 1629 m/sec, and "dense cataract" for the velocity computation using 1660 m/sec. If the selection of the dioptric power of an intraocular lens would be affected by the difference in the computations, then the surgeon, after examining the cataract at the time of surgery, could decide which value for the implanted lens is more applicable.

Third, after surgery the eye may have a flatter cornea than that in the presurgical state. Depending upon the surgical technique, this could indicate a corrective factor in the selection of lens power. Patients selected for keratoprosthesis commonly have such significant scarring of the cornea that their axial length is substantially shorter than normal.[93]

Once the axial length is obtained, the selection of intraocular lens power can be determined by use of keratometry and a nomogram such as that published by Worst,[98] or by calculation of the intraocular lens power using a formula such as that published by Binkhorst.[85] Binkhorst's formula for calculation of the intraocular lens power required to render a given eye emmetropic is:

$$D = \frac{1336\,(4r - a)}{(a - d)(4r - d)}$$

where D = the dioptric power in aqueous or vitreous (refractive index 1.336) of the intraocular lens

where r = the radius of curvature of the anterior surface of the cornea in mm

where a = the axial length in mm

where d = the distance between the anterior vertex of the cornea and the intraocular lens in mm

With a programmable hand calculator, lens power for emmetropia or desired myopia or hyperopia can be quickly ascertained.

Ultrasound Velocity of Tissue

Techniques for measuring tissues to determine their inherent velocity of sound conduction have been described by Jansson[125] and by Oksala.[35] A method that we have found reliable uses a knowledge of the velocity of sound in saline to compute tissue velocity.[130] A transducer is fixed in a saline bath, and the time for the sound beam to traverse a given thickness of tissue (Fig. III-21) is measured. In this technique, a measurement of the sound transmission time from transducer to anterior tissue surface is made (T1), as well as the time from the anterior surface of the tissue to the posterior surface of the tank (T2). When the tissue is then removed, the transmission time is measured from the transducer to the posterior surface of the tank (T3). Subtraction of the initial measurement of transducer to anterior tissue from the new total measurement will provide the total thickness of fluid that has "replaced" the tissue. With knowledge of the velocity of sound in saline and the measured ratio of transit times, (T3–T1)/T2, the velocity of sound in the "unknown" tissue is easily derived. These three measurements thus allow computation of the tissue velocity.

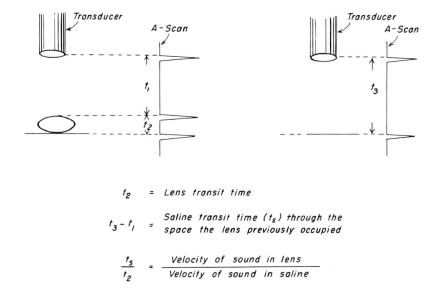

I. Lens in position beneath fixed transducer   *II. Lens removed, transducer unchanged*

$$t_2 = \text{Lens transit time}$$

$$t_3 - t_1 = \begin{array}{l}\textit{Saline transit time } (t_s) \textit{ through the}\\ \textit{space the lens previously occupied}\end{array}$$

$$\frac{t_s}{t_2} = \frac{\textit{Velocity of sound in lens}}{\textit{Velocity of sound in saline}}$$

FIG. III-21. Method of determining tissue velocity illustrated here with the human lens.

The identification and location of intraocular tumors are of the greatest importance diagnostically; therefore, most tumors require only a gross estimation of their size. Ultrasonography, however, provides reproducible and highly accurate measurements of tumor elevation. The observation of intraocular tumors is often enhanced by the use of ultrasound to determine the rate of growth or regression. In addition, calculation of optimum tumor radiation dosage and the proper selection of external cobalt plaques are aided by accurate measurement of tumor height.

The height of a tumor can be adequately measured by either A- or B-scan methods. The two main problems in obtaining a proper measurement are: (1) maximizing the height of a tumor and aligning the transducer appropriately, and (2) discerning the acoustic separation of tumor from underlying choroid or sclera.

The transducer must be carefully positioned to intercept the peak of the tumor while maintaining a normal or perpendicular orientation to the scleral base. This is a visual correlation made by the examiner during the scanning procedure. On the B-scan, the photograph should be taken utilizing gray scale in order to select the tissue plane of tumor-sclera separation. This plane is usually detectable by the high-amplitude leading edge of the sclera, but occasionally may be indistinguishable even on the A-scan.

Since the accuracy required in measurements of tumor elevation prior to placement of external cobalt plaques is generally acceptable within half a millimeter, a velocity correction factor for tumor tissue is not usually required. For determination of growth or regression, however, the comparative time for tumor traverse is the essential fact and conversion to millimeter measure is superfluous. Nevertheless, the tissue thickness can be computed by using a velocity constant. At present, we use a velocity constant of 1600 m/sec for choroidal malignant melanoma.

B-scan Biometry

Weinstein and Baum[131] early reported on the advantages of B-scan as compared to A-scan measurements. While their comparison of B-scan to A-scan has not been widely accepted, due to the velocity constant they used, the use of B-scan to provide measurements of different structures is uniquely applicable in many situations.[4] Not only does B-scan provide an easier way of measuring distances between structures that are not along the visual or optical axis but it also allows estimation of volume and curvatures.[132-134]

The curvature of the anterior and posterior lens can be obtained with compass measurements of these curved surfaces from photographs. A photographic transparency with enlargement on a suitable screen expedites this measurement. Whereas various formulas can in some instances be used to calculate volume based on curvatures obtained by ultrasound, the eye structures would require complex geometric equations. The measurement of volume is best obtained from a series of B-scans taken with parallel planes.[135] A planimeter can be used to outline the area to be evaluated, and then volume is computed. Total volume equals cross-section area times depth increase between each scan (Fig. III-22).

Volume measurement from B-scans provides a suitable means of estimating the lens, anterior chamber and vitreous volume. It must be remembered that, unless serial sections are made, a single scan through the maximum anterior-to-posterior diameter may provide measurements from a scan plane that is not perfectly sagittal or normal to the tissue. Consequently, if the plane is slightly off axis, a substantial error can be obtained in estimating volumes and in comparing this volume to volumes determined on subsequent measurements.

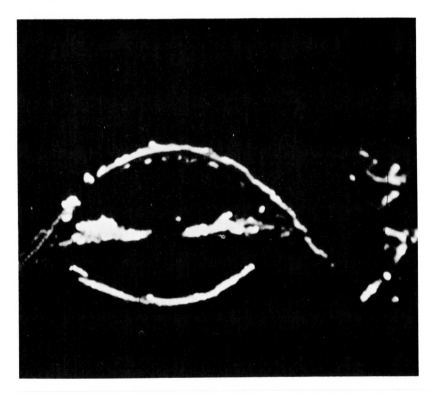

FIG. III-22. An anterior segment of an eye on B-scan, graphically demonstrating how the anterior chamber or lens can be measured for area. Serial measurements can be used to provide an estimate of volume.

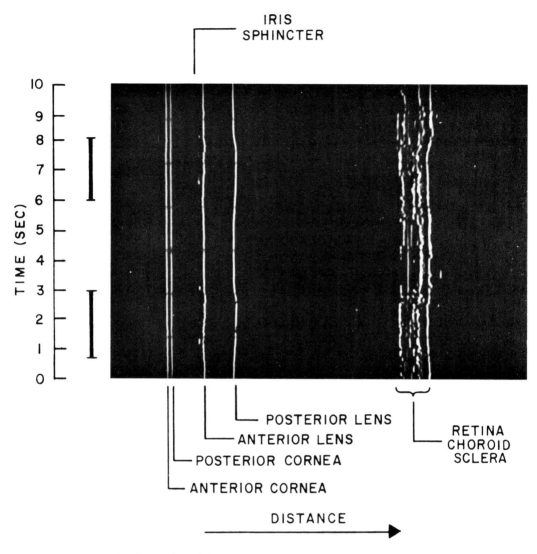

FIG. III-23. M-scan showing motion of the lens surface during accommodation in the eye.

M-scan Measurements

Biometry using M-scan has achieved little clinical use to date since alignment problems make it difficult to be completely sure that the measurements are being simultaneously recorded from identifiable surfaces.[136] Secondly, small movements of the patient's eye are greatly magnified, so that many M-scans of precise physiologic function require anesthesia. Measurement through the lens, for example, which would seem an easy way to demonstrate variations in lens thickness, have to be continually compared to the velocity

Vitreo-
Retinal
Interface —

Posterior —
Scleral
Wall

R

C

CA

O

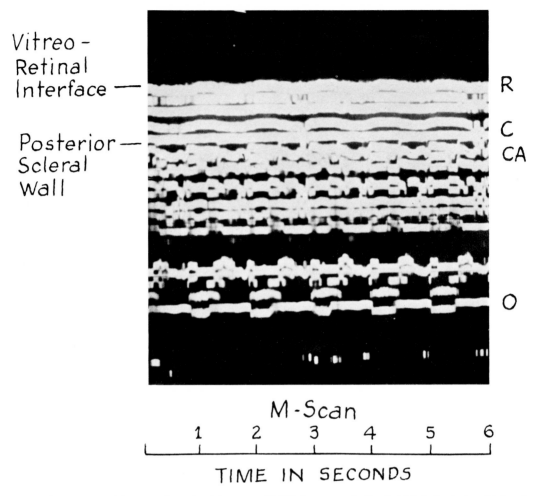

M-Scan

1   2   3   4   5   6

TIME IN SECONDS

FIG. III-24. M-scan of the posterior pole of the eye at 20 MHz in an anesthetized child. Retinal, choroidal and retrobulbar vascular pulsations are shown. (R = retina, C = choroid, CA = ciliary artery, O = ophthalmic artery.)

variations through the lens in order to determine the true motions of the posterior lens surface (Fig. III-23).

Nevertheless, estimates of vascular pulsations and accommodative changes of the lens can be graphically and precisely shown with this technique[137] when the experimental conditions are carefully controlled (Fig. III-24).

This technique is a graphic way of demonstrating movement of vascular surfaces and will surely be of great interest in future biometric studies.

A summary of some of the points discussed above is listed here for convenience:

Transducer	Higher frequency gives better accuracy. Focused transducers give better lateral resolution.
Display	Radio frequency display preserves highest axial resolution. Video displays should use full wave rectification.
Receiver	Proper bandwidth should be selected for transducer used. Automatic gain control allows correction for sound attenuation in measurement of deeper tissues.
Patient alignment	Transducer should be "stood off" from eye so main bang does not mask the initial signal. Transducer should not compress globe. Optical or visual axis alignment is possible by different techniques.
Measurement	In order of preference: (1) electronic interval counter, (2) standard distance comparator, (3) oscilloscope time markers.
A-mode	Best for tissue thickness measurements
B-scan	Can provide area and volume measurements
M-mode	Can provide measurement of rate and excursion of tissue motion, e.g., vascular and respiratory changes.

References Cited

1. Mundt, G. H., and Hughes, W. F.: Ultrasonics in ocular diagnosis. Am. J. Ophthalmol., 41:488–498, 1956.
2. Baum, G.: The effect of ultrasonic radiation upon the eye and ocular adnexa. Am. J. Ophthalmol., 42:696–706, 1956.
3. Buschmann, W.: Ultrasonic measurement of the axial length of the eye. Klin. Monatsbl. Augenheilkd., 144:801–815, 1964.
4. Coleman, D. J.: Ophthalmic biometry using ultrasound. Int. Ophthalmol. Clin., 9(3):667–683, 1969.
5. Coleman, D. J.: Unified model for accommodative mechanism. Am. J. Ophthalmol., 69:1063–1079, 1970.
6. Franceschetti, A.: Clinical importance of measurement of ocular components. Am. J. Ophthalmol., 59:1139, 1965.
7. Francois, J.: Ultrasonic biometry of the eye. In: Ultrasonics in Medicine. Edited by M. DeVlieger, et al. Amsterdam, Excerpta Medica, 1974, pp. 128–139.

8. Franken, S.: Measuring the length of the eye with the help of ultrasonic echo. Ophthalmologica, 143:82–85, 1962.
9. Gernet, H., and Franceschetti, A.: Ultrasound biometry of the eye (review). *In:* Ultrasonics in Ophthalmology. Edited by A. Oksala and H. Gernet. Basel, S. Karger, 1967, pp. 175–200.
10. Gernet, H.: Biometry of the eye by means of ultrasound. Klin. Monatsbl. Augenheilkd., 146:863–869, 1965.
11. Giglio, E., and Ludlam, W. M.: High resolution ultrasonic equipment to measure intra-ocular distances. J. Am. Optom. Assoc., 38:367–370, 1967.
12. Giglio, E. J., and Ludlam, W. M.: Ultrasound—A diagnostic tool for the examination of the eye. Am. J. Optom., 43:687–731, 1966.
13. Jansson, F.: Measurement of intraocular distances by ultrasound and comparison between optical and ultrasonic determinations of the depth of the anterior chamber. Acta Ophthalmol., 41:25–61, 1963.
14. Kanki, K., et al.: Measurement of the axial length of the eye by the application of ultrasonic waves. Acta Soc. Ophthalmol. Jap., 65:1877–1883, 1961.
15. Leary, G. A., et al.: Ultrasonographic measurement of the components of ocular refraction in life. I. Technical considerations. Vision Res., 3:487–498, 1963.
16. Lowe, R. F.: Linear A-scan ultrasonography in the measurement of intra-ocular distances: A stand-off technique. Trans. Ophthalmol. Soc. Aust., 26:72–77, 1967.
17. Nover, A., and Grote, W.: On the determination of the length of the axis of the human eye with ultrasound in the living person. Graefe. Arch. Ophthalmol., 168:405–418, 1965.
18. Purnell, E. W., and Sokollu, A.: Ultrasonic measurements of eye length. Acta Ophthalmol., 40:219–222, 1962.
19. Ricci, A.: Discussion of H. Gernet: Analytical considerations of the optical dimensions of emmetropic eyes resulting from ultrasonic examination. Bull. Soc. Ophtalmol. Fr., 652–655, 1964.
20. Rivara, A.: Research on using ultrasound for measurement of the anterior-posterior ocular axis. Otti Soc. Oftal. Lombarda, 18:48–50, 1963.
21. Sorsby, A., Leary, G., Richards, M., and Chaston, J. C.: Ultrasonographic measurement of the components of ocular refraction in life. 2. Clinical procedures: ultrasonographic measurements compared with phakometric measurements in a series of 140 eyes. Vision Res., 3:499–505, 1963.
22. Trier, G., Hammerla, O., and Reuter, R.: A high resolution TAU-system for eye biometry. *In:* Diagnostica Ultrasonica in Ophthalmologia. Edited by M. Massin and J. Poujol. Paris, Centre National d'Ophtalmologie des Quinze-Vingts, 1973, pp. 51–58.
23. Yamamoto, Y., et al.: A study on the measurement of ocular axial length by ultrasound echography. Acta Soc. Ophthalmol. Jap., 64:1333–1341, 1960.
24. Stenstrom, S.: Research on variation and covariation of the optical elements of the human eye. Acta Ophthalmol. (Suppl.), 26, 1946.
25. Sorsby, A., and O'Connor, A.: Measurement of the diameters of the living eye by means of X-ray. Nature, 156:779, 1945.
26. Araki, M.: Studies on refractive components of human eye by ultrasonic wave. Part I. Accuracy of the measurement of ocular axial length by ultrasonic echography. Jap. J. Clin. Ophthalmol., 15:111–119, 1961.
27. Coleman, D. J., and Carlin, B.: A new system for visual axis measurements in the human eye using ultrasound. Arch. Ophthalmol., 77:124–127, 1967.
28. Freeman, M. H.: Measurement of ocular distances. Factors affecting accuracy. Wiss. A. Humboldt-Univ. Berlin, Math.-Nat. R., 14:209–211, 1965.
29. Gernet, H.: Basic values in clinical oculometry. Bull. Mem. Soc. Fr. Ophtalmol., 83:379, 1970.
30. Grignolo, A., Rivara, A., and Zingirian, M.: An evaluation of errors of optical and ultrasonographic methods to oculometry. *In:* Ultrasonics in Medicine. Edited by M. DeVlieger, et al. Amsterdam, Excerpta Medica, 1974, pp. 154–160.

31. Jansson, F.: Determination of the axis length of the eye roentgenologically and by ultrasound. Acta Ophthalmol., 41:236–246, 1963.
32. Kimura, T., Yamazaki, M., Nakajima, A., Hayashi, C., and Nagata, Y.: Analysis of errors in ultrasound biometry and phacometry. In: Ophthalmic Ultrasound. Edited by K. Gitter, et al. St. Louis, C. V. Mosby Co., 1969, pp. 190–200.
33. Massin, M., Poujol, J., and Hieronimus, M.: Statistical study of the different factors influencing the precision of biometric measurements. In: Ultrasonographia Medica. Vienna, Verlag der Wiener Med. Akad., 1971, pp. 467–472.
34. Merlin, U., and Rossi, A.: Critical evaluation of the value of functional biometry formulas. In: Ultrasonography in Ophthalmology. Edited by J. Francois and F. Goes. Basel, S. Karger, 1975, pp. 301–309.
35. Oksala, A., and Salminen, L.: Experimental observation on the accuracy of the method in the measurement of the axial diameter of the lens by ultrasound. Acta Ophthalmol., 46:826–830, 1968.
36. Oksala, A.: Experimental research in the significance of amplification, distance and beam width in the measurement of lens thickness by ultrasound. Acta Ophthalmol., 46:821–825, 1968.
37. Rivara, A., Zingirian, M., and Grignolo, A.: An evaluation of errors of optical and ultrasonographic methods applied to oculometry. In: Ultrasonography in Ophthalmology. Edited by J. Francois and F. Goes. Basel, S. Karger, 1975, pp. 310–319.
38. Rivara, A., and Zingirian, M.: On the error of measuring the antero-posterior axis of the eye by means of ultrasound when adopting a propagation speed constant. Ophthalmologica, 150:431–440, 1965.
39. Gernet, H.: Axial length and refraction of the emmetropic living eye. Graefe. Arch. Ophthalmol., 166:424–431, 1964.
40. Gernet, H.: A contribution to the question of emmetropia. Ophthalmologica, 147:235–243, 1964.
41. Gernet, H.: Clinical ultrasonic studies in emmetropes; emmetropia and spread of accommodation. Wiss. Z. Humboldt Univ. Berlin (Math. Naturwiss), 14:201–204, 1965.
42. Franceschetti, A., and Luyckx, J.: Study of the emmetropization effect of the crystalline lens by ultrasonic echography. Am. J. Ophthalmol., 61:1096–1100, 1966.
43. Gernet, H., and Boateng, A.: On the dimension of the vitreous body. Ber. Dtsch. Ophthalmol. Ges., 68:31–36, 1968.
44. Coleman, D. J., Wuchinich, D., and Carlin, B.: Accommodative changes in the axial dimension of the human eye. In: Ophthalmic Ultrasound. Edited by K. Gitter, et al. C. V. Mosby Co., St. Louis, 1969, pp. 134–141.
45. Reference deleted.
46. Cherkasov, I. S., et al.: Effect of ultrasound on the hydrodynamics of the eyes of healthy persons and patients with glaucoma. Oftalmol. Zh., 28:587–589, 1973.
47. Delmarcelle, Y., Luyckx-Bacus, J., and Weekers, R.: Biometric study of the anterior segment of the eye in angle closure glaucoma. Bull. Soc. Belge Ophtalmol., 153:638–650, 1969.
48. Fahmy, J. A., and Fledelius, H.: Yoga induced attacks of acute glaucoma. Acta Ophthalmol., 51:80–84, 1973.
49. Gernet, H., and Jurgens, V.: Echographic findings in chronic simple glaucoma. Graefe. Arch. Ophthalmol., 168:419–422, 1965.
50. Gernet, H. and Hollwich, F.: Oculometry of infantile glaucoma. Ber. Dtsch. Ophthalmol., Ges., 69:341, 1969.
51. Hollwich, F., and Boateng, A.: Ultrasonographic measurements in primary glaucomas. In: Ophthalmic Ultrasound. Edited by K. Gitter, et al.: St. Louis, C. V. Mosby Co., 1969, pp. 187–189.
52. Koretskaia, I. M., et al.: Ultrasonic biometry of the vitreous body with the ophthalmotonus fluctuations. Vestn. Oftalmol., 2:42–44, 1974.

53. Lowe, R.: Time amplitude ultrasonography for ocular biometry. Am. J. Ophthalmol., 66:913–918, 1968.

54. Lowe, R. F.: Central corneal thickness. Ocular correlation in normal eyes and those with primary angle closure glaucoma. Br. J. Ophthalmol., 53:824–826, 1969.

55. Lowe, R. F.: Causes of shallow anterior chamber in primary angle-closure glaucoma. Ultrasonic biometry of normal and angle-closure glaucoma eyes. Am. J. Ophthalmol., 67:87–93, 1969.

56. Lowe, R. F.: Corneal radius and ocular correlations in normal eyes and with primary angle-closure glaucoma. Am. J. Ophthalmol., 67:864–868, 1969.

57. Lowe, R. F.: Aetiology of the anatomical basis for primary angle-closure glaucoma. Biometrical comparisons between normal eyes and eyes with primary angle-closure glaucoma. Br. J. Ophthalmol., 54:161–169, 1970.

58. Luyckx, J., and Weekers, J.: Ultrasonographic contributions to the study of glaucoma. Ann. Ocul., 200:489–504, 1967.

59. Luyckx-Bacus, J.: Contribution of A-scan echography to the study of angle closure glaucoma. In: Ultrasonographia Medica. Edited by J. Bock and K. Ossoinig. Vienna, Verlag der Wiener Med Akad., 1971, pp. 573–577.

60. Machekhin, V. A.: Ultrasonic biometry in unilateral glaucoma. Vestn. Oftalmol., 5:7–10, 1972.

61. Machekhin, V. A., and Protasov, A. I.: Ultrasonic biometry of the eyes in patients with glaucoma. Vestn. Oftalmol., 3:35–39, 1972.

62. Tane, S., and Takemoto, N.: The studies on the ultrasonic diagnosis in ophthalmology. 6. Echographic findings of glaucomatous eye. Folia Ophthalmol. Jap., 24:49–53, 1973.

63. Weekers, R., Luyckx, J., and Weekers, J. F.: Narrow-angle glaucoma due to a congenital anomaly of the lens thickness. Klin. Monatsbl. Augenheilkd., 155:625–629, 1969.

64. Abramson, D. H., Coleman, D. J., Forbes, M., and Franzen, L. A.: The effects of pilocarpine on anterior chamber and lens thickness. Arch. Ophtalmol., 87:615–620, 1972.

65. Abramson, D. H., Chang, S., and Coleman, D. J.: Pilocarpine therapy in glaucoma. Arch. Ophthalmol., 94:914–918, 1976.

66. Abramson, D. H., Franzen, L. A., and Coleman, D. J.: Pilocarpine in the presbyope. Arch. Ophthalmol., 89:100–102, 1973.

67. Axelsson, U.: Glaucoma, miotic therapy and cataract. 3. Visual loss due to lens changes in glaucoma eyes treated with parazon (mintacol), echothiophate (phospholine iodine) or pilocarpine. Acta Ophthalmol., 46:831, 1968.

68. Chang, S., Abramson, D. H., Coleman, D. J., and Smith, M. E.: Pilocarpine induced lens changes: an ultrasonic biometric evaluation of dose-response. Arch. Ophthalmol.: 92:464–469, 1974.

69. Francois, J., and Goes, F.: Comparative study of the effect of pilocarpine and aceclidine on the eye components. In: Ultrasonography in Ophthalmology. Edited by J. Francois and F. Goes. Basel, S. Karger, 1975, pp. 320–327.

70. Bonnac, J. P., Massin, M., and Poujol, J.: Comparison between the measures of length of a myopic eye in the axis and in the para-axial regions. In: Ultrasonography in Ophthalmology. Edited by J. Francois and F. Goes. Basel, S. Karger, 1975, pp. 283–286.

71. Curtin, B., and Karlin, D.: Axial measurements and fundus changes of the myopic eye. Am. J. Ophthalmol., 71:42–53, 1971.

72. Fledelius, H.: Ultrasound oculometry and exophthalmometry in high myopia with reference to the occurrence of retinal detachment. Acta Ophthalmol., 49:707–714, 1971.

73. Fledelius, H.: Ultrasound oculometry and exophthalmometry in high myopia with reference to the occurence of retinal detachment. In: Diagnostic Ultrasonica in Ophthalmologia. Edited by M. Massin and J. Poujol. Paris, Centre National d'Ophtalmologie des Quinze-Vingts, 1973, pp. 307–312.

74. Franceschetti, A., and Gernet, H.: On optical values in mild and severe myopia on the basis of echographic findings. Graefe. Arch. Ophthalmol., 168:1–16, 1965.

75. Francois, J., and Goes, F.: Comparative study of ultrasonic biometry of emmetropes and myopes, with special regard to the heredity of myopia. *In:* Ophthalmic Ultrasound. Edited by K. Gitter, et al. St. Louis, C. V. Mosby Co., 1969, pp. 165–180.

76. Francois, J., and Goes, F.: Echography of the myope. Bull. Soc. Belge Ophtalmol., 154:415–430, 1970.

77. Francois, J., and Goes, F.: Biometry of juvenile myopia. *In:* Ultrasonica Diagnostica in Ophthalmologia. Edited by M. Massin and J. Poujol, Paris, Centre National d'Ophtalmologie des Quinze-Vingts, 1973, pp. 277–285.

78. Francois, J., and Goes, F.: Oculometry of progressive myopia. *In:* Ultrasonography in Ophthalmology. Edited by J. Francois and F. Goes. Basel, S. Karger, 1975, pp. 277–282.

79. Gernet, H.: Biometric findings in retinal detachment due to tears of the myopic eye. Contributions to its pathogenesis. Ophthalmologica, 150:386–400, 1965.

80. Grignolo, A., and Rivara, A.: An attempt to classify infant myopia based on biometric findings. *In:* Ophthalmic Ultrasound. Edited by K. Gitter, et al. St. Louis, C. V. Mosby Co., 1969, pp. 158–164.

81. Pallin, O., and Ericsson, R.: Ultrasound studies in a case of Hygroton-induced myopia. Acta Ophthalmol., 43:692–696, 1965.

82. Perez-Llorca, R., Torres, J., and Unzurrunzaga, A.: Echographic biometry in myopia. *In:* Ultrasonography in Ophthalmology. Edited by J. Francois and F. Goes. Basel, S. Karger, 1975, p. 276.

83. Rivara, A., and Cambiaggi, A.: Rapporto tra entita, della refrazione, lunghezza dell'asse oculare antero-osteriore egravita del delle alterazioni corioretiniche in soggetti miopi. Atti Soc. Oftal. Ital., 22:267–271, 1964.

84. Rivara, A., and Grignolo, A.: Réfraction ocularre totale et réfraction du cristallin par rapport au degré de myopie. *In:* Ultrasonographia Medica. Vienna, Verlag der Wiener Med. Akad., 1971, pp. 521–530.

85. Binkhorst, R. D.: The optical design of intraocular lens implants. Ophthalmic Surg., 6:17–31, 1975.

86. Suzuki, K.: Studies on myopia considering hereditary tendency. I. Correlation between changes of refractive components and development of myopia. Acta Soc. Ophthalmol. Jap., 73:333–348, 1969.

87. Suzuki, K.: Studies on myopia considering hereditary tendency, II. New device to measure accommodative changes of optical components of the human eye by ultrasonic echography. Acta Soc. Ophthalmol. Jap., 73:349–362, 1969.

88. Suzuki, K.: Studies on myopia considering hereditary tendency. 3. Correlation between accommodative changes in intraocular distance and annual changes in refractive components. Acta Soc. Ophthalmol. Jap., 73:2262–2271, 1969.

89. Young, F.: The development of simple myopia. Eye Ear Nose Throat Mon., 47:171–174, 1968.

90. Young, F., and Leary, G.: A comparison of the development of myopia in humans and chimpanzees. Invest. Ophthalmol., 7:114–115, 1968.

91. Schwartz, J. T.: A monozygotic cotwin control study of a treatment for myopia. Acta Genet. Med Gemellol., in press.

92. Barraquer, J., and Henao, H.: Functional exploration in refractive keratoplasty. Arch. Soc. Am. Oftalmol. Optom., 7:195–206, 1969.

93. Coleman, D. J., Jack, R. L., and Cardona, H.: Ultrasonic evaluation of keratoprosthetic eyes. Am. J. Ophthalmol., 74:543–554, 1972.

94. Elstein, J. K., Sehgal, V. N., and Kaplan, M. M.: Instrumentation and techniques for refractive keratoplasty. Am. J. Ophthalmol., 68:282, 1969.

95. Gernet, H., and Worst, J.: Clinical ocular biometry and Binkhorst lens implants. *In:* Diagnostica Ultrasonica in Ophtalmologia. Edited by M. Massin and

J. Poujol. Paris, Centre National d'Ophtalmologie des Quinze-Vingts, 1973, pp. 247–256.

96. Leary, G. A.: Ultrasonographic assessment of the implant lens required to produce emmetropia after implantation. Invest. Ophthalmol., 10:745–749, 1971.

97. Oguchi, Y.: The ultrasonic study of the refraction of the patient with pseudo-phakia. Presented at Second World Congress on Ultrasonics in Medicine, Rotterdam, 1973.

98. Worst, J. G. F.: A simplified procedure for clinical echographic determinations of the axial length of the eye for the purpose of calculation of the power of artificial lenses. *In:* Ultrasonography in Ophthalmology. Edited by J. Francois and F. Goes. Basel, S. Karger, 1975, pp. 269–272.

99. Bronson, N. R.: Nonmagnetic foreign body localization and extraction. Am. J. Ophthalmol., 58:133–134, 1964.

100. Bronson, N. R.: Intraocular foreign bodies—Ultrasonic localization. Int. Ophthalmol. Clin., 8:199–203, 1968.

101. Coleman, D. J., and Trokel, S. L.: A protocol for B-scan and radiographic foreign body localization. Am. J. Ophthalmol., 71:84–89, 1971.

102. Cowden, J. W., and Runyan, T. E.: Localization of intraocular foreign bodies. Further experience in ultrasonic vs. radiologic methods. Arch. Ophthalmol., 82:299, 1969.

103. Nover, A., and Stallkamp, H.: Possibilities and limitations of ultrasonic diagnosis of intraocular foreign bodies. Ber. Dtsch. Ophthalmol. Ges., 63:251–256, 1960.

104. Oksala, A., and Lehtinen, A.: Use of the echogram in the location and diagnosis of intraocular foreign bodies. Br. J. Ophthalmol., 43:744–752, 1959.

105. Coleman, D. J., Abramson, D. H., Jack, R. L., and Franzen, L. A.: Ultrasonic diagnosis of tumors of the choroid. Arch. Ophthalmol., 91:344–354, 1974.

105a. Hamard, H., Massin, M., and Poujol, J.: Echography of the eye and orbit, bibliography. Bull. Soc. Ophtalmol. Fr. (Suppl.), 185–222, 1973.

106. Vanysek, J., Preisova, J., and Obraz, J.: Ultrasonography in Ophthalmology. London, Butterworths, 1969, pp. 213–218.

107. Gitter, K., et al.: Ophthalmic Ultrasound. St. Louis, C. V. Mosby Co., 1969, pp. 350–367.

108. Buschmann, W., and Schwaar, R.: On exophthalmometry 1. The relation between the middle of the globe and the orbital apex in emmetropia. Graefe. Arch. Ophthalmol., 173:261, 1967.

109. Buschmann, W.: Ultrasonic exophthalmometry. *In:* Diagnostica Ultrasonica in Ophthalmologia. Edited by M. Massin and J. Poujol. Paris, Centre National d'Ophtalmologie des Quinze-Vingts, 1973, pp. 303–306.

110. Cherasov, I. S., and Marmur, R. K.: The use of ultrasonics in the diagnosis and assessment of the efficacy of therapy and hydrophthalmos. Oftalmol. Zh., 22:361–366, 1967.

111. Flament, J., and Gerhard, J. P.: Biometrical effect of some technics of chorio-retinal surgery. A comparative study. *In:* Ultrasonography in Ophthalmology. Edited by J. Francois and F. Goes. Basel, S. Karger, 1975, pp. 328–336.

112. Fledelius, H.: Ultrasound A-mode in a case of nasal posterior scleral ectasy. Acta Ophthalmol., 48:502–507, 1970.

113. Francois, J., and Goes, F.: Biometric study of a peripapillary scleral ectasia, a true congenital posterior staphyloma. Bull. Soc. Belge Ophtalmol., 144:945–952, 1966.

114. Francois, J., and Goes, F.: Unilateral echography A and exophthalmos. Bull. Soc. Belge Ophtalmol., 155:475–486, 1970.

115. Gernet, H., and Ostholt, H.: Optics of an only eye. A new area for clinical ocular biometry. Klin. Monatsbl. Augenheilkd., 162:114, 1973.

116. Gernet, H.: Clinical ultrasonic ocular biometry and optics of single eyes. *In:* Ultrasonics in Medicine. Edited by M. DeVlieger, et al. Amsterdam, Excerpta Medica, 1974, p. 127.

117. Herrmann, U., and Buschmann, W.: Combination of exophthalmometry and ultrasonic length measurement. *In:* Diagnostica Ultrasonica in Ophthalmology. Edited by J. Vanysek. Brno, University of Brno, 1968, pp. 245–250.

118. Itin, W.: Axial length of the eye in two brothers with peripheral sclero-cornea and cornea plana, one presenting with high myopia, the other with strong hypermetropia. Ophthalmologica, 152:369–377, 1966.

119. Itin, W.: Echographic study of axial length in 2 brothers with sclerosing corneas and cornea planata. Klin. Monatsbl. Augenheilkd., 148:454, 1966.

120. Luyckx, J.: Relation between the rigidity coefficient and eye length measured by echography. Ophthalmologica, 153:321–400, 1967.

121. Miettinen, P., and Ursin, K.: Ultrasound studies on changes in the length of cerclage operated eyes. *In:* Diagnostica Ultrasonica in Ophthalmologia. Edited by J. Vanysek. Brno, University of Brno, 1968, pp. 239–243.

122. Nakijima, A., Konyama, K., Yamazaki, M., Kimura, T., and Magatani, H.: The changes in optical elements of the eye and contact lens wear. *In:* Contact Lenses. Edited by O. Dabezies and A. Schlossman. Basel, S. Karger, 1967. pp. 139–148.

123. Weekers, R., Luyckx-Bacus, J., and Weekers, J. F.: Etude ultrasonique des dimensions respectives des segments antérieur et postérieur du globe oculaire dans diverses affections génétiques. *In:* Ultrasonics in Ophthalmology. Edited by A. Oksala and H. Gernet. Basel, S. Karger, 1967, pp. 215–225.

124. Gernet, H., and Ostholt, H.: Objective measurement of aniseiconia. Principles and possibilities. *In:* Ultrasonography in Ophthalmology. Edited by J. Francois and F. Goes. Basel, S. Karger, 1975, pp. 287–293.

125. Jansson, F.: Measurements of intraocular distances by ultrasound. Acta Ophthalmol. (Suppl.), 74:1–51, 1963.

126. Coleman, D. J., and Carlin, B.: Transducer alignment and electronic measurement of visual axis dimensions in the human eye using time-amplitude ultrasound. *In:* Ultrasonics in Ophthalmology. Edited by A. Oksala and H. Gernet. Basel, S. Karger, 1967, pp. 207–213.

127. Gernet, H.: Measurement of the eye in vivo. Graefe. Arch. Ophthalmol., 166:402–411, 1963.

128. Yamamoto, Y., Namiki, R., Baba, M., and Kato, M.: A study on the measurement of ocular axial length by ultrasonic echography. Jap. J. Ophthalmol., 5:134–139, 1961.

129. Giglio, E., and Ludlam, W.: Eye measurement device. New York Times, July 11, 1969.

130. Coleman, D. J., Lizzi, F. L., Franzen, L. A., and Abramson, D. H.: A determination of the velocity of ultrasound in cataractous lenses. *In:* Ultrasonography in Ophthalmology. Edited by J. Francois and F. Goes. Basel, S. Karger, 1975, pp. 246–251.

131. Weinstein, G., Baum, G., Binkhorst, R., and Troutman, R.: A comparison of ultrasonographic and optical methods for determining the axial length of the aphakic eye. Am. J. Ophthalmol., 62:1194–1201, 1966.

132. Rivara, A., and Zingirian, M.: Globe volume and scleral rigidity. Ophthalmologica, 156:394–398, 1968.

133. Rivara, A., and Zingirian, M.: Measure of ocular volume in the living by means of ultrasonics. Description and statistical evaluation of the method. Ann. Ottal., 91:387–393, 1965.

134. Rivara, A., and Zingirian, M.: Biometrical results on the length of various ocular axes and the ocular volume obtained with the echographic method. Ann Ottal., 91:1233–1238, 1965.

135. Sterns, G. K., Coleman, D. J., Franzen, L. A., and Smith, M.: Ultrasonic volume determination in ophthalmology. Seattle, American Institute of Ultrasound in Medicine, 1974.

136. Coleman, D. J., and Weininger, B. S.: Ultrasonic M-mode technique in ophthalmology. Arch. Ophthalmol., 82:475–479, 1969.

137. Coleman, D. J.: Measurement of choroidal pulsation with M-scan ultrasound. Am. J. Ophthalmol., 71:363–365, 1971.

Additional References

Biometry of the Cornea

Itin, W.: Axial length of the eye in 2 cases of microcornea measured by means of ultrasonic echography (microcornea with and without microphthalmia). Ann. Ocul., 198:465–471, 1965.

Luyckx-Bacus, J., and Delmarcelle, Y.: Biometric research on eyes presenting with microcornea and megalocornea. Study of 84 cases. Bull. Soc. Belge Ophtalmol., 149:433–443, 1968.

Luyckx, J., and Delmarcelle, Y.: Contribution of ultrasonography to the study of microcornea and megalocornea. *In:* Ophthalmic Ultrasound. Edited by K. Gitter, et al. St. Louis, C. V. Mosby Co., 1969, pp. 149–157.

Ricci, A.: Discussion de la communication de H. Gernet sur: Microcornee sans microphtalmie. Bull. Mem. Soc. Fr., Ophtalmol., 78:372–374, 1965.

Rivara, A., and Grignolo, A.: Microphthalmos and microcornea: a biometric investigation. *In:* Ophthalmic Ultrasound. Edited by K. Gitter, et al. St. Louis, C. V. Mosby Co., 1969, pp. 181–186.

Soriano, H., and Psilis, K.: Marchesani syndrome associated with megalocornea and iris atrophy; an echographic study. Ophthalmologica, 161:268–272, 1970.

Biometry of the Lens

Babel, J., Psilis, K., and Itin, W.: Echographic measures of the thickness of the lens in unilateral cataracts, *In:* Ultrasonographia Medica. Edited by J. Bock and K. Ossoinig. Vienna, Verlag der Weiner Med. Akad., 1971, pp. 547–555.

Delmarcelle, Y., and Luyckx-Bacus, J.: Influence of senile cataracts on the thickness of the lens and anterior chamber depth. Bull. Soc. Belge Ophtalmol., 155:465–474, 1970.

Delmarcelle, Y., and Luyckx-Bacus, J.: Biometry of the anterior segment with senile cataracts. Acta Ophthalmol., 49:454–456, 1971.

Itin, W., and Brawand, L.: Echographic study of the long axis of the eye before and after extraction of the lens. Ophthalmologica, 156:256, 1968.

Lowe, R. F.: Anterior lens displacement with age. Br. J. Ophthalmol., 54:117–121, 1970.

Luyckx, J., and Delmarcelle, Y.: Biometry of the eye for refraction in infants. *In:* Diagnostica Ultrasonica in Ophthalmologia. Edited by M. Massin and J. Poujol. Paris, Centre National d'Ophtalmologie des Quinze-Vingts, 1973, pp. 269–275.

Luyckx-Bacus, J., and Delmarcelle, Y.: Influence of biometric alterations on the lens and depth of the anterior chamber. Bull. Soc. Ophtalmol. Fr., 152:507–513, 1969.

Massin, M., Poujol, J., and Svilarich, J.-C.: Uses and value of echography of globes with cataracts. Bull. Soc. Ophtalmol. Fr., 67:1094–1098, 1967.

Psilis, K., and Itin, W.: Some problems in biometry of the clear and cataractous lens. *In:* Diagnostica Ultrasonica in Ophthalmologia. Edited by M. Massin and J. Poujol. Paris, Centre National d'Ophtalmologie des Quinze-Vingts, 1973, pp. 257–260.

Schum, U., et al.: Echographic measurements of the vitreous space before and after cryoextraction of the lens. Klin. Monatsbl. Augenheilkd., 163:369–375, 1973.

Storey, J., and Phillips, C.: Ultrasonic investigations on mobility of crystalline lens. *In:*

Diagnostica Ultrasonica in Ophthalmologia. Edited by M. Massin and J. Poujol. Paris, Centre National d'Ophtalmologie des Quinze-Vingts, 1973, pp. 261–264.

Yakimenko, S. A.: Study of the accuracy of ultrasound biometry of the lens. Oftalmol. Zh., 26:373–375, 1971.

Biometry in Studies of Refraction, Emmetropia and Aniseiconia

Avetisov, E. S., Fridman, F., and Shapiro, Z.: Research on aniseiconia with convergent strabismus with the aid of ultrasound biometry. Vestn. Oftalmol., 5:17–20, 1966.

Belkin, M., et al.: Ultrasonography in the refraction of aphakic infants. Br. J. Ophthal., 57:845–848, 1973.

Elenius, V., and Sopanen, V.: Power of the correcting lens of the aphakic eye as calculated from the keratometric measurement of the corneal radius and the ultrasonically-measured axial length of the eye. Acta Opthalmol., 41:71–74, 1963.

Franceschetti, A., and Gernet, H.: Ultrasonic diagnosis of microphthalmia without microcornea with macrophakia, high hypermetropia associated with tapetoretinal degeneration, glaucomatous disposition and dental anomalies (new familial syndrome). Arch. Ophtalmol., 25:105–116, 1965.

Franceschetti, A., and Gernet, H.: Importance of ultrasonic echography for measurements of the optical components of the eye. Trans. Am. Acad. Ophthalmol. Otolaryngol., 69:465–473, 1965.

Franceschetti, A.: Ultrasonic biomeasuration (echography) of the optical components of the eye and its value for the interpretation of refractive anomalies. Bull. Soc. Ophtalmol. Fr., 66:239–246, 1966.

Franceschetti, A., and Luyckx, J.: Study of the effect of emmetropization on the lens by ultrasound. Ann. Ocul., 200:177–190, 1967.

Francois, J., and Goes, F.: Oculometry in emmetropia and ametropia. In: Ultrasonigraphia Medica (SIDUO III). Edited by J. Bock and K. Ossoinig. Vienna, Verlag der Weiner Med. Akad., 1971, pp. 473–515.

Francois, J., and Goes, F.: Echographic study of the lens thickness as a function of the axial length in emmetropic eyes of the same age. In: Ultrasonographia Medica (SIDUO III). Edited by J. Bock and K. Ossoinig. Vienna, Verlag der Weiner Med. Akad., 1971, pp. 531–538.

Fridman, F. B.: The significance of ultrasound biometry in the determination of anatomic-optical parameters in ametropia. In: Diagnostica Ultrasonica in Ophthalmologia (SIDUO II). Basel, S. Karger, 1968, pp. 259–267.

Gernet, H.: Compensatory behavior of corneal refraction and globe length in buphthalmus, Klin. Monatsbl. Augenheilkd., 144:429–431, 1964.

Gernet, H., and Franceschetti, A.: On the prognosis of refraction and the magnifying effect following Fukala operation by means of ultrasonic examination. Ophthalmologica, 148:393–404, 1964.

Gernet, H.: For calculation of theoretical total refractive index in the non-accommodated living eye. Graefe. Arch. Ophthalmol., 166:415–423, 1964.

Gernet, H.: Analytical study concerning the optical dimensions in emmetropic eyes based on ultrasonic examinations. Bull. Soc. Ophtalmol. Fr., 77:644–658, 1964.

Gernet, H.: On calculating the average refractive index in human lenses. Klin. Monatsbl. Augenheilkd., 147:288–289, 1965.

Gernet, H., and Olbrich, E.: Excess of the human refraction curve and its cause. In: Ophthalmic Ultrasound. Edited by K. Gitter, et al. St. Louis, C. V. Mosby Co., 1969, pp. 142–149.

Gernet, H.: Objective measurement of aniseiconia. First clinical applications. In: Ultrasonography in Ophthalmology. Edited by J. Francois and F. Goes. Basel, S. Karger, 1975, pp. 294–300.

Grignolo, A., Rivara, A., and Zingirian, M.: Determination de la grandeur de l'image retinienne dans l'oeil emmetrope au moyen de la biometrie ultrasonique dans le but d'obtenir une evaluation objective de l'aniseiconie. *In:* Diagnostica Ultrasonica in Ophthalmologia. Edited by M. Massin and J. Poujol. Paris, Centre National d'Ophtalmologia des Quinze-Vingts, 1973, pp. 293–298.

Kožoušek, V.: Objective determination of aniseikonia by means of ultrasonics. Cesk. Oftalmol., 19:162–165, 1963.

Leary, G., and Young, F.: A set of equations for computing the components of ocular refraction. Am. J. Optom., 45:743–759, 1968.

Luyckx, J., and Weekers, J.: Biometric studies of the human eye by ultrasound. Part I. The ametropic eye. Bull. Soc. Belge Ophtalmol., 143:552–567, 1967.

Machekhin, V. A.: Ultrasonic biometry of eyes with varied refraction. Oftalmol. Zh., 27:204–207, 1972.

Nakajima, A., and Kimura, T.: Ultrasonography and phacometry in the study of refractive elements of the eye. *In:* Ultrasonics in Ophthalmology. Edited by A. Oksala and H. Gernet. Basel, S. Karger, 1967, pp. 226–237.

Oksala, A.: Some thoughts on the significance of ultrasonic diagnosis in myopia research. J. Pediatr. Ophthalmol., 2:45–52, 1965.

Otsuka, J., et al.: Comparison of phacometry with ultrasonic method in the measurement of human refractive elements. Acta Soc. Ophthalmol. Jap., 65:1777–1792, 1961.

Otsuka, J., Tokoro, T., and Araki, A.: A correction to the article: Comparative studies of phacometry with ultrasonic method on refractive elements of the human eyes. Acta Soc. Ophthalmol. Jap., 66:85–86, 1962.

Rivara, A., and Gemme, G.: Measurement of the anterior-posterior ocular axis and dioptric power in the premature. Ann. Ottal., 91:1328–1334, 1965.

Rivara, A., and Zingirian, M.: Calculation of total refractive ocular power and refractive lens power: An ultrasonic-optical procedure. Ophthalmologica, 159:202–210, 1969.

Zingirian, M., and Rivara, A.: On the use of echography to find the refractive index of the vitreous and lens. *In:* Ultrasonographia Medica. Edited by J. Bock and K. Ossoinig., Vienna, Verlag der Wiener Med. Akad., 1971, pp. 517–520.

Zingirian, M., and Rivara, A.: Prediction of the aphakic correction, before cataract extraction by means of ultrasound biometry. Boll. Ocul., 48:563–568, 1969.

Zingirian, M., Rivara, A., and Grignolo, A.: Objective measurement of aniseikonia in ametropia with ultrasonic biometry with and without optical correction. *In:* Diagnostica Ultrasonica in Ophthalmologia. Edited by M. Massin and J. Poujol. Paris, Centre National d'Ophtalmologie des Quinze-Vingts, 1973, pp. 299–302.

Velocity Determinations

Barone, A., and Scafati, A.: Measure of the propagation velocity of ultrasound in biological tissue with an interferometer method. Rend. Inst. Supiore di Sanita Roma, 23:15–31, 1960.

Bell, D. S.: Approximate determination of the speed of sound through liquids and solids. J. Acoust. Soc Am., 44:656, 1968.

Bradley, E., and Sacerio, J.: The velocity of ultrasound in human blood under varying physiological parameters. J. Surg. Res., 12:290–297, 1972.

Buschmann, W., Voss, M., and Kemmerling, S.: Acoustic properties of normal human orbit tissues. Ophthalmol. Res., 1:354–364, 1970.

Cristmann, C., and Ehler, E.: Velocity of sound waves, acoustic impedence and absorption in human long bones of upper extremity. Beitr. Orthop. Traumatol., 18:324–334, 1971.

Freese, M., and Makow, D.: High-frequency ultrasonic properties of freshwater fish tissue. J. Acoust. Soc. Am., 44:1282–1289, 1968.

Frucht, A. H.: The velocity of ultrasound in human and animal tissue. Naturwissenschaften, 39:491–492, 1952.

Frucht, A. H.: The velocity of sound in human and animal tissue. Z. Ges. Exp. Med., 120:526–557, 1953.

Gaertner, M. C.: Comparative measurements of the velocity of ultrasound in various organs of in vitro animals. Med. Diss. Leipzig, 1951.

Goldman, D. E., and Hueter, T. F.: Errata: Velocity and absorption of high frequency sound in mammalian tissues. J. Acoust. Soc. Am., 29:655, 1957.

Goldman, D. E., and Hueter, T. F.: Tabular data of the velocity and absorption of high-frequency sound in mammalian tissues. J. Acoust. Soc. Am., 28:35–37, 1956.

Goldman, D. E., and Richards, J. R.: Measurement of high-frequency sound velocity in mammalian soft tissues. J. Acoust. Soc. Am., 26:981–983, 1954.

Jansson, F., and Sundmark, E.: Determination of the velocity of ultrasound in ocular tissues at different temperatures. Acta Ophthalmol., 39:899–910, 1961.

Jansson, F., and Kock, E.: Determination of the velocity of ultrasound in the human lens and vitreous. Acta Ophthalmol., 40:420–433, 1962.

Kossoff, G., Robinson, D. E., and Garrett, W. J.: Acoustic properties of materials. Report 31, C. A. L. Sydney, 1965, p. 9.

Oksala, A., and Lehtinen, A.: Measurement of the velocity of sound in some parts of the eye. Acta Ophthalmol., 36:633–639, 1958.

Nover, A., and Glanschneider, D.: Studies on the transmission rate and absorption of ultrasonics in tissue. Experimental contributions to ultrasonic diagnosis of intraocular tumors. Graefe. Arch. Ophthalmol., 168:304–321, 1965.

Ludwig, G. D.: The velocity of sound through tissues and the acoustic impedance of tissue. J. Acoust. Soc. Am., 22:862–866, 1950.

Rivara, A., and Sanna, G.: Determination of the speed of ultrasound in ocular tissues of humans and swine. Ann. Ottal., 88:675–682, 1962.

Rudiger, W.: The velocity of sound in human fat tissue under the influence of water content and temperature. Med. Diss., Leipzig, 1953.

Tschewnenko, A. A.: Velocity of ultrasound in ocular tissues. Wiss. Z. Humboldt Univ. Berlin [Math. Naturwiss.], 14:67–69, 1965. (International Symposium on Diagnostic Ultrasound in Ophthalmology, Berlin, 1964.)

Van Venrooij, G. E.: Measurement of ultrasound velocity in human tissues. Ultrasonics, 9:240–242, 1971.

Vanysek, J., Preisova, J., and Obraz, J.: Ultrasonography in Ophthalmology. London, Butterworths, 1969, p. 11.

General Biometry

Abe, K.: Dimensions of the pupil. Jap. J. Ophthalmol., 19:1227–1235, 1965.

Araki, M.: Studies on refractive components of human eye by ultrasonic wave Report II. Measurement of chamber depth and lens thickness by ultrasonic method. Acta Soc. Ophthalmol. Jap., 66:886–892, 1961.

Araki, M.: Studies on refractive components of human eye by means of ultrasonic wave: III. The correlation among refractive components. Acta Soc. Ophthalmol. Jap., 66:128–147, 1962.

Baum, G.: An evaluation of ultrasonic techniques used in measurements of eye size. Am. J. Ophthalmol., 64:926–936, 1967.

Boateng, A., and Hollwich, F.: Ultraschallmessungen bei primarem Blaukom. *In:* Ultrasonographia Medica. Edited by J. Bock and K. Ossoinig. Vienna, Verlag der Wiener Med. Akad., 1971, pp. 563–572.

Delmarcelle, Y., Luyckx-Bacus, J.: Biometric evolution of the anterior chamber in infants. Study of 1,960 globes. Bull. Soc. Belge Ophtalmol., 158:451–465, 1971.

Delmarcelle, Y., Collignon-Brach, J., and Luyckx-Bacus, J.: The role of the cornea and lens in biometry of the anterior chamber in normal subjects. Arch. Ophtalmol., 30:291–300, 1970.

Delmarcelle, Y., Collignon-Brach, J., and Luyckx-Bacus, J.: The depth of the anterior chamber in the normal eye and its constituent factors. Bull. Soc. Belge Ophtalmol., 152:447–454, 1969.

Flament, M. J.: Value of ultrasonic method in measurement of the thickness of the sclera. Bull. Soc. Ophtalmol. Fr., 70:911–917, 1970.

Fledelius, H., and Alsbirk, P. H.: Results of ultrasound oculometry with three different standard equipments. *In:* Ultrasonography in Ophthalmology. Edited by J. Francois and F. Goes. Basel, S. Karger, 1975, pp. 263–268.

Franceschetti, A-Th., Linder, A., and Franceschetti, A.: New results concerning the problem of axial length of the eye in anisometropia. *In:* Diagnostica Ultrasonica in Ophthalmologia (SIDUO II), Edited by J. Vanysek. Brno, University of Brno, 1968, pp. 235–238.

Franken, S.: Length measurements of the eye with the aid of an ultrasonic echo. Ned. Tijdschr. Geneeskd., 105:1803–1804, 1961.

Franken, S.: Measurements of dimensions of the human eye by means of ultrasound echography. Thesis, Utrecht, 1961.

Gernet, H.: Axis length and refraction of the living eye in newborn infants. Graefe. Arch. Ophthalmol., 166:530–536, 1964.

Gernet, H.: Biometry of the eye by means of ultrasound. Bull. Soc. Belge Ophtalmol., 140:327–339, 1965.

Gernet, H.: Recent advances in ultrasound biometry of the eye. *In:* Diagnostica Ultrasonica in Ophthalmologia (SIDUO II), Edited by J. Vanysek. Brno, University of Brno, 1968, pp. 217–234.

Gernet, H.: Data collection in clinical oculometry. Doc. Ophthalmol., 27:42, 1969.

Giglio, E., Ludlow, W., and Wittenberg, S.: Improvement in the measurement of intraocular distances using ultrasound. J. Acoust. Soc, Am., 44:1359–1364, 1968.

Giglio, E.: Ultrasonic system for measurement of intraocular distances. *In:* Ophthalmic Ultrasound. Edited by Gitter, K., et al. St. Louis, C. V. Mosby Co., 1969, pp. 122–133.

Grignolo, A., and Rivara, A.: Biometry of the human eye from the sixth month of pregnancy to the tenth year of life (measurements of the axial length, retinoscopy refraction, total refraction corneal refraction. *In:* Diagnostica Ultrasonica in Ophthalmologia (SIDUO II), Edited by J. Vanysek. Brno, University of Brno, 1968, pp. 251–257.

Grignolo, A., and Rivara, A.: Biometric observations of eyes in infants born at full term and prematurely up to the first year. Ann. Ocul., 201:817–725, 1968.

Jansson, F.: Intraocular measurements with ultrasonics. Wiss. Z. Humboldt Univ. Berlin [Math. Naturwiss.], 14:205–208, 1965.

Kawagoe, M.: The studies of the ultrasonic measurements in ophthalmology. I. The results of the ultrasonic axial measurements in normal human eye. Acta Soc. Ophthalmol. Jap., 77:743–52, 1973.

Kimura, T.: Developmental change of the optical components in twins. Acta Soc. Ophthalmol. Jap., 69:963–969, 1965.

Larsen, J. S.: The sagittal growth of the eye. 1. Ultrasonic measurement of the depth of the anterior chamber from birth to puberty. Acta Ophthalmol., 49:239–262, 1971.

Larsen, J. S.: The sagittal growth of the eye. II. Ultrasonic measurement of the axial diameter of the lens and the anterior segment from birth to puberty. Acta Ophthalmol., 49:427–440, 1971.

Larsen, J. S.: The sagittal growth of the eye. III. Ultrasonic measurement of the posterior segment (axial length of the vitreous) from birth to puberty. Acta Ophthalmol., 49:441–453, 1971.

Leary, G. A.: Ultrasonographic measurement of the components of ocular refraction in life. Wiss. Z. Humboldt Univ. Berlin [Math. Naturwiss.], 14:217–219, 1965.

Leary, G. A.: Ophthalmological biometrics. Ultrasonics, 7:138, 1969.

Leary, G. A., and Young, F. A.: Reliability and validity of ultrasonographic measurements in primates. *In:* Ophthalmic Ultrasound. Edited by K. Gitter et al. St. Louis, C. V. Mosby Co., 1969, pp. 117–122.

Lehtinen, A., and Oksala, A.: A new quick method for measuring distances between ultrasonic echoes on echograms of the eye. Acta Ophthalmol., 39:50–54, 1961.

Lewis, G. W.: Ultrasonic measurements of the living primate eye: The effects of transducer manipulations. Ultrasonics, 10:267–275, 1972.

Luyckx-Bacus, J., and Weekers, J. F.: Biometric studies of the human eye by ultrasound. Bull. Soc. Belge Ophtalmol., 143:552–567, 1966.

Luyckx, J.: Measurement of the optic components of the eye of the newborn by ultrasonic echography. Arch. Ophtalmol., 26:159–170, 1966.

Nakijima, A.: Measurement of the axial length of the eye by ultrasonic device. Jap. J. Clin. Ophthalmol., 14:1594, 1960.

Nakijima, A., Kimura, T., and Yamazaki, M.: Applications of ultrasound in biometry of the eye. *In:* Ultrasonics in Ophthalmology. Edited by R. Goldberg and L. Sarin, Philadelphia, W. B. Saunders, 1967, pp. 124–144.

Oksala, A., and Varonen, E.-R.: Experimental and clinical studies regarding the measurement of the thickness of the sclera by means of ultrasound. Wiss. Z. Humboldt Univ. Berlin [Math. Naturwiss.], 14:193–197, 1965.

Oksala, A., and Varonen, E.-R.: Experimental and clinical investigations concerning the measurement of scleral thickness with ultrasound. Acta Ophthalmol., 43:75–84, 1965.

Pallin, O.: The influence of the axial length of the eye on the size of the recorded B-potential in the clinical single-flash electroretinogram. Acta Ophthalmol. (Suppl.), 101:1–57, 1969.

Perez-Llorca, R.: Statistical echographic biometry of the anterior segment and the axial length of the living human eye from premature birth to old age in the inhabitants of Cadiz. Bull. Mem. Soc. Fr. Ophtalmol., 84:275–281, 1971.

Preisova, J.: Measurement of the eye by ultrasonics. Cesk. Oftalmol., 24:13–19, 1968.

Rivara, A.: Measurement of the antero-posterior ocular axis by means of ultrasonics. Ann. Ottal., 89:195–206, 1963.

Saraux, H., and Bechetoille, A.: Biometric study of the growth of the adolescent eye. *In:* Diagnostica Ultrasonica Ophthalmologia. Edited by M. Massin and J. Poujol. Paris, Centre National d'Ophtalmologie des Quinze-Vingts, 1973, pp. 265–268.

Sorsby, A.: Measurement of the optical components of the globe. *In:* Modern Trends in Ophthalmology, 2nd ed. London, Butterworths, 1967, pp. 30–33.

Stepanik, J., and Ossoinig, K.: Measurement of the sagittal axis of the human eye during applanation of the cornea. Graefe. Arch. Ophthalmol., 173:114–124, 1967.

Stepanik, J., and Ossoinig, K.: Measurements of the sagittal axis of the human eye in vivo during applanation of the cornea. Br. J. Ophthalmol., 52:801–807, 1968.

Szczypinski, J.: Ultrasound ophthalmobiometry I. Techniques. Klin. Oczna, 43:1055–1059, 1973.

Szczypinski, J.: Ultrasonic ophthalmobiometry II. Results of anatomical and functional biometry. Klin. Oczna, 43:1381–1384, 1973.

Tomlinson, A. and Phillips, C.: Applanation tension and axial length of the eyeball. Br. J. Ophthalmol., 54:548–553, 1970.

Vanysek, J., Preisova, J., and Obraz, J.: Measurement of the distances in the eye. *In:* Ultrasonography in Ophthalmology. London, Butterworths, 1969, pp. 203–209.

Weekers, R., Grieten, J., and Lavergne, G.: Study of anterior chamber dimensions in the human eye. Ophthalmologica, 142:650, 1961.

Young, F. A.: Ultrasound and phakometry measurements of the primate eye. Am. J. Optom., 43:370–386, 1966.

Young, F., and Leary, G.: Comparison of the optical characteristics of the human, ape and monkey eye. Proceedings 75th Annual Congress APA, 1967, pp. 89–90.

Young, F., and Leary, G.: Comparative optical characteristics of the major primates. Invest. Ophthalmol., 8:234, 1969.

Young, F., and Leary, G.: Ocular biometry of eskimo families. *In:* Diagnostica Ultrasonica in Ophthalmolgia. Edited by M. Massin and J. Poujol. Paris, Centre National d'Ophtalmologie des Quinze-Vingts, 1973, pp. 287–292.

IV

Introduction to
Diagnostic Ultrasound

THE earliest diagnostic equipment for ophthalmic evaluation was a hand-held transducer with A-mode display. Oksala of Finland, a pioneer, was prolific in describing his techniques and observations with A-mode.[1] More currently, Ossoinig has developed the A-mode techniques to a high degree of sophistication, using tissue standards that allow quantification of echo amplitudes to aid in identifying tissue.[2]

The two-dimensional B-scan display for ophthalmology was first described by Baum and Greenwood,[3] a short time after Oksala's initial observations. The original B-scan equipment was extremely expensive and the special face mask required for a water bath standoff (Fig. IV-1) limited widespread clinical use. Nevertheless, Baum made numerous early observations with this technique. Purnell and Sokollu dramatized the essential value of B-scan ultrasonic diagnosis by their thorough and original investigations.[4] Purnell devised a simpler coupling apparatus between the transducer and the eye (Fig. IV-2) which preserved optimum resolution, and with Sokollu and Holasek devised the first hand scanner for use in ophthalmic evaluation[5] (Fig. IV-3).

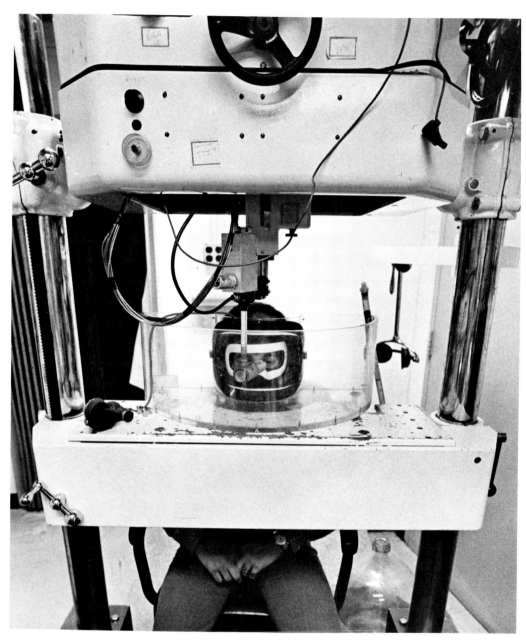

FIG. IV-1. The original mask and water bath immersion technique described by Baum. Excellent standoff properties and the ability to scan one or both eyes are provided.

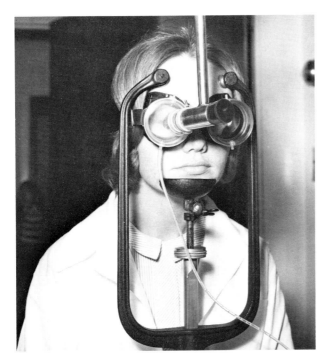

FIG. IV-2. A simplified immersion standoff system devised by Purnell, which allows automatically spaced horizontal scanning as utilized in Baum's method, but which also allows a smaller, more easily controlled volume of water to be used and reduces the problems of face mask adaptation.

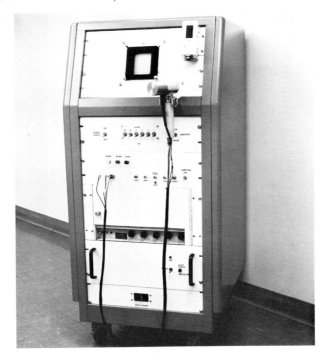

FIG. IV-3. The original contact B-scan equipment developed by Purnell, Sokollu and Holasek.

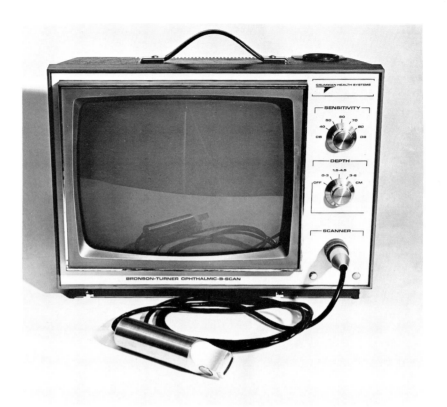

FIG. IV-4A. The first commercially available contact B-scan equipment designed by Bronson and Turner. The display is a television picture tube.

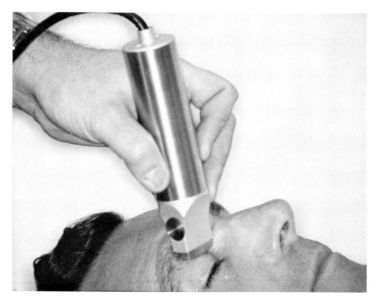

FIG. IV-4B. A close-up view of the hand-held contact B-scan device shown in Figure IV-4A.

Color Plates

Plate 1

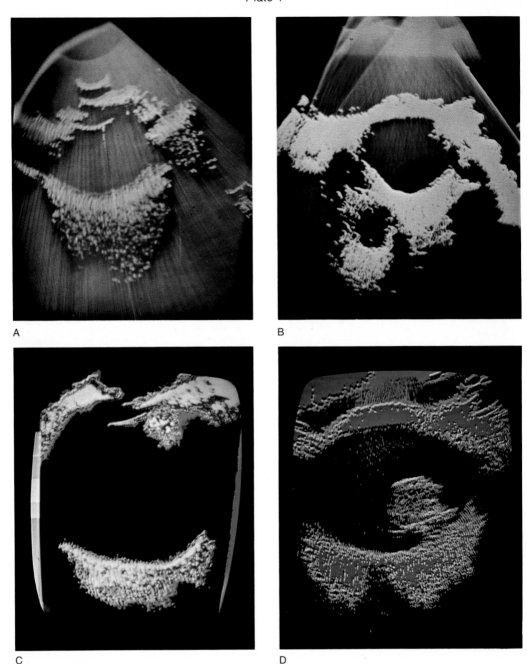

A

B

C

D

Color Plate A. B-scan ultrasonogram of a normal globe used to demonstrate gray scale. Note that the deeper orbital structures are less dense than the scleral echoes.

Color Plate B. Orbital cyst as shown with compound scanning rather than sector scan alone. While gray scale is degraded, more of the equatorial regions can be seen to complete the contour of ocular and orbital structures.

Color Plate C. Color B-scan ultrasonogram of a globe with a malignant melanoma of the ciliary body. The cornea is not well seen on the top because of obliquity of section. The tumor adjoins the lens and iris. Color coding here is eight levels and allows visual perception of the amplitude variation within the tumor.

Color Plate D. Color B-scan ultrasonogram of a malignant melanoma in which an irregularity of the choroidal outline directly posterior to the mass is seen. Additionally, the high leading edge characteristic of a malignant melanoma is denoted by the high (red) color level and the interspaced high color levels within the tumor probably relate to vascular channels.

Plate 2

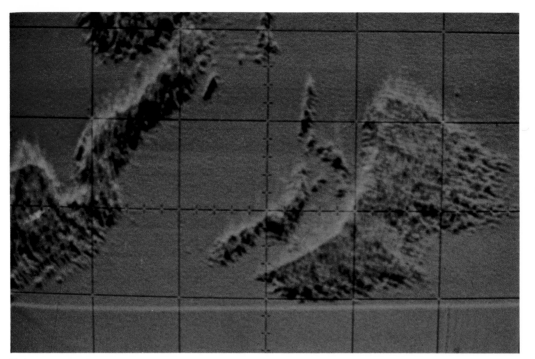

E

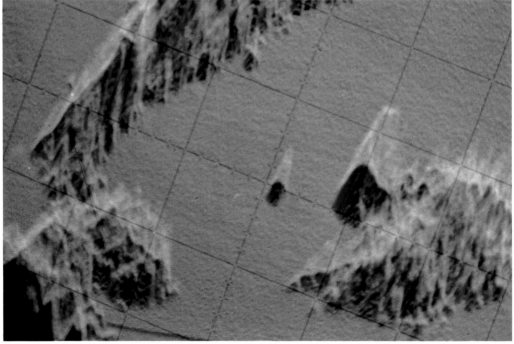

F

COLOR PLATE E. Isometric presentation of an intraocular vitreous membrane, demonstrating the comparative thickness and echo amplitude of sections of the membrane. Identification of the membrane may be more easily accomplished with this display technique.

COLOR PLATE F. An isometric scan showing an intraocular foreign body in mid-vitreous, preceded by scattered vitreous debris. This means of display presents the spatial relationship of such abnormalities far more graphically than either A- or B-scan alone.

Plate 2 (cont'd)

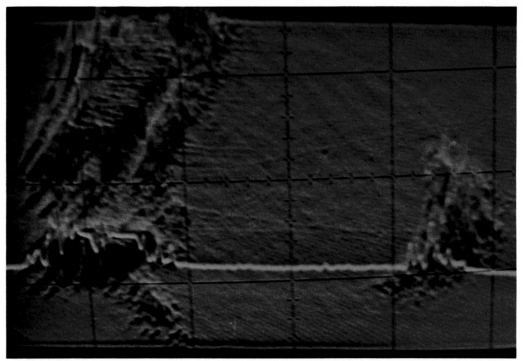

G

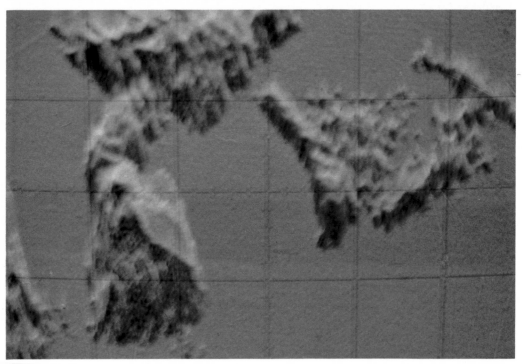

H

COLOR PLATE G. Isometric view of a globe and orbit with cursor line cutting through a region where a metallic foreign body rests against the sclera. The isometric view allows rapid visual appreciation of high-amplitude echoes (as seen with foreign bodies) extending above normal orbital echoes.

COLOR PLATE H. Isometric scan of an orbital tumor which graphically portrays the lower amplitude of the intraorbital echoes, while allowing the examiner to readily appreciate the well-delineated borders of this mass.

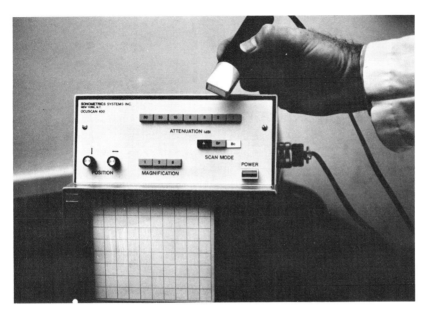

FIG. IV-5A. Commercially available contact scanner produced by Sonometrics Systems, Inc.

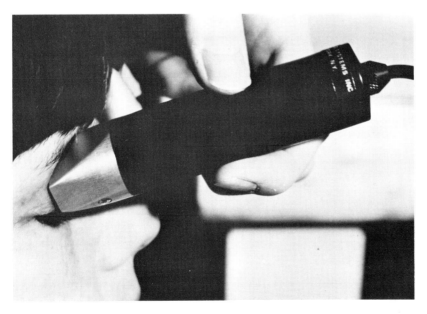

FIG. IV-5B. The hand scanner shown in Figure IV-5A may be placed directly upon the closed lid, eliminating the need for a water bath at the expense of the better resolution available with the immersion method.

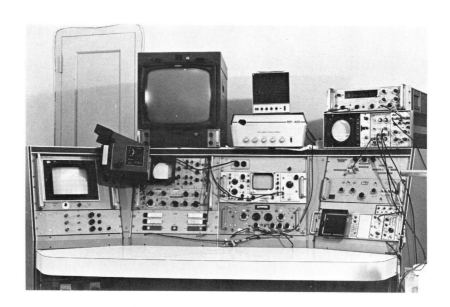

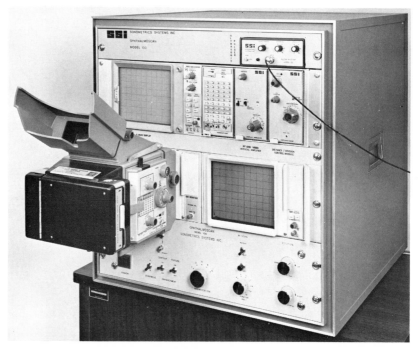

FIG. IV-6. *Top:* The equipment console used by Coleman for clinical ultrasonic evaluation. Two separate interchangeable A- and B-scans are used with several simultaneous oscilloscope displays. An electronic interval counter and color and isometric display functions can be utilized. This equipment is more complex than required for routine clinical use. *Bottom:* A commercially available adaptation of our laboratory's equipment console (top), devised by Sonometrics Systems, Inc. In this equipment, both A- and B-scan modes may be observed simultaneously by the examiner, with a separate oscilloscope available for photography of implementation of the M-mode in required instances.

TABLE IV-1. Immersion Advantages

1. Permits serial scans
2. Has greater stability than hand-held methods
3. Permits resolution of anterior ocular structures
4. Gives improved resolution of all ocular structures
   (adjustment of a transducer focal zone)
   (no lid attenuation)
5. Allows interchange of transducers
6. Allows observation during B-scan
7. Allows M-scan
8. Avoids globe compression

Our own laboratory, which had initially applied itself to high-resolution A-scan techniques for accurate measurements of ocular dimensions, developed a relatively simple hand-operated B-scanner in 1967 which preserved resolution and reduced equipment cost.[6] More recently, Bronson has developed a contact B-scanner (Fig. IV-4A,B) that allows the ophthalmic practitioner recourse to ultrasonic evaluation.[7] While present contact B-scan techniques provide less resolution than the immersion method, and frequency flexibility is restricted, their availability and usefulness are of great merit (Fig. IV-5A,B).

In our technique, we prefer the immersion method in order to allow selection of appropriate examining frequencies and for placement of the transducer a proper distance from the area of interest, maximizing resolution (Table IV-1). The hand-operated immersion technique (Fig. IV-6) also allows A- and B-scan to be used concurrently. In addition, we feel that the 1 cm of overlying saline places less stress on the globe, particularly in traumatized eyes, than may be induced with a contact system (Figs. IV-7, -8).

Conversely, the immersion technique is more time consuming, and is not as easily performed on children as are the contact methods. For this reason, we utilize contact A- and B-mode evaluation to complete the examination of children and for evaluation during a surgical procedure.

In all thorough examinations, both the A- and B-modes are required. The B-mode provides topographic information while the A-mode provides relative echo amplitude comparisons that are also critical to tissue identification. The combined method—using the same equipment—allows areas that are specifically identified from the B-scan to be simultaneously studied with the A-scan. In contrast, sequential A- and B-mode examinations require more time to assure that the same area is being examined by each technique and to

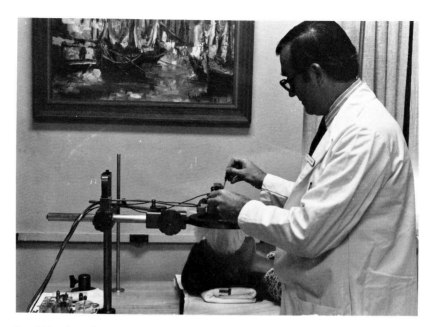

FIG. IV-7. Scanning is performed while the patient is supine on an examination table. This reduces the patient's head movement and permits the examiner to observe the relationship of transducer to eye while also observing the scan display on the oscilloscope.

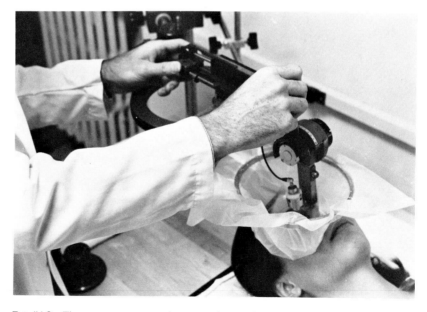

FIG. IV-8. The scanner arm may be swung into various positions to obtain vertical or oblique scans.

reduce the continuous correlation inherent in the combined immersion method.

An additional major advantage of immersion examinations is the ability to provide parallel, spaced "slices" or tomographic cuts with the B-scan, thus facilitating three-dimensional conceptualization. The random sectioning provided by contact B-scan methods is less easily assimilated than spaced tomograms. Conversely, the contact B-scan unit can provide tangential perspectives, i.e., the transducer can be aimed more perpendicular to certain ocular and orbital structures such as the globe equator, especially at 12:00 and 6:00, and the superior and inferior orbital walls.

A-mode equipment and displays also vary. For diagnostic work, a means of comparing echo amplitudes should be available either with a standard or with a fiducial echo such as the posterior scleral wall.

A-mode equipment also varies primarily in terms of the frequencies provided and the type of amplification employed. For example, linear, logarithmic or amplifiers with S-shaped characteristics are available.

For biometry, the ability to use high frequencies such as 15 and 20 MHz is essential for highly accurate measurements. The commonly used examining frequency of 10 MHz may be adequate for more coarse estimations.

Thus, depending on the information sought, the type of both A- and B-scan equipment may vary. In all instances, equipment designed for ophthalmic use is strongly recommended over equipment designed for general body scanning, which uses lower frequencies and resolution than are required for ophthalmic studies.

References Cited

1. Oksala, A., and Lehtinen, A.: Diagnostic value of ultrasonics in ophthalmology. Ophthalmologica, 134:387–395, 1957.
2. Ossoinig, K. C.: Quantitative echography—the basis of tissue differentiation. J. Clin. Ultrasound, 2:33–47, 1974.
3. Baum, G., and Greenwood, I.: The application of ultrasonic locating techniques to ophthalmology, Part I. Reflective properties. Am. J. Ophthalmol., 46:319–329, 1958.
4. Purnell, E. W.: Ultrasound in ophthalmological diagnosis. *In:* Diagnostic Ultrasound. Edited by C. Grossman, et al. New York, Plenum Press, 1966, pp. 95–109.
5. Holasek, E., and Sokollu, A.: Direct contact, hand-held, diagnostic B-scanner. Proceedings IEEE Ultrasonics Symposium, 1972.
6. Coleman, D. J., Konig, W. F., and Katz, L.: A hand operated, ultrasound scan system for ophthalmolic evaluation. Am. J. Ophthalmol., 68:256–263, 1969.
7. Bronson, N. R.: Development of a simple B-scan ultrasonoscope. Trans. Am. Ophthalmol. Soc., 70:365–408, 1972.

V

Ocular Diagnosis

Introductory Discussion and Background Material

Historical Survey

The first use of ultrasound in ophthalmic diagnosis was reported in 1956 by Mundt and Hughes,[1] who used industrial ultrasound equipment to examine enucleated normal eyes and eyes with intra-ocular tumors. The first clinical use of A-scan in ocular diagnostic problems was presented in 1957 by Oksala,[2] in the first of many pioneering papers. Slightly later, Jansson of Sweden described the use of ultrasound for ocular measurement[3] and determined velocity constants for ocular tissues.[4] Oksala also made early measurements of velocities of tissues.[5] In 1958, Baum, with Greenwood, described the clinical use of B-scan for ophthalmic diagnosis and measurement.[6] Coleman, with Weininger,[7] in 1967 described the use of M-scan in ophthalmic application.

In the area of ocular diagnosis, Oksala's initial descriptions were followed by many subsequent papers on A-scan for clinical diagnosis.[8] Later, Bronson developed the first ultrasonically directed intra-ocular forceps,[9] and Ossoinig popularized specific A-scan equipment and described clinical results.[10] Ossoinig has made many original observations on the A-scan properties of specific tissues. He has evolved a sophisticated diagnostic technique which involves the quantification of echo amplitudes in A-scan patterns, and kinetic A-scans in which movement of both the transducer and the examined structures are used to characterize tissues.[11]

Other investigators who have contributed greatly to A-scan diagnosis include Buschmann[12] and Gernet[13] of West Germany, Massin and Poujol[14] of France, Francois and Goes[15] of Belgium, Vanysek and Preisova[16] of Czechoslovakia, Bertenyi[17] of Hungary and Gallenga[18] of Italy. In the United States, in the hospital-based laboratory at the Wills Eye Institute, Gitter, Meyer and Sarin,[19] under the direction of Keeney,[20] made early contributions regarding A-scan evaluation. At the Walter Reed Army Hospital, Penner and Passmore[21] and Cowden and Runyon[22] have described the uses of A-scan in the diagnosis of foreign bodies.

B-scan diagnosis was first developed by Baum,[6] who made numerous original observations on B-scan evaluation of the eye and orbit.[23,24] His efforts have been primarily devoted toward the development of equipment with increased accuracy and better resolution. Purnell, with Sokollu,[25] made early observations which had a major influence on B-scan diagnosis. His laboratory described orbital B-scan evaluation, and provided the first systematic classification of orbital disease with B-scan ultrasonography.[26] He and his co-workers,[25] simultaneously with Penner and Passmore,[21] were the first to utilize the magnetic properties of a foreign body in ultrasonic evaluation. Purnell also described special techniques for using continuous wave ultrasound,[27] early experiments for the treatment of retinal detachment with ultrasound,[28] and development of the first hand scanner for use in ophthalmic ultrasound.[29] Coleman, with Konig and Katz, described the first simplified hand-operated B-scan.[30] Coleman has presented an evaluation of the reliability of ocular[31] and orbital[32] diagnosis with A-, B- and M-scan ultrasound, and a systematic description of ocular and orbital diagnosis. The use of color monitoring and encoding[33] and isometric viewing[34] were first described by Coleman and co-workers.

Other areas of B-scan ophthalmic investigations have been explored by Hughes of Australia, who, with Kossoff, using Commonwealth Acoustic Laboratory equipment, has shown excellent resolution of ocular structures.[35] Recently Bronson, with Turner, developed a hand-held B-scanner, which was the first of many easily used contact B-scanners available.[36]

M-scan diagnosis, first described by Coleman and Weininger,[7] has been used to study physiologic changes during accommodation, and the magnetic properties of foreign bodies.[37] It has also been used for examining the vascular[38] and respiratory pulsations in ocular and orbital tumors.

As has been discussed in Chapter II, there are three available techniques for ocular ultrasonic examination: A-, B- and M-scan. With these techniques, several different systems for ultrasonically evaluating patients have evolved. It is important to mention at this point that A-scan and B-scan are not mutually exclusive methods of diagnosis. A thorough knowledge of either A-scan or B-scan ocular ultrasonography will provide reliable diagnostic information, but a combination of both A- and B-scan diagnostic methods is optimal. The two modes are not competitive, but are instead complementary. In our laboratory, we rely primarily upon B-scan; however, we use a constant A-scan monitor to obtain maximum quantitative echo amplitude information.

B-scan provides a two-dimensional display which presents a more complete total picture than is available with A-scan. The third dimension of amplitude levels can be displayed on certain types of B-scan, but in less sophisticated equipment is more easily obtained by observing the A-scan monitor simultaneously with the B-scan. Ideally, B-scan ultrasound can present a tomogram, or a thin cross section of the eye, with highly accurate resolution of tissue surfaces such as the cornea or the anterior chamber. It also displays reflectivity patterns within the tissue being observed. These are used to characterize the particular tissue once it has been accurately localized and outlined. M-scan has been of primary benefit in demonstrating consistent or reproducible pulsations, such as the respiratory or vascular pulsations of certain tissues, or the magnetic properties of foreign bodies.

Ossoinig has properly emphasized the value of A-scan ultrasonography in providing quantitative echo information. However, most ophthalmologists can more readily interpret two-dimensional B-scan patterns. Clinical analogies to ultrasonic B-scan are numerous (e.g., pathologic sections, X-ray tomograms, slit-lamp section), as has been pointed out by Baum.[39] The B-scan technique, because of its clinically demonstrated value and its recent commercial availability, has aroused great interest in the ophthalmic community. The following portions of the book describe diagnostic methods developed in these laboratories in which B-scan images provide the primary diagnostic information, which is supplemented by specific data acquired from the A- and M-mode techniques.

Regardless of the presentation used (whether A-, B- or M-scan), the information available with ultrasound is the same, that is, the relative amount of energy reflected back to the transducer from each tissue interface. By studying the patterns of reflected sound, ana-

TABLE V-1. Diagnostic Parameters

GROSS MORPHOLOGIC FEATURES
  Location
  Size
  Outline/contour/shape
  Associated ocular changes
  Changes with time

FINE MORPHOLOGIC FEATURES
  Boundary layer properties
    a. Acoustic impedance
    b. Roughness of surface
  Internal tissue properties
    Internal texture (homogeneous or heterogeneous)
    Type of internal structural elements
    Spatial distribution of internal structural elements
    Acoustic absorption coefficient (rate of absorption)

tomic or morphologic characteristics of the tissue can be determined, providing information not obtainable with any other technique.

This book will outline our method of diagnosis, which uses the B-scan to provide the broad, topographic conceptualization of tissue morphology and the A- and M-scans to provide specific comparative information regarding the tissues of greatest diagnostic interest.

Diagnostic Parameters

Ophthalmic examinations proceed in two stages aimed at studying the morphologic features listed in Table V-1. First, gross tissue features such as size and position are established. Second, various tissues, particularly anomalous structures, are identified by examining echo characteristics that are indicative of finer morphologic features.

While gross tissue features are readily discerned in B-scans, finer features can be interpreted only with an understanding of how tissue structure influences ultrasonic reflectivity. Different tissues transmit, absorb and reflect in various manners, depending upon factors such as density, rigidity and internal structural features. The ultrasonic echoes received from tissues can be used to delineate features which characterize their boundaries and their interiors.

At boundaries between tissues, ultrasound is reflected to a degree determined by the acoustic impedance mismatch between the tissues and by the size, orientation, and roughness of the boundary. To use an analogy, a mirror that is very smooth and that lies perpendicular to a flashlight beam will reflect most of the energy back to the flashlight. If the mirror is roughened, or smaller than the total beam, or angled away from the beam, it will reflect proportionately less light back to the flashlight. Similarly, a tissue interface that is smaller than the incident ultrasonic beamwidth or that is not perpendicular to the beam axis will reflect little energy back to the transducer.

Internal tissue characteristics also influence ultrasonic transmission and reflection. If a tissue has a homogeneous structure (e.g., lens, vitreous or a solid tumor such as a malignant melanoma), there are few internal reflective surfaces, giving a "cystic" or hollow appearance on B-scans. This appearance contrasts sharply with the dense speckled appearance generated by reflections from internal features of heterogeneous structures such as hemangioma, angioma and vitreous hemorrhage. In these hetereogeneous structures, echo amplitude and spatial distributions depend on the type and distribution of the internal structural elements (e.g., blood vessels, calcific deposits, necrotic regions). In addition, the falloff of echo amplitude with increasing depth is indicative of absorptivity. (In homogeneous structures, absorptivity is manifested by a "shadowing" of posterior tissues.)

In many cases, tissue can be identified by a close examination of boundary and interior features as ascertained from ultrasonograms. This ultrasonic identification of tissues is analogous to that made possible by light microscopy where structural and chemical characteristics influence affinities for various stains and, thereby, permit tissue differentiation.

Specific tissue absorption of ultrasound and frequency-related variations in tissue absorptions and reflectivity are intimately related to a variety of tissue characteristics. Current research in these areas promises to provide even more information than is presently available for tissue diagnosis.

Types of Diagnostic Information

We have found it convenient to consider ultrasonic diagnosis in terms of: (1) the *unique* information that is available from ultrasound, (2) *supplemental* information available from ultrasound, and (3) *documentary* information available from ultrasound. Unique information indicates that which is obtained in the presence of opaque ocular media, or in the orbit (where there are few other reliable methods of outlining soft tissue surfaces). Supplemental information may be exemplified by tumor diagnosis. Although a mass may be

TABLE V-2. Indications for Ocular Ultrasonography

Opaque media
  (corneal leukoma, hyphema, hypopyon, cataract, vitreous hemorrhage)
Occluded or markedly miotic pupil
Ophthalmoscopically visible mass lesion
Suspicion of tumor underlying retinal detachment
Ocular trauma
Ocular foreign body

visualized ophthalmoscopically, differentiation by means of clinical appearance is often inaccurate. The ultrasonic characteristics of a mass (e.g., shape, height, and acoustic transmission properties) may be added to information which is obtained visually. Documentary information refers to the ability of ultrasound to measure accurately the thickness of the lens, the length of the globe, the dimensions of a tumor, the motion of the lens during accommodation, or ocular properties which vary under the influence of drugs. All of these are measurements which are not easily or not at all obtainable by other means. While the unique information is the most dramatic and often described utilization of ultrasound, (e.g., detection of tumors in opaque eyes), the supplemental and documentary uses, such as in characterizing tumors, are of equal importance.

Indications for Ocular Ultrasound

A summary of the indications for the ophthalmic use of ultrasound is presented in Table V-2. In addition, there are other specific uses of ultrasound, such as detecting loci of choroidal effusion in patients with flat chamber, preoperatively studying the character and form of vitreous hemorrhages prior to vitrectomy, measuring the size and volume of tumors prior to cobalt plaque treatment, and measuring axial lengths to determine keratoprosthetic or intraocular lens dioptric powers.

In general, where visual techniques fail to provide sufficient information as to the structural configuration of the eye, ultrasonic evaluation is indicated.

The Normal Eye

A-Scan

AXIAL A-SCAN ULTRASONOGRAPHY. The axial ultrasonogram is obtained by using the visual or optical axis as the path of the

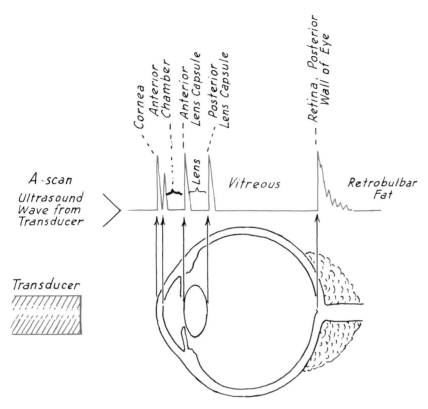

Cornea

Anterior
Chamber

Anterior
Lens Capsule

Posterior
Lens Capsule

Retina, Posterior
Wall of Eye

A-scan
Ultrasound
Wave from
Transducer

Lens

Vitreous

Retrobulbar
Fat

Transducer

FIG. V-1. An axial A-scan is obtained by aligning the transducer beam with the optic or visual axis. Maximum amplitude echoes from the cornea, lens, and retina indicate optic axis alignment. The posterior lens echo is the most critical, yet the most difficult to maximize.

examining ultrasound beam, so that echoes are obtained from structures along the path of the central cornea posteriorly. Echoes arise from ocular tissue interfaces which give rise to acoustic impedance mismatches. These echoes are displayed as vertical deflections on an oscilloscope screen. In the axial echogram of the normal eye (Figs. V-1, V-2), high echoes are produced by the two corneal surfaces, by the two lens surfaces, and by the vitreoretinal interface. The vitreoretinal interface echo is followed by a complex of echoes representing retina, choroid, sclera, and retrobulbar fat. The echoes in the retrobulbar fat diminish gradually to baseline. Certain parts of the eye are normally acoustically homogeneous. These include the anterior chamber, the lens, and the vitreous. These areas appear as baseline (zero echo or anechoic) segments between echo groups.

DIASCLERAL (OFF-AXIS) A-SCAN ULTRASONOGRAPHY. To obtain the diascleral ultrasonogram, the examining ultrasound beam must pass

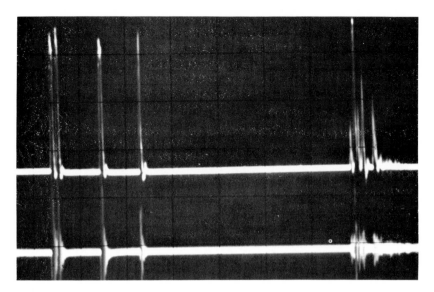

FIG. V-2. An axial A-scan with a video tracing (*top*) and a simultaneous radio-frequency tracing (*bottom*), taken at 20 MHz. Both corneal surfaces, the lens surfaces and the retrobulbar echo complex are shown. If present, a small pupil will give an echo preceding the anterior lens. This echo can easily be distinguished at 20 MHz. The radio-frequency trace provides more information than the video tracing alone.

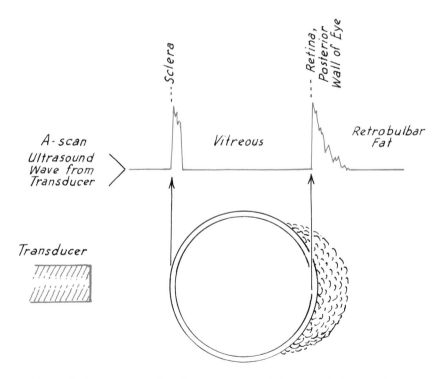

FIG. V-3. An A-scan across the vitreous cavity, avoiding the anterior chamber and lens, gives high-amplitude posterior ocular and retrobulbar echoes.

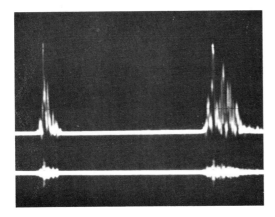

FIG. V-4. A diascleral A-scan taken over the pars plana at 20 MHz. Note that the decay pattern of echoes from the anterior sclera trail into the anterior vitreous, obscuring details along the zonule-anterior hyaloid region.

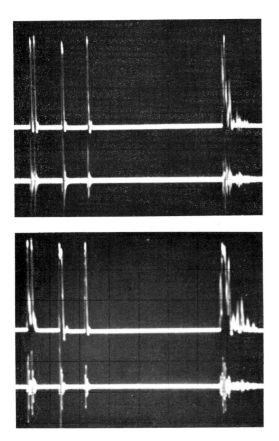

FIG. V-5. A-scans along the optic axis at 20 MHz (*top*) and 10 MHz (*bottom*), to demonstrate the better sensitivity and penetration to the orbit at 10 MHz, while better resolution, especially of anterior structures, is produced at 20 MHz. Note that the anterior corneal echo returns to baseline at 20 MHz, and not at 10 MHz.

peripheral to the cornea and the lens. The transducer is placed on or anterior to the sclera, and angled backward so the ultrasound beam will reach the posterior structures. The normal diascleral ultrasonogram (Figs. V-3, V-4) consists of a high-amplitude echo complex, representing sclera, followed by a long acoustically empty (sonolucent) interval, representing the normal vitreous cavity. The final echo complex produced by retina, choroid, sclera, and retrobulbar fat is similar to that seen in the axial ultrasonogram. Oksala[40] has pointed out that the echoes from the posterior ocular wall in the diascleral ultrasonogram are higher and broader than those obtained in the axial ultrasonogram, since there is no sound absorption from the lens.

FREQUENCY-RELATED VARIATION. As we have discussed in Chapters I and II, there is a balance, or "trade-off," between resolution and penetration. Figure V-5 shows A-scans of the same normal eye taken at 10 and 20 MHz, to illustrate the high resolution obtainable with the 20-MHz transducer. The penetration of the ultrasound beam from a 20-MHz transducer, however, is much less than that obtained with a 10-MHz transducer, which depicts more of the orbital fat and optic nerve. In general, the 10-MHz examining frequency is the best compromise for initial examination, with higher or lower frequency transducers then substituted for the study of specific tissues.

B-scan

B-mode ultrasonographic systems have been described in Chapter II. B-scan ultrasonography provides a two-dimensional "acoustic section" of the globe along any desired scan plane. As in A-scan ultrasonography, the appearance of the normal eye varies according to the scan plane selected.

AXIAL B-SCAN ULTRASONOGRAPHY. A typical B-scan ultrasonogram along an axial scan plane (Fig. V-6) shows both the anterior and posterior surfaces of the cornea, separated by a sonolucent interval representing the corneal stroma. The anterior chamber appears as a uniformly acoustically clear (black) area. The anterior surface of the iris is usually demonstrable. The echoes from the posterior iris surface usually merge with those from the anterior lens surface. However, with a dilated pupil, the anterior lens curvature is more prominently seen. The interior of the lens appears as an acoustically homogeneous space. The posterior curvature of the lens is usually well demonstrated, but the equator is not seen because of its alignment to the beam. The vitreous compartment appears as a sono-

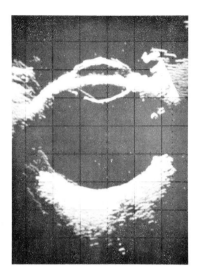
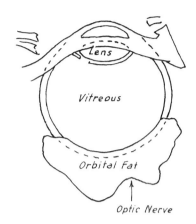

FIG. V-6. A B-scan at 10 MHz through the midline of the globe in horizontal section (*left*) with a schematic drawing of the section (*right*). A B-scan produces a thin tomographic section of the eye which can be repeated at spaced, selected intervals to section the globe completely, much as in a histologic preparation.

lucent cavity with no internal sound reflections. The vitreoretinal interface forms a smooth, concave curvature. Echoes from the retina merge with echoes from the choroid and the sclera, and in the normal eye these contiguous echoes cannot be separated at normal examining frequencies of 10 and 15 MHz. Often, in B-scan ultrasonography, the area between the ora serrata and the equator of the globe is poorly demonstrated, since, as with the equator of the lens,

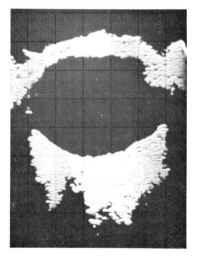
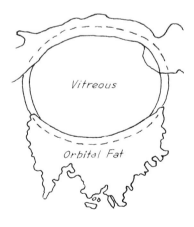

FIG. V-7. B-scans at 10 MHz obtained through a plane external to the anterior chamber-lens axis show better orbital penetration since the ultrasound energy is not subject to absorption by the lens.

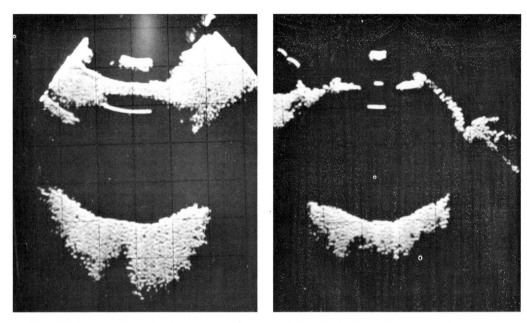

FIG. V-8.   B-scans at 10 MHz (*left*) and 20 MHz (*right*) demonstrate the better resolution available at the higher frequency and the better sensitivity and penetration available at the lower frequency.

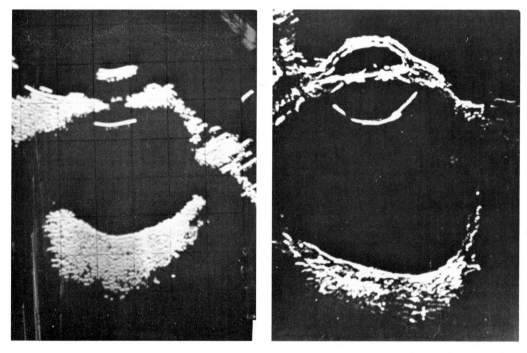

FIG. V-9.   A sector B-scan (*left*) shows less detail of the cornea and anterior segment since only the central area is tangent to the beam. Posterior ocular and orbital structures are well seen. The compound scan (*right*) fills in more topographic detail, especially anterior and equatorial structures, but at the expense of gray scale since the overlapped areas can no longer be easily compared to areas where only a "single" pass is shown. This compound scan is of a staphylomatous eye at 20 MHz.

these areas are parallel to the sound beam. In an axial B-scan, the retrobulbar fat forms a W-shaped pattern, with a black notch formed by the optic nerve. The normal orbital B-scan appearance will be discussed further in Chapter VI on orbital diagnosis.

DIASCLERAL (OFF-AXIS) B-SCAN ULTRASONOGRAPHY. A diascleral ultrasonogram of the normal eye (Fig. V-7) shows a rounded echo complex representing the scleral curvature anteriorly, followed by an acoustically clear (black) space representing the vitreous cavity and a concave echo pattern from the posterior globe wall. The retrobulbar fat pattern above and below the nerve appears as a white crescent behind the globe.

FREQUENCY-RELATED VARIATION. As discussed in the section on A-scan ultrasonography, there is always a trade-off between resolution and penetration. Figure V-8 shows a comparison of B-scan ultrasonograms of the same normal eye obtained with 10- and 20-MHz transducers. The anterior structures are much better delineated with the 20-MHz transducer; however, the penetration into the orbital fat is better with the 10-MHz transducer.

EFFECT OF SCANNING MODE (CHAPTER II). Figure V-9 shows the difference between a sector scan and a compound scan of the eye utilizing a 10-MHz transducer. A compound scan is better at outlining the contours of the anterior segment and the equator of the globe than is the sector scan.

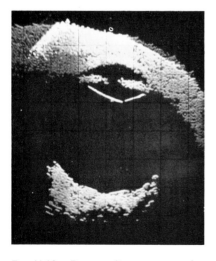
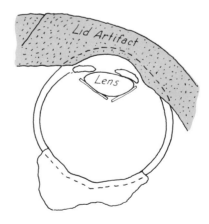

FIG. V-10. B-scan ultrasonogram of a normal globe performed through the lid, demonstrating the loss of definition of the cornea and attenuation of the sound beam by the lid, and producing a foreshortened retrobulbar fat pattern.

EFFECT OF LID ATTENUATION. We prefer to use a water bath standoff in all diagnostic work; however, both immersion and contact B-scan ultrasonography can be performed through the closed eyelid. Figure V-10 demonstrates the marked attenuation of ultrasound energy caused by passage through the lids. In addition to the marked absorption of the sound beam, ocular structures immediately posterior to the lid are obscured. For optimum B-scan ultrasonography, a water bath standoff with lids open is recommended.

Artifacts Encountered in Ocular Ultrasonography

Occasionally, artifacts arise in the course of ultrasonic evaluation of the eye and familiarity with their appearance will avoid erroneous interpretation. Artifacts may be classified into four groups: (1) electronic artifacts, (2) reduplication echoes, (3) refraction artifacts, and (4) absorption effects. The sources of these artifacts are treated in Chapter II. Clinical examples of each type of artifact are presented below.

ELECTRONIC ARTIFACTS. In certain scan situations, artifacts may arise from unsatisfactory electronic processing of the ultrasonic echoes. Typical artifacts are mentioned here.

"Snow." Snow is produced by background noise ("grass" on the A-scan trace) and resembles interference on a television screen (Fig. V-11). Background noise can usually be eliminated electronically by requiring incoming echo-generated energy to exceed a certain threshold level before triggering the B-scan presentation, thus rejecting low-amplitude background noise.

"Swiss Cheese." High-amplitude echoes or excessive gain can cause receiver saturation. In this case A-scan signals reach a plateau where they remain until the echo level returns below the saturation threshold. B-scans obtained in a pulsed mode are insensitive to echoes returned during this plateau and the corresponding tissue areas appear as cystic or spongy spaces resembling Swiss cheese (Fig. V-12).

Overlap Failure. Overlap is seen only in the compound B-scan and indicates that the angular alignment of the potentiometer or the resolver correlating the transducer and display alignment is faulty or misaligned (Fig. V-13). This problem is not seen when sector scanning is used alone.

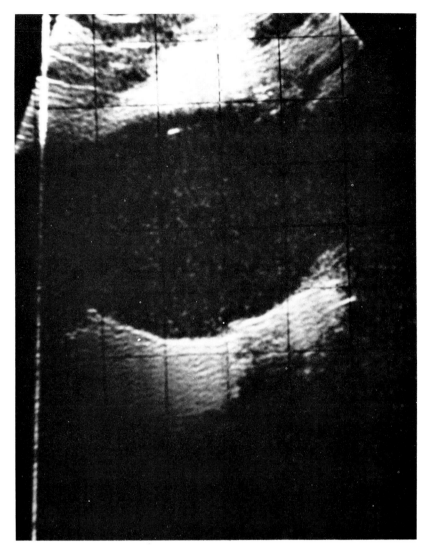

Fig. V-11. B-scan ultrasonogram of a normal eye, demonstrating the electronic artifact of "snow" caused by an overload of background noise which appears as scattered specks in the normally anechoic areas such as the vitreous.

REDUPLICATION ECHOES. These echoes (also known as multiple echoes) occur commonly and have been analyzed by Kossoff.[41] They usually appear along the axis of the cornea and lens. They occur when the transducer is aligned perpendicular to a tissue surface and high-amplitude echoes are reflected back to it. These echoes can then be reflected from the transducer back to the tissue and then rereflected, producing what is called a reduplication echo or a multiple of the distance between the transducer and the reflecting surface. An echo of this type is often seen in mid-vitreous

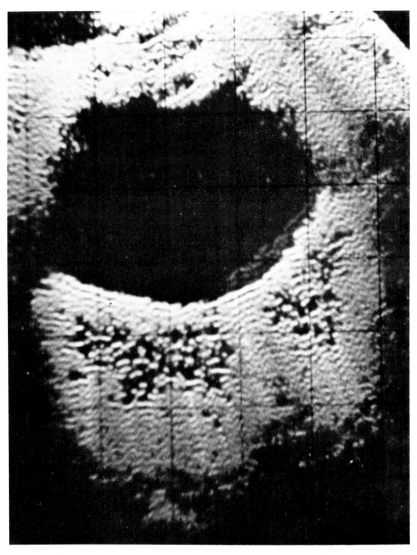

FIG. V-12. Apparent cystic structures resembling Swiss cheese can be produced on the B-scan when excessive amplitude echoes saturate the amplifiers.

when, utilizing a water bath standoff, the transducer is positioned a short distance (e.g., 1 cm) from the eye. The artifact would then appear in mid-vitreous, although this artifactual echo can be displaced into the orbit fat by positioning the transducer farther away from the eye. Echoes bouncing back and forth between the transducer and the cornea may mimic abnormal tissue or foreign bodies. These echoes may be distinguished from real echoes by moving the transducer either toward or away from the eye. This causes more rapid movement of the reduplication echo relative to tissue, allowing it to be identified (Fig. V-14).

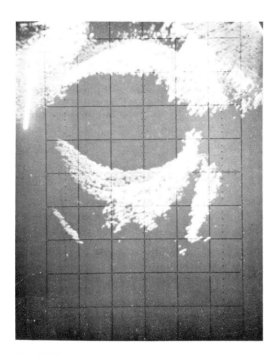

FIG. V-13. Compound B-scans may show overlap failure when the potentiometers are not adjusted, the transducer is not properly positioned, or the patient moves. Compound scans may appear out of alignment due to wide transducer beamwidth. Posterior lens echoes are especially prone to this apparent artifact.

REFRACTION ARTIFACTS. Other artifacts relating to the transducer position are produced by refraction of ultrasound within ocular tissues. On B-scan, the relatively high lenticular propagation velocity can produce apparent abnormalities of the posterior pole that resemble tumor formations or thickening of the choroid (Fig. V-15). Purnell has referred to these refraction abnormalities of the posterior pole as "Baum's bumps," since they were originally described by Baum.[42] In general, if a mass is seen at the posterior pole, scans should be made through different planes of preceding tissue to ascertain that the abnormality is not a reduplication echo, or caused by refraction through the lens. Scans of the posterior pole should be made through the limbus or a more peripheral position so that only normal sclera and vitreous precede the area of interest (Fig. II-16).

ABSORPTION EFFECTS (SHADOWING). Absorption of sound energy by anteriorly located structures may cause abnormal ocular ultrasonic patterns. The absorption of sound energy by an anteriorly located structure may result in the absence or attenuation of echoes

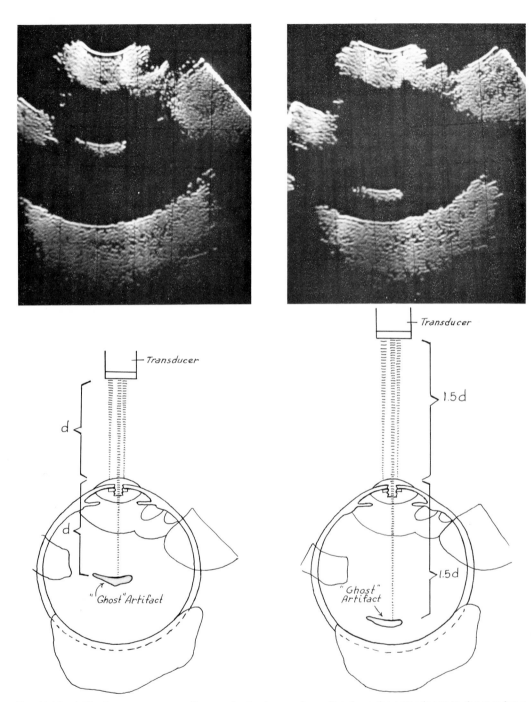

FIG. V-14. Artifacts may appear as the result of echoes rebounding from the transducer to the eye for a second or third "trip." Usually only multiple trips of the corneal echoes have sufficient energy to be displayed and appear as structures within the vitreous cavity. They can easily be detected by moving the transducer closer or farther away from the eye. Real echoes move with the transducer. Multiple echoes move faster than the tissue since the round trip distances should assure a different relation to the transducer-cornea separation.

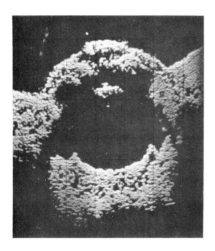 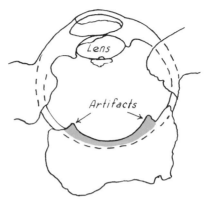

FIG. V-15. B-scan ultrasonogram demonstrating tumor-like artifactual elevations (Baum's bumps) at the posterior pole of the eye. These artifacts are caused by refraction of sound through the margins of the lens, and may be avoided by selecting a scan plane through an area outside the limbus and transecting the same region of the posterior pole.

in the posterior segment, giving an appearance of a defect in the ocular wall. Commonly encountered causes of such defects are dense cataract (Fig. V-16) and organized hemorrhage.

Whenever an abnormal ocular B-scan pattern is encountered, the above artifacts should be ruled out. Recognition of these artifacts is aided by (1) careful monitoring of the A-scan, which permits recognition of many electronic artifacts, (2) repositioning of the transducer if a reduplication echo is suspected, and (3) analysis of any ocular abnormality which may cause absorption defects in the acoustic pattern.

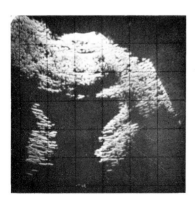 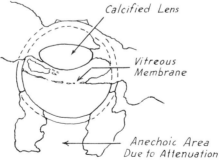

FIG. V-16. B-scan ultrasonogram demonstrating artifactual loss of definition of the posterior pole of the eye caused by marked attenuation of the echoes within a calcified lens. A similar pattern may be produced by dense organized vitreous hemorrhage or ocular tumor.

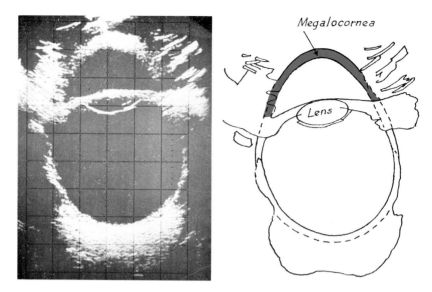

FIG. V-17. B-scan ultrasonogram of an abnormally large globe demonstrating megalocornea and an unusually deep anterior chamber.

Abnormalities of Ocular Size and Shape

B-scan ultrasonography graphically portrays anomalies of ocular size and contours. A-scan can provide the same information; however, B-scan ultrasonography, with its capability for two-dimensional, cross-sectional display, allows more information to be derived from a

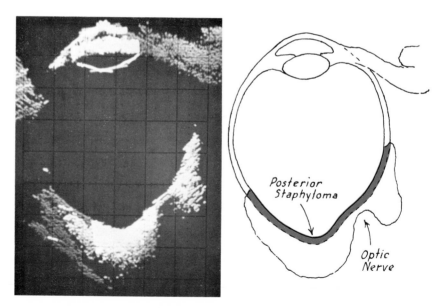

FIG. V-18. B-scan ultrasonogram of an abnormally long globe in a patient with myopia, demonstrating a staphyloma at the posterior pole.

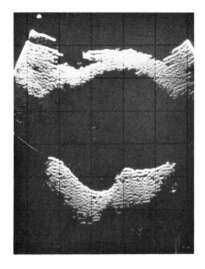
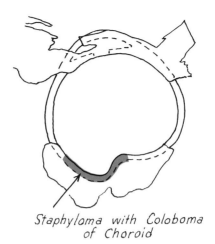

Staphyloma with Coloboma
of Choroid

FIG. V-19. B-scan ultrasonogram of an eye showing a staphyloma at the posterior pole with a cleft or coloboma of the choroid, demonstrating a pronounced, localized irregularity at the posterior pole.

single scan plane. Figure V-17 shows the B-scan ultrasonogram of a patient with megalocornea, demonstrating steepness of the corneal curvature and enlargement of the globe and anterior segment structures. Figure V-18 is a B-scan ultrasonogram of a patient with a posterior staphyloma due to high myopia. This aberration from the normal posterior contour of the globe appears acoustically as a concave dip in the globe wall. Figure V-19 is the ultrasonogram of a patient with a coloboma of the choroid in addition to a posterior staphyloma. The coloboma gives an even more pronounced aneurysm-like defect in the ocular wall, with a sharply defined rim.

B-scan portrayal of an enlarged globe and A-scan axial measurement documenting increased axial length allow differentiation of pseudoproptosis from true proptosis. This feature will be discussed further in Chapter VI.

Anterior Segment Abnormalities

Cornea

SIZE AND SHAPE ABNORMALITIES. As has been discussed above, anomalies of corneal size, such as megalo- or microcornea, may be demonstrated with B-scan ultrasonography. Corneal curvatures can be directly measured from the B-scan display and abnormalities of corneal shape (such as keratoconus) are demonstrable.

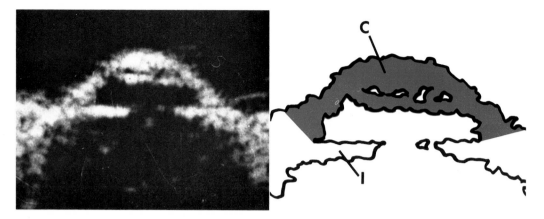

FIG. V-20. B-scan ultrasonogram through a thickened edematous cornea. The eye is aphakic. (Courtesy of Dr. E. Purnell.)

CORNEAL THICKENING. Thickening of the cornea is best determined by A-scan ultrasonic biometry (Chapter III). B-scan ultrasonographic techniques, however, may also be utilized. Figure V-20, courtesy of Dr. E. Purnell, shows an expanded B-scan view of a centrally thickened edematous cornea in an aphakic eye in which thickened and indistinct echoes precede the iris plane. Figure V-21 is a B-scan ultrasonogram of the eye of a patient with surgical aphakia, iris touch to the corneal endothelium, and a thickened edematous cornea. The ultrasonic demonstration of iris adherence or of a

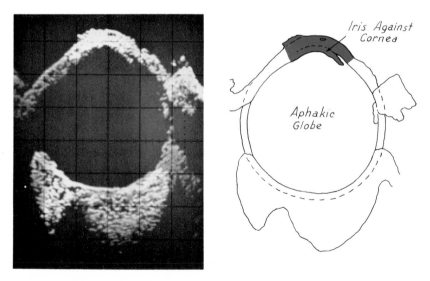

FIG. V-21. B-scan ultrasonogram demonstrating a markedly thickened central cornea and iris touch in an aphakic eye. Scans made through an aphakic eye, with loss of definition of the iris plane, may resemble a diascleral section (see Fig. V-7).

shallow anterior chamber may be of benefit when corneal edema is so severe that the retrocorneal structures cannot be visualized. Ultrasonic evaluation of the cornea and anterior segment in this manner is of assistance.

KERATOPROSTHESES. In addition to the examination of the globe prior to keratoplasty, ultrasound is of great value in the evaluation of eyes prior to prosthokeratoplasty. As previously mentioned, clinical evaluation of eyes with opaque corneas is difficult, whereas ultrasound permits accurate determination of the status of the posterior segment of the globe. The axial length of the eye can be obtained ultrasonically, allowing the placement of accurate dioptric correction in the optic cylinder of the prosthesis. Although most eyes proposed for keratoprosthesis insertion are known to be aphakic, in some cases a lens or lens remnant may be present. Ultrasonography determines the presence or absence of a lens, and prepares the surgeon for a lens extraction at the time of keratoprosthesis placement should the eye be phakic. If a cyclitic membrane is found ultrasonically prior to prosthokeratoplasty, it may be surgically excised during prosthesis placement.

Postprosthokeratoplasty evaluation of a globe is extremely difficult because of the very limited field of view (2 disk diameters) through the keratoprosthesis. The two-dimensional acoustic section of the globe provided by B-scan ultrasonography facilitates recognition of pathologic changes.

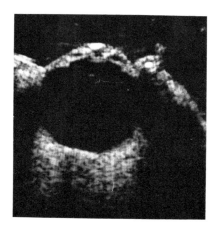
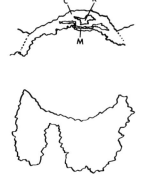

FIG. V-22. B-scan of an eye containing a keratoprosthesis. The outline of the keratoprosthesis (K) can be seen, as can a membrane (M) behind the prosthesis. The high acoustic reflectivity of plastic often complicates interpretation of the anterior segment in these eyes because of multiple echoes and acoustic refraction. (Courtesy of Dr. E. Purnell.)

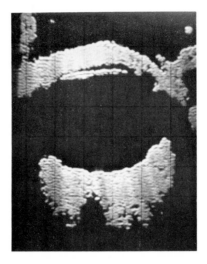
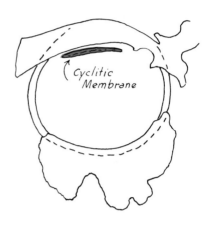

FIG. V-23. B-scan ultrasonogram of an eye with a keratoprosthesis in place. The anterior segment echoes are obscured by a thickened cornea, but a cyclitic membrane can be seen just posterior to the anterior echo complex.

Normal Eye with Cardona Keratoprosthesis. An eye with a keratoprosthesis in place is shown in Figure V-22. In scans made through the keratoprosthesis, acoustic artifacts are commonly produced, giving rise to possible confusion in interpretation (see Fig. V-14). To avoid these artifactual echoes, B-scans of eyes with keratoprosthesis in place are best made on a plane above or below the prosthesis. The normal globe then appears as an acoustically dense (white) ring, enclosing the acoustically empty circular area representing the vitreous cavity.

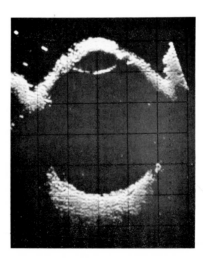
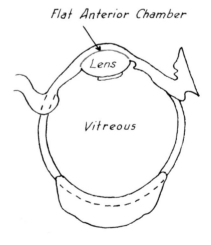

FIG. V-24. B-scan ultrasonogram of a phakic globe outline showing a flat anterior chamber.

Abnormal Eye with Cardona Keratoprosthesis. Coleman, Jack and Cardona[43] have described results in twenty-two patients who were referred for ultrasonography because of unexplained visual loss after months or years with a satisfactory result from keratoprosthesis insertion. Nineteen of these patients were found to have ultrasonically demonstrable posterior segment abnormalities accounting for their visual loss. These abnormalities were classifiable into four groups: (1) cyclitic membrane (Fig. V-23), (2) choroidal detachment, (3) vitreous hemorrhage, and (4) retinal detachment. In some of these eyes, two of these conditions coexisted.

Anterior Chamber

ANTERIOR CHAMBER DEPTH. Accurate measurement of anterior chamber depth is obtained by A-scan ultrasonic biometry (Chapter III). The A-scan beam should be positioned along the visual or optical axis to obtain a central representative and repeatable measurement. B-scan ultrasonography can also provide accurate two-dimensional information as to anterior chamber depth. Figure V-24 is the B-scan ultrasonogram of a phakic patient with a flat anterior chamber. The lens is displaced anteriorly and the iris is seen to lie against the corneal surface. The echoes from the posterior cornea and anterior iris merge, and the interface between these two structures cannot be outlined. Figure V-25, conversely, demonstrates a very deep anterior chamber in a phakic eye.

HYPHEMA. See discussion on page 249.

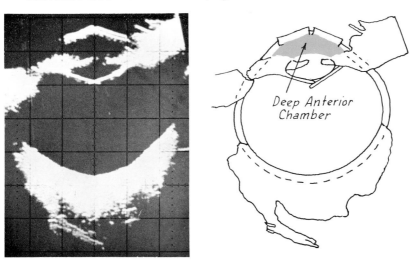

FIG. V-25. B-scan ultrasonogram of a normal phakic globe with an unusually deep anterior chamber.

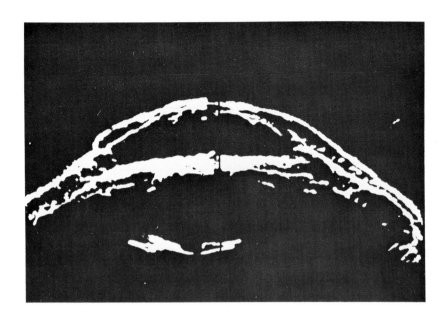

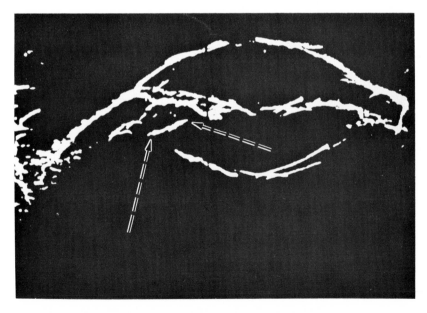

FIG. V-26. Electronically expanded view of a B-scan of the anterior chamber of a phakic eye, showing the variation in scan planes and transducer angulation required to demonstrate an iris cyst (arrows). (Courtesy of Dr. R. Dallow.)

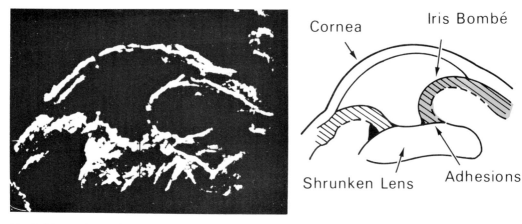

Cornea   Iris Bombé

Shrunken Lens   Adhesions

FIG. V-27. An electronically expanded view of the anterior segment demonstrating iris bombé. (Courtesy of Dr. R. Dallow.)

Iris

TUMORS. Iris tumors can be detected with ultrasonography if they are more than one millimeter in size. Preceding scleral echoes mask smaller lesions and may make the A-scan pattern difficult to interpret. Generally, these lesions are small and only a "solid" versus "cystic" differentiation can be made. Of greater worth, however, is the evaluation of possible extension of the tumor into the ciliary region.

IRIS CYSTS. Iris cysts are seen ultrasonically as rounded sonolucent areas and may be differentiated from iris tumors, which appear solid or acoustically opaque. The B-scan ultrasonogram of a patient with an iris cyst, courtesy of Dr. R. Dallow, is shown in Figure V-26.

IRIS BOMBÉ. A B-scan ultrasonogram of a patient with iris bombé, courtesy of Dr. R. Dallow, is shown in Figure V-27. This iris is pushed forward in a convex fashion, and lies against the posterior corneal surface.

ANIRIDIA. B-scan ultrasound can demonstrate the absence of an iris or can be used to measure the pupillary size.

EFFECT OF PHARMACOLOGIC AGENTS. Dilation, and the degree of dilation or contraction of the pupil, can be demonstrated with B-scan ultrasound, and ordinarily the pupillary size can be roughly estimated. Positioning the transducer parallel to the iris in contact B-scan ultrasonography can show the actual movement of the iris sphincter in a graphic manner.

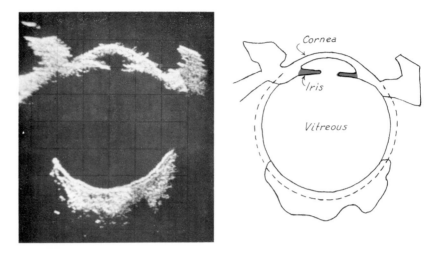

FIG. V-28. B-scan ultrasonogram of an normal aphakic eye demonstrating the cornea, pupillary opening and ciliary region.

Lens

ABSENCE AND DISPLACEMENT. Variations of normal lens position may be depicted ultrasonically. Figure V-28 is a B-scan ultra-sonogram of a patient with surgical aphakia, with the iris and ciliary body well outlined. Figure V-29 is a B-scan ultrasonogram of a patient with homocystinuria and a subluxated lens. The absence of the lens from its proper position in patients suffering from trauma should initiate a thorough search of the vitreous compartment for a displaced lens, as seen in Figure V-30.

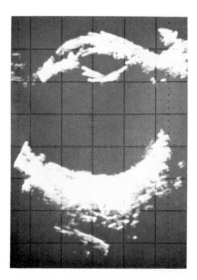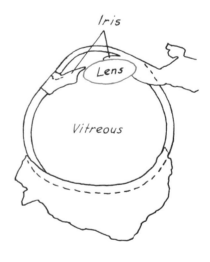

FIG. V-29. B-scan ultrasonogram showing a displaced lens in a patient with homo-cystinuria in an otherwise acoustically normal globe.

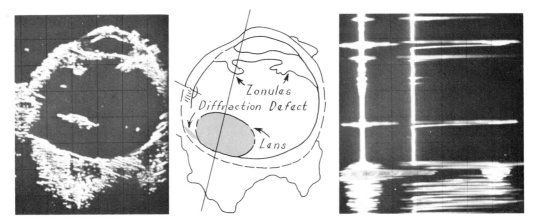

FIG. V-30. B-scan ultrasonogram showing a lens displaced to the posterior vitreous following trauma. When the lens rests on the retina, careful kinetic examination will determine its motility. Distortion of the globe posterior to a dislocated lens can aid in its identification.

CATARACT. Oksala[44] and Metz[45] have described the ultrasono- graphic appearance of a cataractous lens. The A-scan trace through the lens changes from a picture of acoustic homogeneity and sonolucence (with echo return only from the anterior and posterior lens surfaces) to an acoustic heterogeneity, where numerous echoes are seen within the nucleus and cortex of the lens. The position of these echoes indicates the area of acoustic change, which usually parallels the optical changes. Figure V-31 demon-

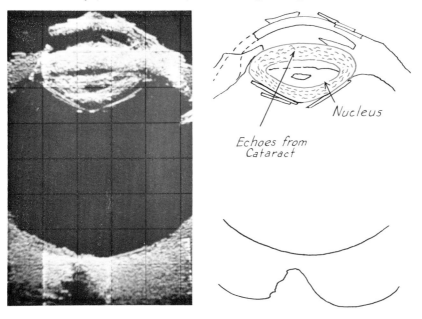

FIG. V-31. B-scan ultrasonographic appearance of a cataractous lens. The separation between nuclear and cortical material is demonstrated and the layered acoustic planes can be discerned.

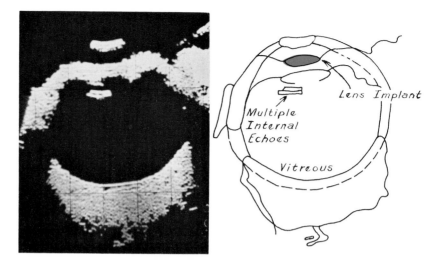

FIG. V-32. B-scan ultrasonogram of an eye with an intraocular lens implant in place. The acoustic artifacts produced by the implant closely parallel the appearance of a normal lens.

strates the separation of nucleus and cortex and shows a posterior cortical cataract. A B-scan ultrasonogram taken in the presence of a cataract demonstrates multiple intralenticular echoes. Pathologic changes responsible for these acoustic alterations include nonuniform lens fiber swelling and water cleft formation.

PREINTRAOCULAR LENS IMPLANT. In this situation, ultrasonography is useful in documentation of the status of the posterior segment of the globe and accurate determination of the axial length of the eye, which, as discussed in Chapter III and in the section on evaluation of eyes for keratoprosthesis, permits placement of accurate dioptric correction in the intraocular lens.

A B-scan ultrasonogram of an eye with an intraocular lens in place is shown in Figure V-32.

Vitreous Abnormalities

Vitreous surgery, particularly those procedures utilizing a pars plana incision, is a rapidly expanding area of ophthalmic surgery. The vitreous surgeon, however, is usually hindered by his inability to evaluate the status of the posterior vitreous and the retina with standard optical evaluation methods, so that he must usually rely upon subjective or indirect examination techniques. Ultrasonography provides a method of direct ocular evaluation which is unhindered by opaque media, and which can demonstrate structural changes in the vitreous and retina in eyes being considered for vitrectomy.

Severe vitreous hemorrhage may produce visual loss by chemical changes (i.e., hemosiderosis of the retina, hemosiderogenic syneresis of the vitreous) and mechanical changes (i.e., formation of strands or membranes producing permanent opacification of the media and retinal detachment). Biological changes occur relatively early and a decision to intervene surgically must be made soon following the initial bleeding. The decision for surgical intervention requires a careful appraisal of the extent of the pathologic changes in the vitreous, including ultrasonic evaluation.

Cibis[46] was a pioneer in demonstrating the changes that take place within the vitreous body secondary to blood and its breakdown products. Cibis and Yamashita[47] documented retinal degeneration secondary to hemosiderogenic changes. Recently, Regnault[48] has supplemented these studies with a description of the temporal relationships in the formation of vitreous membranes. Fibroblasts, which spread along the path of hemorrhage into the solid vitreous, organize the vitreous along the hemorrhagically disrupted plane into membranes. These membranes, as they contract, tend to produce stress on the retina that may lead to retinal detachment. Even if detachment does not ensue, the eye may remain visually useless because of optically dense membranes.

Therefore, to prevent or treat serious changes resulting from hemosiderogenic syneresis and membrane formation, the vitreous body must be evaluated from the time of onset of hemorrhage. In most cases of vitreous hemorrhage optical evaluation is inadequate. With the development of ophthalmic ultrasound, adequate determination of the extent of vitreous hemorrhage is now possible. The A-scan ultrasonographic findings in vitreous hemorrhage were first reported by Oksala and Lehtinen in 1958.[49] The B-scan ultrasonographic appearance of vitreous hemorrhage has been reported by Baum,[39] Purnell[25] and Coleman.[50]

In the normal eye, the vitreous appears as an acoustically clear cavity. On the A-scan, no echoes are seen above baseline between the posterior lens capsule and the retina. On B-scan, the vitreous appears as a uniformly sonolucent area. The retina in the normal eye appears on B-scan ultrasonograms as a smooth, concave, acoustically opaque (white) surface formed by echoes arising from the vitreoretinal interface. These echoes are contiguous with, and inseparable from, the choroid and sclera. In many cases, hemorrhagic

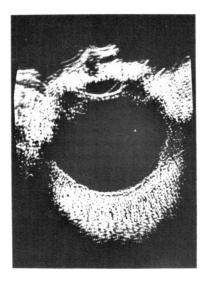 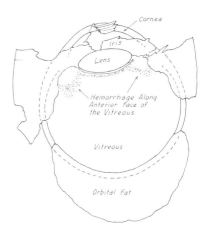

FIG. V-33. B-scan ultrasonogram of a vitreous hemorrhage showing light scattering of low-amplitude echoes along the anterior hyaloid face of the vitreous, seen just posterior to the lens in the vitreous fossa. The rest of the vitreous is acoustically clear and the retina is seen to be in place.

vitreous which is opaque to optical examination methods remains acoustically clear on B-scan at low gain. Denser hemorrhages appear as irregular opaque areas (Figs. V-33, V-34, V-35 and V-36). The location, extent and density of vitreous hemorrhage can be shown by ultrasonography.

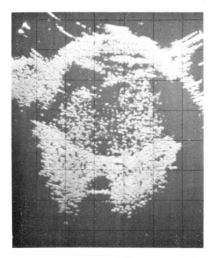 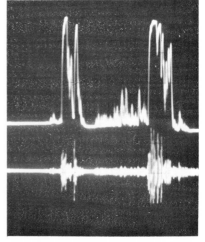

FIG. V-34. B-scan ultrasonogram of diffuse vitreous hemorrhage with an accompanying A-scan to emphasize the use of amplitude analysis in differentiating hemorrhage from tumor. Vitreous hemorrhage echoes are of low amplitude compared to the retinal and scleral echoes.

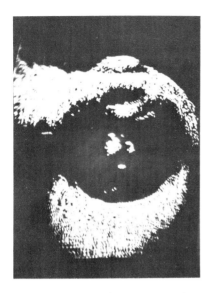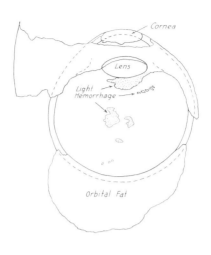

FIG. V-35. B-scan ultrasonogram of a more densely organized vitreous hemorrhage appearing as conglomerates of moderate-amplitude echoes in the retrolental space and mid-vitreous. The retina is seen to be in place.

EXTENT AND DENSITY OF VITREOUS HEMORRHAGE. Light, diffuse, unclotted blood produces little or no echo response, so that the vitreous may appear sonolucent (Fig. V-33). Clumps of cells will produce echoes higher than the normal baseline echo of the vitreous. Low-amplitude echoes are usually best seen on the A-scan

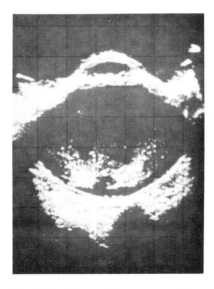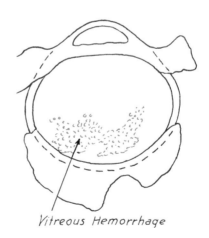

FIG. V-36. B-scan ultrasonogram of an organized hemorrhage along the posterior limiting membrane of the vitreous. The retina is close to the membrane but is in place.

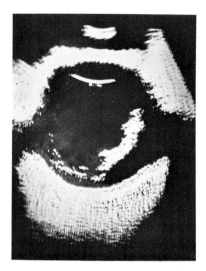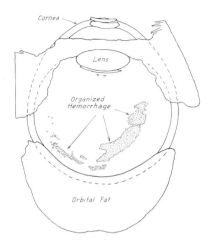

Cornea

Lens

Organized
Hemorrhage

Orbital Fat

FIG. V-37. B-scan ultrasonogram of an organized hemorrhage along the posterior limiting membrane of the vitreous with early vitreous veil formation. In this eye the vitreous is beginning to contract, but the scans show clear separation of the membrane from the retina, which is in position.

display, since the amplitude of the echoes from small clumps of cells is low compared to that of retina or membrane[50] (Fig. V-34). The density of hemorrhage is estimated from the character of A-scan echoes and the area of vitreous involvement as determined from the B-scan. Comparison of A- and B-scans is thus critical. Movement of the eye causes these low-amplitude echoes to move freely within the globe and helps to distinguish them from more fixed vitreous membranes. A more damped, lesser movement is apparent when the clumps are restrained by the solid vitreous.

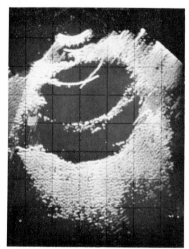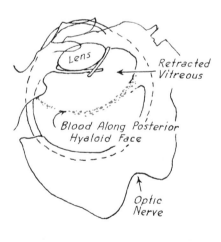

Lens

Retracted
Vitreous

Blood Along Posterior
Hyaloid Face

Optic
Nerve

FIG. V-38. B-scan ultrasonogram showing remnants of blood along the posterior hyaloid membrane in a patient with a contracted vitreous. The retina is in place.

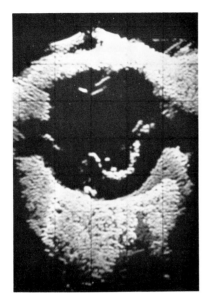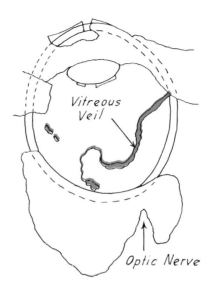

FIG. V-39. B-scan ultrasonogram of coagulated blood along the posterior aspect of the solid vitreous, producing a relatively tortuous appearance similar to that seen in retinal detachment. Kinetic B-scans (i.e., scans made while the patient voluntarily turns his eye from side to side and up and down) demonstrate the gossamer-like wafting typical of vitreous veils and the lack of attachment to the optic nerve head.

The extent of clotted blood is more easily appreciated on the B-scan (Figs. V-35 and V-36), and serial sectioning can be used to delineate the hemorrhage. A coagulum within the hemorrhage is indicated by moderately high-amplitude, closely spaced echoes, giving the appearance of a solid mass.

LOCATION AND SOURCE OF VITREOUS HEMORRHAGE. The localization of hemorrhage to areas of solid or fluid vitreous is based on the position and movement of the hemorrhage. Hemorrhage localized in the anterior vitreous compartment is usually interpreted as residing in the solid vitreous. Often blood along the posterior limiting membrane or "hyaloid face" of the solid vitreous will form a "veil" or membrane that separates and outlines the fluid and solid compartments (Figs. V-37 and V-38). This veil may be studied with kinetic B-scanning. Kinetic scans are obtained by asking the patient to move his eye while fast sector scanning is performed. The "after" movements of hemorrhage and membranes are observed after the eye has come to rest in its new position. Motion of hemorrhage in the solid vitreous is damped much more quickly than that of hemorrhage in the fluid vitreous. The final or resting position of an area of hemorrhage varies with gravity in fluid vitreous but remains quite constant in solid vitreous.

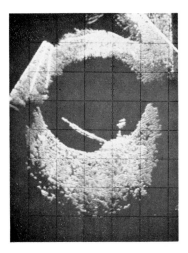 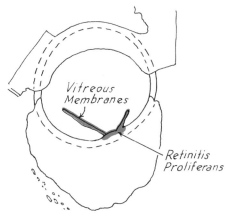

Fig. V-40. B-scan ultrasonogram of retinitis proliferans with tenting of the proliferans extending into the vitreous. Kinetic scans will often show wafting of the ends of these sections. These membranes do not extend anteriorly and are unlikely to attach at the ora serrata.

The importance of localizing the hemorrhage in the solid or fluid vitreous is indicated in a recent study by Coleman and Franzen.[50] Their data suggest that patients with spontaneous hemorrhage of light density limited to the posterior vitreous have a better than 50 per cent chance of clearing. Patients with dense hemorrhage into the solid vitreous, whether anterior or posterior, regardless of etiology, have only about a 33 per cent chance of clearing.

The position of hemorrhage relative to the limbus-iris plane, lens, and optic nerve can be determined with B-scan ultrasound. In younger patients with a solid vitreous, the source of bleeding can frequently be recognized as the point where echoes extend to the globe wall on the B-scan display.[37] A kinetic or fast sector scan of the moving eye can aid in tracing the point of origin of a vitreous hemorrhage. The vitreous attachments to the optic nerve and/or to the macula can often be seen (Fig. V-39). When only attachment to the nerve is noted, vitreous membranes along the posterior limiting membrane of the vitreous may resemble retinal detachment.

VITREOUS MEMBRANES. Vitreous membranes are usually discernible from hemorrhagic clots by their pattern (Figs. V-40, V-41 and V-42) and echo height (which is moderately high but usually lower than that of the retina). Occasionally, vitreous membranes may be difficult to distinguish from a localized retinal detachment, particularly when retinitis proliferans is present (Fig. V-40). Tracing the membranes to their attachment on the globe wall may be of help: if the attachment is anterior to the ora serrata (Fig. V-41), a vitreous

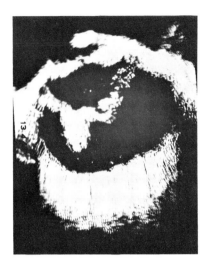
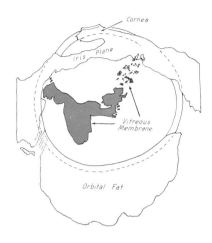

FIG. V-41. B-scan ultrasonogram of a densely organized membrane extending from the ciliary region along the posterior aspect of the vitreous to the region of the ciliary muscle and ora serrata. The retina is in place.

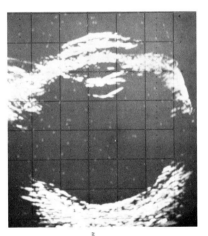
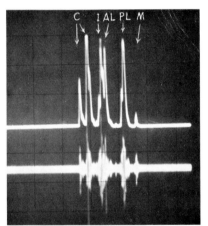

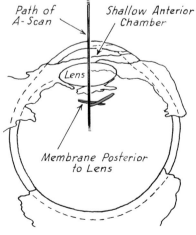

FIG. V-42. B-scan ultrasonogram of a membrane just posterior to the lens. The accompanying A-scan of this anterior segment shows a low-amplitude echo typical of a membrane rather than of retina.

membrane is indicated, whereas if attachment to the ora serrata and the optic nerve head is demonstrable, usually a retinal detachment is present. The B-scan is essential for tracing membranes, as it provides the topographic pattern of amplitude contours that is not readily apparent from the A-scan alone (Fig. V-42). Kinetic B-scanning may graphically illustrate a membrane by showing its failure to attach at the optic nerve. On A-scan, echoes from a retinal detachment are of higher amplitude than most vitreal membranes. The retina echo is of equivalent height to the sclera while membranes are usually about 50 per cent or less of the scleral echo height.

Proliferative Diabetic Retinopathy with Vitreous Hemorrhage

Vitreous hemorrhage secondary to proliferative diabetic retinopathy is the most common indication for pars plana vitrectomy. Presurgical evaluation of such patients with opaque media is greatly enhanced by ultrasound. B-scan ultrasonography in an eye with diabetic retinopathy can demonstrate (1) vitreous hemorrhage, (2) retinitis proliferans, (3) vitreous membranes, and (4) retinal detachment.

VITREOUS HEMORRHAGE. As has been mentioned in the previous section, vitreous filled with diffuse hemorrhage often appears acoustically clear on B-scan ultrasonograms. A nonfocused 10-MHz transducer is best to demonstrate diffuse low-amplitude vitreous hemorrhage. The A-scan trace through the vitreous may stay at

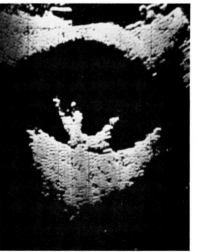 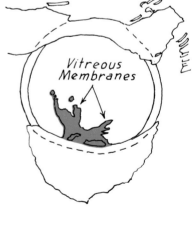

FIG. V-43. B-scan ultrasonogram of a relatively dense proliferative membrane. Orthogonal scans are advised to help in differentiation of this variety of membrane from retinal detachment.

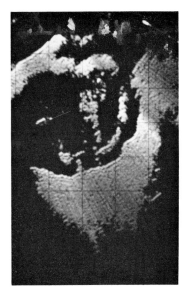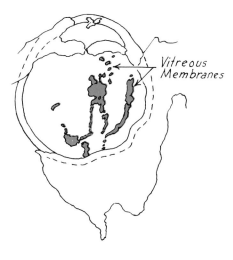

Vitreous Membranes

FIG. V-44. B-scan ultrasonogram of vitreous membranes which have assumed a linear, parallel configuration.

baseline at low gain. Denser vitreous hemorrhages present an ultrasonic picture varying from scattered dots throughout the vitreous to a dense sheet of white opacities filling the vitreous compartment. They have indistinct borders and a relatively amorphous appearance. In simple vitreous hemorrhage, the lens is in its normal position and the retina is in place.

RETINITIS PROLIFERANS. An area of retinitis proliferans appears on the B-scan ultrasonogram as an echo configuration forming a stalk which arises from the retina (Fig. V-43). The echoes often tend to diverge as the stalk extends forward in the vitreous. At the distal end of retinitis proliferans, areas of vitreous hemorrhage and vitreous membranes may be demonstrable ultrasonically.

VITREOUS MEMBRANES. Whereas vitreous hemorrhages have indistinct borders and irregular shapes, vitreous membranes on B-scan ultrasonography appear as more regular, linear echo configurations (Fig. V-44). They have a much more structured appearance than do vitreous hemorrhages. A vitreous membrane may lie along the posterior surface of a retracted formed vitreous. This finding is common in diabetic patients (Fig. V-45). The sites of vitreous membrane attachment to the retina may be ultrasonically demonstrable in eyes with diabetic retinopathy and traction retinal detachments (Fig. V-46).

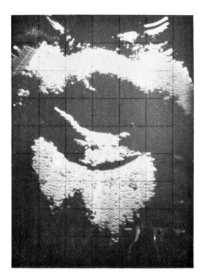 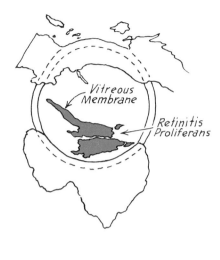

FIG. V-45. B-scan ultrasonogram demonstrating a dense membrane along a retracted formed vitreous, overlying an area of retinitis proliferans.

A vitreous membrane formation which may be encountered is that of two doubled linear echo configurations extending from the region of the ora serrata on each side of the eye to the posterior pole. These double lines of echoes cross in the posterior central vitreous in an "X" shape, always at a distance anterior to the nerve head (Fig. V-47).

A-scan ultrasonography can provide important quantification information regarding the density of vitreous membranes. It is our clinical impression that the density of the membrane as shown by A-scan is roughly correlated with the "toughness" of the membrane at surgery. Certain membranes are very dense and their echo amplitude can simulate that of detached retina.

RETINAL DETACHMENT (SEE ALSO RETINAL ABNORMALITIES). A-scans and kinetic B-scans are both useful in differentiating vitreous membranes from retinal detachment. The kinetic B-scan will often show the vitreous body and membranes floating away from the disk while the retina remains attached. It should be remembered, however, that solid vitreous *may* be firmly attached to the disk and/or the macula and thus, with hemorrhagic collection along the hyaloid, a detachment may be mimicked on the static and kinetic B-scans.

Traumatic Vitreous Hemorrhage

Vitreous hemorrhage as a result of trauma is discussed at length under *Ocular Trauma,* below.

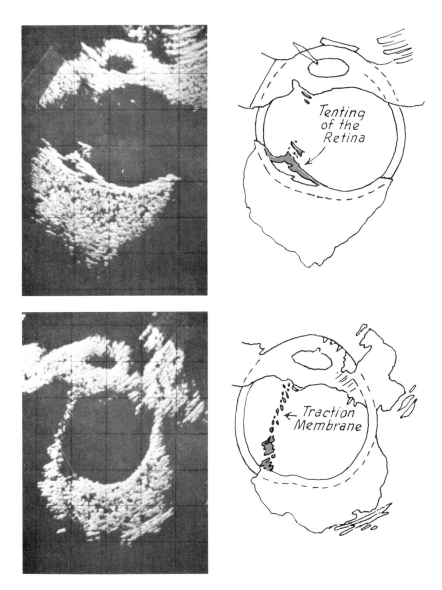

FIG. V-46. B-scan ultrasonogram of a traction detachment seen in both horizontal and vertical sections, demonstrating the connection of a vitreal or proliferative membrane to the leaf of the retina.

Miscellaneous Vitreous Abnormalities

ASTEROID HYALOSIS. Goldberg et al.[51] originally described the A-scan ultrasonographic pattern in asteroid hyalosis. These calcium soap particles show widely scattered low-amplitude spikes on the A-scan. On kinetic A-scans, they can be seen to "dance" or move quickly. On the B-scan, asteroid hyalosis appears as a plethora of echoes in the vitreous cavity (Fig. V-48). As Jaffe[52] has noted,

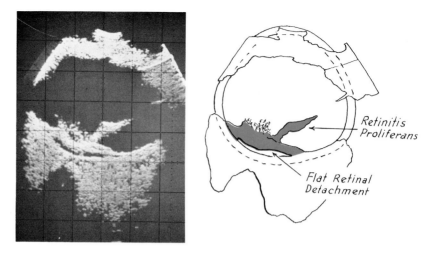

FIG. V-47. B-scan ultrasonogram of retinitis proliferans in a characteristic X shape overlying a flat retinal detachment.

asteroid hyalosis tends to occur preferentially in the primary vitreous, and thus is often best seen between the lens and optic nerve. The peripheral vitreous may be acoustically clear.

AMYLOIDOSIS OF THE VITREOUS. Extensive experience with ultrasonography in patients with amyloidosis of the vitreous, a rare abnormality, has not been obtained. We have examined one patient with pathologically confirmed amyloidosis of the vitreous in the

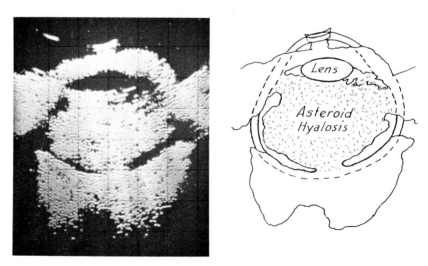

FIG. V-48. B-scan of asteroid hyalosis demonstrating the dense vitreal echoes and the connection of the central vitreous to the optic nerve head with a clear area posterior to the central diseased vitreous. On the A-scan, the echoes are of relatively high amplitude and show marked movement with small motion of the globe.

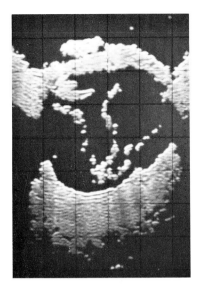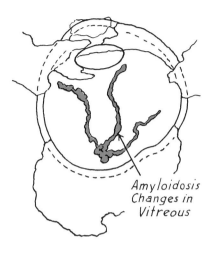

FIG. V-49. B-scan ultrasonogram of a patient with proven amyloidosis showing central vitreal membranes in a strand-like pattern which indicates organization.

fellow eye, and the ultrasonogram is shown in Figure V-49. There are irregular strand-like echoes in the vitreous, which are of low amplitude on the A-scan. This pattern is similar to that seen in vitreous hemorrhage and endophthalmitis.

ENDOPHTHALMITIS. Oksala[53] described the A-scan ultrasonographic appearance of endophthalmitis. The B-scan pattern seen in

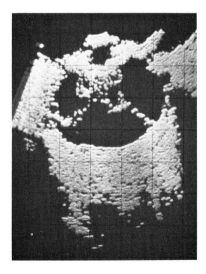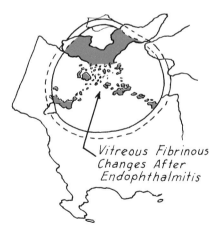

FIG. V-50. B-scan ultrasonogram of a patient after endophthalmitis. The acoustic pattern of central constriction and strands extending into the vitreous has been seen consistently in such patients.

patients with endophthalmitis has been characteristic. This is an H-shaped pattern, where the crossbar of the H is a markedly thickened central vitreous echo pattern, and the limbs of the H are usually curved lines of scattered echoes (Fig. V-50). In one patient examined, the uprights of the H pattern were convex curves straddling the ora serrata, and resembled a choroidal detachment. This particular acoustic pattern has not been noted in the presence of any other ocular abnormality.

Ultrasonography and Vitreous Surgery

ULTRASONIC CLASSIFICATION OF VITREOUS HEMORRHAGE. Since the prognosis and treatment of eyes with vitreous hemorrhage are dependent on the extent and severity of hemorrhage and associated structural changes, we have found it convenient to classify vitreous hemorrhage into four categories:[54]

1. Vitreous hemorrhage without fibrinous change or retinal detachment.
2. Vitreous hemorrhage with fibrinous vitreous density or structural change such as a dislocated lens, or both, but without retinal detachment.
3. Vitreous hemorrhage with organized membranes such as cyclitic membranes or retinal detachment without evidence of organization, or both.
4. Vitreous hemorrhage with total retinal detachment and apparent organization of the retina.

This classification was developed primarily to correspond to the types of treatment, surgical or medical, that can be offered to patients. The class I patient has the best prognosis of clearing. Surgical intervention, when indicated in this group, is often only a vitreous exchange. The presence of membranes and/or lens dislocation in a patient in class II creates a more ominous prognostic situation. Surgical intervention here requires special instrumentation for severing and removing the membranes or the lens. Patients in this category, however, may benefit significantly from vitrectomy. Patients in the third category, where a retinal detachment is also present, are less likely to benefit from surgery, but may be helped with combined vitreoretinal techniques. Patients in the fourth category (those with retinal organization) must be considered poor candidates for surgery.

ACCURACY OF PREOPERATIVE ULTRASONIC DIAGNOSIS. Jack, Hutton and Machemer[55] have published the results of preoperative ultrasonography in a series of 35 eyes with opaque media prior to pars plana vitrectomy. Confirmation or refutation of results was obtained at the time of surgery. Ultrasonographic diagnosis of the status of the retina was correct in 30 of 35 cases, or 85 per cent. With further knowledge of ultrasonic patterns in diabetic retinopathy (an extremely challenging area to the ultrasonographer because of the coexistence of vitreous hemorrhage, vitreous membranes, vitreous detachment, preretinal gliosis, retinitis proliferans, and retinal detachment), and with the use of horizontal, vertical and oblique B-scan tomography and quantitative A-scan ultrasonography, this accuracy can be improved.

PRACTICAL ROLE OF ULTRASONOGRAPHY. The practical role of ultrasonography prior to vitrectomy can be summarized as follows: First, it aids in determining the operability in borderline cases. Second, it is useful in planning the operative procedure. If ultrasound indicates the possibility of a retinal detachment, additional care must be taken at surgery to prevent an iatrogenic retinal hole. If a retinal detachment is suspected, detachment equipment and additional operating room time must be available. Finally, ultrasonic demonstration of vitreous disease located temporally suggests modification of the standard insertion site of the vitrectomy instrument (which is usually on the temporal side).

Vitreous surgery, of course, can be performed without the benefit of preoperative ultrasonographic examination. We feel that ultrasonography provides accurate supplemental information about the status of the vitreous and the retina, and is of significant value to the vitreous surgeon, much as the indirect ophthalmoscope aids the retinal surgeon.

We feel that the ultrasonography should be performed, or at least observed, by the operating surgeon or his assistant. The actual dynamic scanning process permits much more information about the status of the eye than does a retrospective review of representative photographs. Also, if the ultrasonographer is present at surgery, precise correlation between ultrasonic and pathologic appearance can be made.

Retinal Abnormalities

Retinal Detachment

Modern surgical techniques for retinal detachment have been considerably influenced by the widespread use of indirect ophthalmoscopy, which permits a thorough evaluation of the peripheral fundus. However, optical evaluation techniques such as indirect ophthalmoscopy are useful in examination of the vitreous and retina only if the ocular media are clear. They are useful in examination of the subretinal space only if the overlying retina is transparent and the subretinal fluid is clear. Ultrasonic evaluation techniques are not subject to these limitations. B-scan ultrasonic evaluation of the vitreous, retina and subretinal space (especially in eyes with clouding or opacification of the ocular media) adds a significant dimension to the diagnosis of retinal detachment and the management of patients with vitreoretinal abnormalities.

The use of A-scan ultrasound in the diagnosis of retinal detachment was first described by Oksala and Lehtinen in 1957.[56] Since then, numerous other reports have appeared. B-scan ultrasonography of retinal detachments has been reported by Baum,[57] Greenwood,[39] Purnell[25] and Coleman and Jack.[58]

RHEGMATOGENOUS RETINAL DETACHMENTS. The retina normally appears on B-scan ultrasonograms as a smooth, concave, acoustically opaque (white) surface formed by echoes from the vitreoretinal interface. These echoes are contiguous with, and inseparable from, echoes from the choroid and the sclera. A detached retina, however, appears on B-scan ultrasonograms as a thin, continuous, acoustically opaque (white) line of echoes separate from, and anterior to, echoes from the wall of the globe (Fig. V-51). A relatively flat

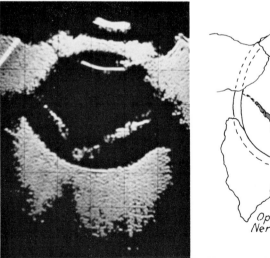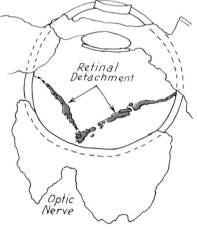

FIG. V-51. B-scan ultrasonogram of a retinal detachment illustrating the leaves of the retina as a thin, continuous, high-amplitude line with connections at the optic nerve head and ora serrata.

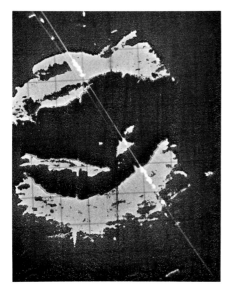 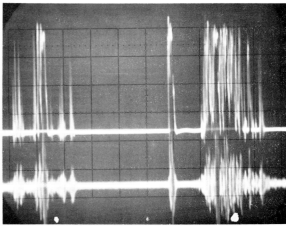

FIG. V-52. Storage B-scan ultrasonogram (*left*) of a retinal detachment. The path of the accompanying A-scan (*right*) appears as bright intensity modulated dots. The A-scan shows a high-amplitude echo in the usually anechoic area of the vitreous cavity. The echo height of the intravitreal membranes suspected of being detached retina is routinely compared to the choroid and scleral echo heights, and when the height is equal or nearly equal to that of the sclera detachment is indicated.

detachment has a narrow, acoustically empty (black) space between detached retina and the globe wall. The subretinal fluid-pigment epithelium acoustic interface has a smooth, concave contour. A highly elevated, totally detached retina appears as convex bullae extending far into the vitreous from attachment points at the nasal and temporal ora serrata and at the optic nerve. The space posterior to the elevated retina is sonolucent.

The extent of a detachment (whether partial or total) is ascertained by performing ultrasonic B-scans in serial, horizontal planes of the eye. Starting above the superior limbus, scans are made at 2-mm intervals along the vertical dimension of the globe. The serial, ocular, acoustic sections thus obtained differentiate a true retinal detachment from a choroidal detachment, which extends anterior to the ora serrata, and from a vitreous veil (hemorrhage along the posterior hyaloid face), which cannot usually be traced back to the optic disk. The amplitude characteristics of returned echoes, best observed on the A-scan, further differentiate retinal detachments from vitreous membranes, as retinal echoes have a higher amplitude than do vitreous membrane echoes (Fig. V-52). Retinal echoes are approximately as high in amplitude as the normal posterior globe wall echoes, while membrane echoes are usually about 50 per cent of this height. If the anterior segment is particularly dense, as in the

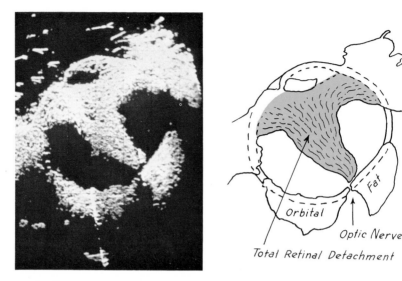

FIG. V-53. B-scan ultrasonogram of an organized retinal detachment with typical morning-glory configuration and high-amplitude central echoes indicative of a contracted vitreous and retinal organization.

presence of a calcified cataract, the amplitude of the retinal echo can be greatly reduced.

B-scan ultrasound indicates the thickness of the detached retina and the extent of retinal organization and shrinkage. A freshly detached retina appears as a thin white line, equal in length to the scleral arc from ora to ora. In long-standing detachments, the retina is thickened and its overall length often shrinks to form a cord from the optic disk to the ora serrata, thus forming a funnel-shaped or "morning-glory" configuration. A contracted retinal detachment of

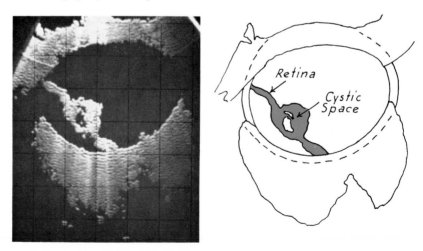

FIG. V-54. B-scan ultrasonogram showing a long-standing detachment of the temporal portion of the retina with a well outlined cystic space in the detached leaf.

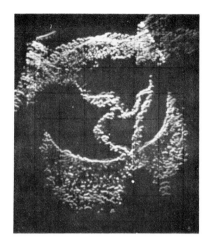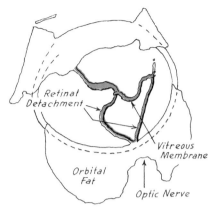

FIG. V-55. B-scan ultrasonogram of a total retinal detachment with a central vitreal membrane connecting the two leaves of the retina.

this type is shown in Figure V-53. Cyst-like structures of the retina in long-standing detachments are indicated ultrasonically by a thickened and convoluted echo pattern (Fig. V-54).

Rhegmatogenous retinal detachments often result from traction of vitreous membranes or bands on the retina. Vitreous membranes and bands, as noted previously, are demonstrable ultrasonically, as are sites of vitreous membrane attachment and their associated traction of the retina (Fig. V-55), indicating the "stress sites" at which retinal holes may be expected to have occurred.

NONRHEGMATOGENOUS RETINAL DETACHMENTS. *Retinal Detachment Secondary to Choroidal Melanoma.* The use of binocular indirect ophthalmoscopy and scleral transillumination significantly aids in the clinical diagnosis of retinal detachment secondary to choroidal malignant melanoma. Mistaken diagnoses do occur, however, and there is a significant incidence of operation of retinal detachment in eyes containing choroidal melanoma (2 per cent in one series).[59] As Norton[60] has emphasized: "The most serious misdiagnosis of retinal separation is the failure to recognize an underlying malignant melanoma of the choroid as the cause of the retinal elevation. Once the patient is subjected to retinal surgery and the integrity of the sclera disrupted, the patient's life is in jeopardy. On the other hand, removal of an eye with an idiopathic retinal detachment because of misinterpretation of the fundus changes is a similar tragedy."

The use of B-scan ultrasonography can reliably demonstrate the presence or absence of a tumor underlying a retinal detachment.

Upon serial sectioning, the profile of a choroidal mass can be detected and characterized. Tumors appear as acoustic solid (white) masses at low examining frequencies, and can be differentiated from hemorrhages or exudative elevations, which are acoustically clear. Since certain detachments overlie tumors, patients with suspected secondary detachments benefit from B-scan ultrasonography to detect the usually obscured etiology of the detachment. All cases of retinal detachment do not necessarily require ultrasonic evaluation. This diagnostic test is most valuable in selected cases of clinically atypical retinal detachment. The following features are clinical suggestive, but not diagnostic, of a nonrhegmatogenous retinal detachment:

1. Absence of breaks: Retinal breaks were not seen by the clinician in 22 of 26 eyes with choroidal melanomas enucleated after detachment surgery.[61] Of the four eyes in this series in which breaks were suspected clinically, they were not found on pathologic examination. The presence of retinal breaks, of course, does not rule out a choridal melanoma.
2. Smooth bullae and shifting fluid.
3. Elevated intraocular pressure: There is a significant incidence of elevated intraocular pressure in eyes with choroidal melanoma. In a recent series, Deneuville[62] found 18 melanomas in 77 eyes having retinal detachment and elevated intraocular pressure.
4. Large iris nevi: The association of iris nevi and melanomas of the choroid has been discussed by Reese.[63]

These and other suggested indications for utilization of B-scan ultrasonography prior to retinal detachment surgery are summarized

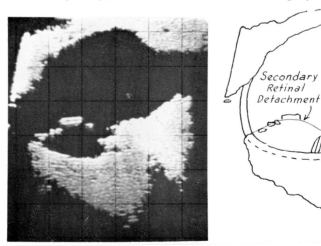

FIG. V-56. B-scan ultrasonogram taken at 10 MHz showing a solid tumor at the posterior pole underlying a secondary retinal detachment. There is no evidence of choroidal excavation by the mass seen in this section.

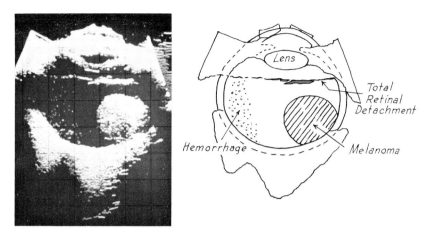

FIG. V-57. B-scan ultrasonogram demonstrating a solid polypoid tumor mass underlying a total retinal detachment. Visualization was further obscured by vitreous hemorrhage anteriorly.

in Table V-2. B-scan ultrasound is an essential test in suspicious or atypical retinal detachment to rule out the presence of a solid tumor under the elevated retina. Serial sections should be employed to localize the tumor, which will often appear as an acoustically opaque mass (Fig. V-56). Associated ocular changes such as hemorrhage can be demonstrated ultrasonically (Fig. V-57).

Other Secondary Retinal Detachments. Retinal detachments may also be secondary to inflammatory (Fig. V-58), exudative (Figs. V-59

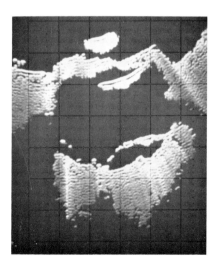

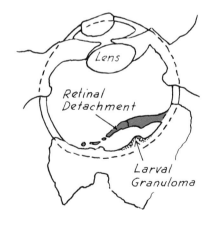

FIG. V-58. B-scan ultrasonogram demonstrating a small mass at the posterior pole underlying a retinal detachment. The absence of choroidal excavation and the height-to-base ratio of the mass militate against tumor and are consistent with a granulomatous reaction.

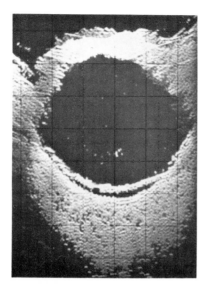
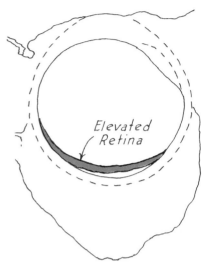

Elevated
Retina

FIG. V-59. B-scan ultrasonogram taken at 10 MHz demonstrating a flatly elevated retina, as commonly seen in choroidal effusion or Harada's disease detachments of nonrhegmatogenous origin. The concavity of the detachment usually follows the choroidal pattern, showing a relatively constant elevation of the retina.

and V-60) and cicatricial (Fig. V-61) conditions. The subretinal space in these conditions is acoustically clear except in the region of the inflammatory focus or cicatrix. That is, the subretinal fluid is acoustically quiet (unless hemorrhagic) but tissue abnormalities may be seen. Evidence of inflammation may be detectable in the overlying sclera and Tenon's space, or in the optic nerve.

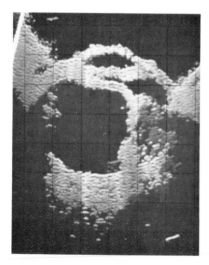
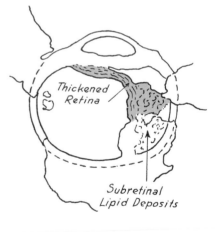

Thickened
Retina

Subretinal
Lipid Deposits

FIG. V-60. B-scan ultrasonogram of a retinal detachment overlying lipid deposit with marked constriction of the retinal funnel, indicating organization and fibrosis of the retina.

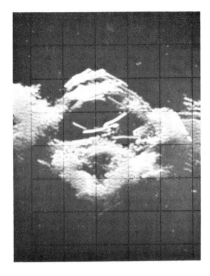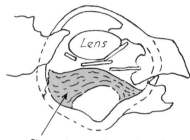

Shrunken, Organized
Retina

FIG. V-61. B-scan ultrasonogram taken at 10 MHz of a phthisical globe showing a relatively normal lens, shallow anterior chamber and markedly shrunken and organized retina with contraction of the sclera posteriorly. When patterns of this type are seen, additional scans at 5 MHz are advised to penetrate to and portray structures obscured by marked attenuation within a densely organized retina. In this instance, the orbital contents are relatively normal and the posterior outline seen is that of the sclera.

POSTOPERATIVE SITUATIONS. After retinal detachment surgery, numerous situations may arise in which management may be facilitated by ultrasonography.

Occasionally after an encircling procedure, especially if extensive cryotherapy has been utilized, choroidal effusion or hemorrhage may occur and cause angle compromise with elevation of intraocular pressure. Usually the choroidal effusion of hemorrhage is visible with the indirect ophthalmoscope. However, a cloudy cornea, a miotic pupil, or a cataract may prevent visualization. B-scan ultrasonography in this condition shows the pathognomonic appearance of a choroidal effusion, i.e., a smooth, convex, circumferential elevation straddling the ora serrata. Choroidal effusion may be differentiated from choroidal hemorrhage with A-scan quantification techniques. Demonstration of a localized choroidal effusion may indicate the site for posterior sclerotomy, should this be clinically warranted.

The extent of settling of the retina after detachment surgery may be impossible to evaluate optically because of cloudy media or a very miotic pupil. In this situation, B-scan ultrasonography can provide accurate information as to the position of the retina (Fig. V-62). Posterior migration of an encircling element can be shown acoustically.

In rare instances, a discolored area may become evident under

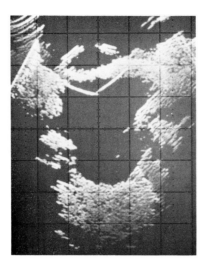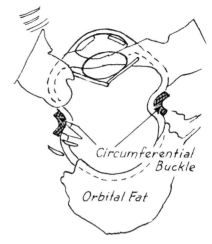

FIG. V-62. B-scan ultrasonogram taken at 10 MHz of a globe demonstrating an encircling element and resultant constriction of the vitreous compartment. In this globe, the retina is in place, but the presence of low-amplitude hemorrhagic change has obscured visualization of the posterior pole.

settled retina following fluid drainage at detachment surgery. Ultrasonography aids in the differentiation of a choroidal tumor from choroidal hemorrhage in such cases.

B-scan ultrasonography can demonstrate the presence of an encircling element or large local implant in patients where the history is unclear and the media are cloudy (Fig. V-63).

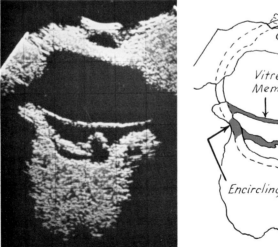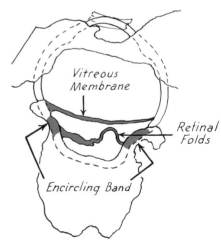

FIG. V-63. B-scan ultrasonogram of a globe with an encircling element, which has apparently slipped posteriorly, demonstrating a vitreous membrane extending from the buckle across the posterior vitreous compartment. A localized retinal detachment is noted behind the vitreous membrane.

The ultrasonographic appearance of retinitis proliferans has been discussed under *Vitreous Abnormalities.* A typical B-scan ultrasonogram of an eye with retinitis proliferans is shown in Figure V-64.

Macular Cysts

In severe macular edema, or in the "sunny-side-up" stage of Best's disease, a cystic structure may be ultrasonically demonstrable. The B-scan shows a convex anterior projection of the vitreoretinal interface echo line in the macular region, followed by a localized sonolucent area. A B-scan ultrasonogram, courtesy of Dr. R. Dallow, is shown in Figure V-65.

Disciform Macular Degeneration

Highly elevated macular lesions of the Kuhnt-Junius type may be extremely difficult to differentiate ophthalmoscopically from small choroidal melanomas underlying the macula. Ultrasonography

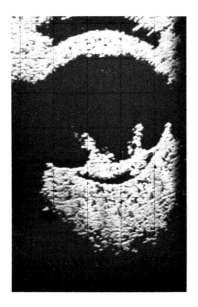
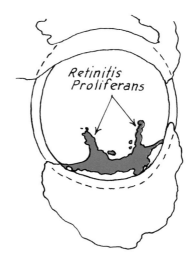

FIG. V-64. B-scan ultrasonogram showing a relatively clear vitreous with the retina in place and a proliferative pattern extending into the vitreous compartment from the posterior pole. These attachments usually emanate from the optic disk, and do not show vascularity with conventional A- or M-scan techniques. A- and B-scanning through such membranes aids in discerning them from localized retinal detachments. The membranes show a lower amplitude on the A-scan than the sclera—usually less than 70 to 80 per cent of the scleral echo height.

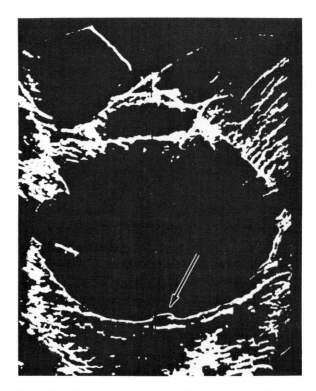

Fɪɢ. V-65. B-scan ultrasonogram showing a normal globe
outline with an elevation of the retina at the posterior pole
and a clear subretinal space, differentiating a macular cyst
from a solid choroidal lesion. (Courtesy of Dr. R. Dallow.)

should be used in conjunction with fluorescein angiography and, in
selected cases, radioactive phosphorus uptake studies to provide
optimum differentiation of these two conditions.

B-scan ultrasonography in cases of advanced, elevated disciform macular degeneration shows an elevated lesion at the posterior
pole (Fig. V-66). The acoustic appearance of the interior of the lesion
may vary. In predominantly hemorrhagic lesions, a cystic appearance with a bright line of front surface echoes separated from the
posterior wall of the globe by a sonolucent zone is noted. An
acoustically opaque (white) appearance is noted in fibrotic, scarred
lesions. This range of appearances is also characteristic of choroidal
melanoma. The phenomenon of choroidal excavation (see discussion of choroidal tumors), often seen with choroidal malignant
melanomas, is not seen, in our experience, with disciform macular
degeneration. Because disciform lesions are restrained by Bruch's
membrane and do not involve the choroid, one would not, on theoretical grounds, expect choroidal excavation to occur in this condition.

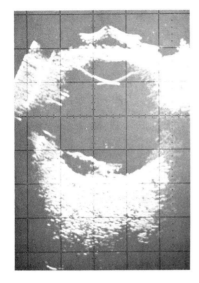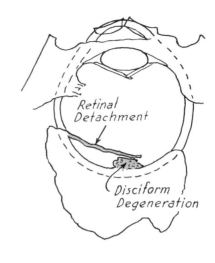

FIG. V-66. B-scan ultrasonogram of a retinal detachment overlying a disciform degeneration of the posterior pole located in the region of the macula. Slight hemorrhagic changes, the low-amplitude echoes beneath the retina and the absence of choroidal excavation are all consistent with disciform degeneration.

Evaluation of the A-scan trace through the lesion is also important for differentiation. In disciform macular degeneration, irregular echoes, often of low amplitude, follow the high-amplitude echo from the retinal surface, and in melanomas gradual echo decay follows the high-amplitude echo from the retinal surface.

Retinoblastoma

Retinoblastoma is the most common malignant intraocular tumor in childhood.[64] Success in its treatment is clearly related to early diagnosis. When the tumor can be seen ophthalmoscopically, the diagnosis is usually straightforward. However, the tumor may be obscured by an overlying retinal detachment, by inflammatory reaction, or by hemorrhage in the vitreous.

Several reports in the literature discuss unusual ophthalmoscopic presentations of this tumor. In these series, misdiagnosis has been reported as 7 to 14.9 per cent.[65-67] The A-scan characteristics of retinoblastoma have been previously reported by others[68-71] as resembling an organized vitreous hemorrhage. In one series, A-scan provided the correct diagnosis in only 25 per cent of proven cases.[72]

We have found B-scan ultrasonography to be of significant value in demonstrating a mass lesion in the eye. This technique combined with the ^{32}P uptake test in certain cases with opaque media may confirm the diagnosis and lead to prompt and effective treatment.

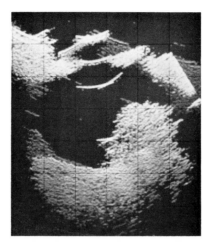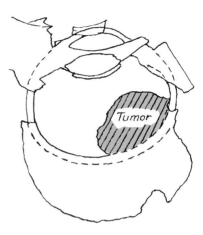

FIG. V-67. B-scan ultrasonogram of a globe with retinoblastoma showing a solid mass at the posterior pole. At 10 MHz, there is little to differentiate this mass from other ocular tumors. In general, retinoblastoma has a lower amplitude profile and often resembles the A-scan pattern of a vitreous hemorrhage.

In all patients with retinoblastoma which we have examined, an intraocular mass lesion was demonstrable. Sterns, Coleman and Ellsworth[73] have described two retinoblastoma configurations: "solid" and "cystic."

The solid tumor is a well-outlined, discrete mass, contiguous with the retina in all sections studied (Fig. V-67). In contrast, cystic lesions may or may not have discrete borders, may contain solid areas interspersed with vacuolated spaces, and may not be contiguous with the retina in all sections examined (Fig. V-68).

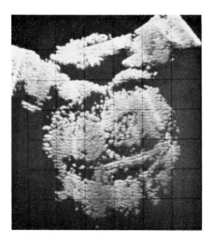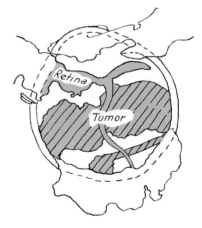

FIG. V-68. B-scan ultrasonogram showing a rounded diffuse tumor underlying a retinal detachment. The tumor shows relatively low-amplitude echoes as compared to a typical choroidal tumor and is difficult to differentiate from an organized vitreous. This mass is classified as a cystic retinoblastoma.

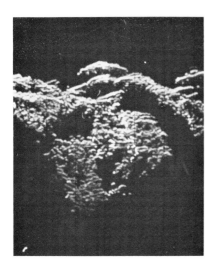

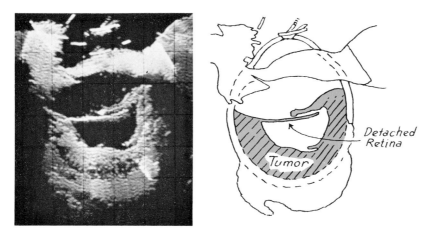

FIG. V-69. B-scan ultrasonogram of a retinal detachment with an underlying cystic tumor mass. This is a placoid retinoblastoma. Differentiation of this tumor from other tumor tissue is aided by the A-scan, but even if differentiation is not possible the outline of a mass in a young child can be helpful in indicating definitive treatment.

Three characteristics common to both solid and cystic retinoblastomas are: (1) little or no sound attenuation (except in heavily calcified tumors), (2) the absence of choroidal excavation, and (3) an associated retinal detachment. Figure V-69 shows a characteristic cystic tumor with an overlying retinal detachment.

A histologic basis for the division of retinoblastoma into two ultrasonic types, solid and cystic, has not been absolutely determined. It is theorized that the solid pattern is characteristic of early

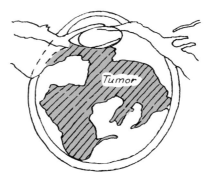

FIG. V-70. B-scan ultrasonogram of a globe containing a retinoblastoma, emphasizing the acoustic similarity to vitreous hemorrhage. There is marked acoustic absorption within this tumor at 10 MHz, typical of this type of retinoblastoma yet also seen in long-standing organized vitreous hemorrhage.

tumors as they arise in the retina as solid tumefactions projecting into the vitreous. The collagenous and vascular stroma of retinoblastoma is not well developed, and, as these tumors grow, large necrotic foci appear; later the tumor may break apart with masses or seeds floating in the vitreous. Apparently, the cystic acoustic pattern relates to this advanced form of the disease. Consistent with this view is the fact that of the three patients who died in Sterns' series of twenty cases, all had the acoustically cystic tumor type.

While the solid acoustic pattern is interpreted with greater confidence, the cystic pattern presents a more difficult problem diagnostically. The B-scan appearance of these cystic tumors (Fig. V-70) is virtually indistinguishable from that of massive, organized vitreous hemorrhage. Figure V-71 shows what was interpreted as a cystic retinoblastoma in an eye that could not be studied ophthalmoscopically. The B-scan demonstrated a mass with vacuolated spaces which was not contiguous with the retina and had indistinct boundaries. Histologic sections of this eye showed vitreous hemorrhage with secondary traction detachment. Unfortunately, therefore, when retinoblastomas present the cystic ultrasonic pattern, we have not been able to distinguish them absolutely from vitreous hemorrhage by present techniques.

In an effort to explain the acoustic similarity of tumor tissue and vitreous hemorrhage, Sterns performed sound velocity determinations on retinoblastoma tumor tissue and on clotted blood.[73] In retinoblastoma tumor specimens, the velocity of sound varied from 1,537 m/sec to 1,600 m/sec, and in all specimens of clotted blood

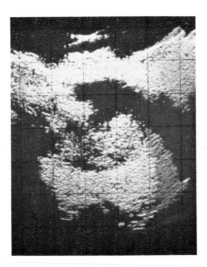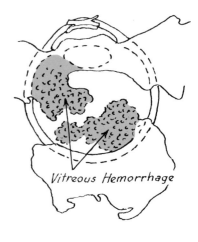

Vitreous Hemorrhage

FIG. V-71. B-scan ultrasonogram of a globe showing diffuse vitreous hemorrhage with organization. This pattern was presented by a child of similar age group as the one with retinoblastoma shown in the preceding illustration.

the velocity of sound was 1,609 m/sec. Thus, the range of sound velocities in retinoblastoma lies between the velocity of sound in normal vitreous (1,532 m/sec) and that of clotted blood. The mean ultrasound velocity value in retinoblastoma tissue is similar to the ultrasound velocity that one would expect with an organized hemorrhage in the vitreous (clot interspersed with vitreous).

However, even if ultrasonography cannot absolutely differentiate between cystic tumor and organized hemorrhage in the vitreous, the demonstration of such organized material rather than a clear vitreous is of clinical value in an eye that cannot be examined by routine methods. This is particularly true if retinoblastoma is known to be present in one eye and visualization of the retina of the fellow eye is impaired. The ultrasonic demonstration of a mass in the eye with opaque media is virtually diagnostic of retinoblastoma. The eye with advanced disease and opaque media would probably then be enucleated and treatment directed to the fellow eye. Also, if vitreous hemorrhage complicates the radiation therapy of retinoblastoma and the tumor mass cannot be visualized, periodic ultrasonography is valuable in following the course of the lesion. Additional therapy can be recommended on this basis, or, if the mass continues to enlarge, enucleation may be advised. In patients without known retinoblastoma, ultrasonography's major value is in distinguishing eyes with mass lesions (which may be either tumor or organized vitreous hemorrhage) from eyes without mass lesions. The latter can then be followed with confidence.

Choroid and Ciliary Body Abnormalities

Choroidal Tumors

Accurate diagnosis of choroidal masses remains a challenge to ophthalmologists. Lesions demanding different therapy may have very similar clinical appearances. Even with the use of indirect ophthalmoscopy and scleral depression,[74] scleral transillumination,[75] fluorescein angiography,[76,77] visual field studies[78,79] and radioactive isotope studies,[80,81] inaccurate diagnosis of ophthalmoscopically visible masses still occurs.

Ultrasound is particularly useful in distinguishing solid choroidal tumors from lesions which they visually resemble filled with serous fluid or blood. Echo amplitude studies with A-scan can usually differentiate an acoustically "solid" ocular tumor from conditions simulating an ocular tumor, such as choroidal detachment or retinal detachment with subretinal hemorrhage or fluid. In addition, A- and

B-scan acoustic criteria may help identify the various types of choroidal tumors (Table V-3).

The A-scan ultrasonographic appearance of a choroidal melanoma was first reported by Oksala in 1959.[82] Further discussions of choroidal tumor patterns were published by Oksala,[83] Ossoinig[84] and Poujol.[85] The B-scan appearance of choroidal tumors has been described in papers by Baum,[86] Purnell[25] and Coleman.[87]

The important role of ultrasonography in choroidal tumor diagnosis in eyes with opaque media has been well documented by the above researchers. Eyes with opaque media often harbor unsuspected malignant melanomas (10 per cent of enucleated eyes in one study from the Armed Forces Institute of Pathology contained malignant melanomas),[88] and thus present a diagnostic problem. Ultrasound is the only test for preoperatively discerning a tumor in such eyes.

In a famous series of 528 eyes with clear media and ophthalmoscopically visible lesions clinically thought to be malignant melanomas which were enucleated, the clinical diagnosis was incorrect in 100 (19 per cent).[89] Combined A-, B- and M-scan ultrasonography of eyes with suspected intraocular tumors provides morphologic and acoustic characteristics which can help significantly in making a correct diagnosis in these cases, just as in those with opaque media.

It is in the area of tumor diagnosis that maximum use of systematic technique and observation of all tissue reflectance parameters must be utilized. While the information presently obtainable with ultrasound does not allow "tissue diagnosis," tumor differentiation can be performed with a high degree of reliability by combining ultrasonic information with a knowledge of tumor characteristics.

In general, there are four tumor types that must be differentiated, as their treatment differs: malignant melanoma, metastatic carcinoma, hemangioma and organized subretinal hemorrhage. Since malignant melanoma is by far the most common neoplastic choroidal tumor, the subsequent discussions of tumor differentiation will be in terms of variation from melanoma patterns.

We have found it useful to describe ultrasonic features of tumors in terms of their morphologic characteristics, primarily two-dimensional analysis, and in terms of their acoustic characteristics, primarily one-dimensional analysis. Obviously, the acoustic properties will affect, indeed produce, the patterns seen in the two-dimensional portrayal.

The use of color,[33] enhanced gray scale, and isometric scan[34] displays accentuates the basic importance of acoustic properties, demonstrating the individual character of tissue much as certain histologic stains demonstrate the tissue types.

TABLE V-3. Differential Diagnostic Criteria for Choroidal Tumors

Characteristic	Malignant Melanoma	Metastatic Carcinoma	Angioma/Hemangioma
Morphologic			
Size	Varies from 0.5 mm to 15 mm in height	Variable	Usual range 0.5 mm to 2 mm in height
Shape	Convex commonest, polypoid infrequent	Convex commonest	Placoid or convex
Location	Anywhere in globe	Usually posterior	Usually posterior pole near optic nerve
Associated ocular changes	Frequent nonrhegmatogenous retinal detachments	Frequent large nonrhegmatogenous retinal detachments	May be associated retinal detachments
Evidence of spread	Extraocular extension can be shown at times	Probably ability to show multiple lesions	None
Changes with time	Growth or regression demonstrable	Growth or regression demonstrable	Growth or regression demonstrable
Acoustic			
Boundary properties	Sharp, smooth leading edge	Sharp, smooth leading edge	Sharp, smooth leading edge
Acoustic quiet zone	Polypoid—solid, no quiet zone; convex—usually has quiet zone at 15 and 20 MHz	Usually solid at 10 and 20 MHz	Quiet zone seen even at 5 and 10 MHz in large lesions; small lesions may appear solid
Choroidal excavation	Prominent	Not seen	Not seen
Absorption defects	Often shows shadowing	Occasionally shows shadowing	Seldom seen
A-scan amplitude	Increasing attenuation through tumor; sharp decay after initial echo	Little attenuation through tumor	Relatively constant, but low amplitude spikes
Texture of A-scan pattern	Relatively close spaced echoes	Relatively close spaced echoes	Relatively wide spaced echoes

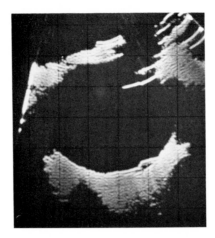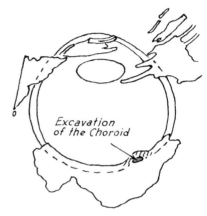

FIG. V-72. B-scan ultrasonogram of a small malignant melanoma at the posterior pole of the globe, showing an elevation of approximately 1.5 mm. The presence of choroidal excavation aids in the evaluation of small tumors, but an A-scan through the tumor is required for more precise tissue differentiation.

The progression of ultrasonic evaluation from morphologic characterization, primarily a B-scan diagnosis, to acoustic characterization, primarily on A-scan diagnosis, proceeds much as histologic evaluations proceed from gross inspection through increasingly higher powers of microscopic examination. Since the evaluation is in vivo, dynamic tissue characteristics, such as vascularity, provide unique insights not comparable to any histologic technique.

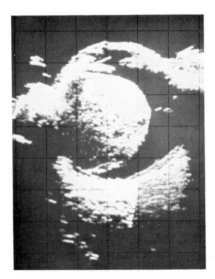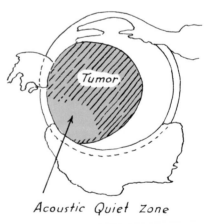

FIG. V-73. B-scan ultrasonogram of a large intraocular tumor, demonstrating a quiet zone in the posterior aspect of the tumor, caused by absorption of sound and tumor homogeneity.

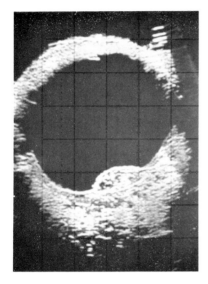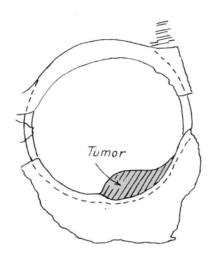

FIG. V-74. B-scan ultrasonogram of a malignant melanoma at the posterior pole showing the typical solid appearance at 10 MHz. A dip in the choroidal outline can be seen, indicating the excavation by the tumor. Scans taken at lower gain and higher frequencies accentuate this acoustic characteristic of excavation. The rounded anterior outline indicates restraint by Bruch's membrane and the height-to-base ratio of approximately 1 to 4 is consistent with malignant melanoma.

MORPHOLOGIC CHARACTERISTICS. *Size.* Malignant melanoma and metastatic carcinoma occur in a continuum of sizes (Figs. V-72 and V-73), ranging from minimally elevated masses to lesions almost filling the globe, all of which can be well shown by B-scan display. Hemangiomas, in our experience, have not typically shown an elevation higher than 5 to 6 mm; however, they can have a very wide cross section. Subretinal hemorrhages sent for ultrasonic evaluation have small elevations, usually less than 4 mm.

With the use of an electronic interval counter, ocular dimensions can be measured to within 0.03 mm at 20 MHz. However, highly accurate tumor measurements are made difficult by the fact that the base of the tumor may not be clearly distinguishable from the scleral echoes, and subsequent measurements may not obtain the same fiducial points. The standard method is to measure maximal tumor thickness (or tumor height). With our equipment, we conservatively consider measurement to be accurate to 0.5 mm for purposes of chronologic comparison.

Shape. Malignant melanomas occur primarily in two characteristic shapes, polypoid or convex, either of which is immediately apparent on B-scan. The most common form of melanoma is an elevated convex mass (Fig. V-74), which occurs when growth of the lesion is

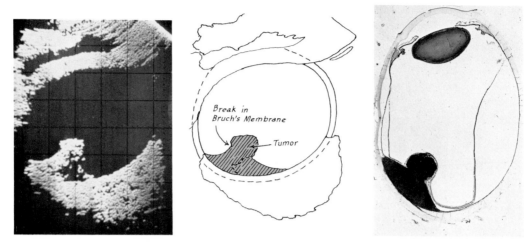

FIG. V-75. B-scan ultrasonogram (*left*) of a malignant melanoma which has broken through Bruch's membrane, producing the characteristic "collar-button" configuration. The histologic section (*right*) emphasizes the correlation between the in vivo appearance and the histologic appearance.

restrained by Bruch's membrane. A polypoid or "collar-button" shape is assumed when the tumor breaks through Bruch's membrane into the vitreous. Ultrasonically, these tumors have a mushroom appearance when the scan plane is passing through the tumor stalk (Fig. V-75). However, when the scan plane does not intersect the stalk, this type of lesion may resemble an isolated intravitreal mass. In such an instance, serial tomographic sections are essential to trace the source of the tumor emanating from the choroid (Fig. V-76).

All metastatic tumors we have examined have appeared as convex masses, and none has exhibited a collar-button shape. In general, metastatic masses have a lower silhouette (i.e., a lower height-to-base ratio) than do malignant melanomas. Choroidal hemangiomas and organized subretinal hemorrhages are usually flattened or slightly convex. In relatively flat lesions, all four types can appear as a simple convex mound.

Location. Localization of the tumor may aid in differentiation, for hemangiomas tend to occur in the posterior pole, particularly near the optic nerve, metastatic tumors at the posterior pole and malignant melanomas throughout the choroid.

Localization of tumors should be done with respect to normal ocular structures (Figs. V-72, V-73, V-74 and V-75), for proximity to the optic nerve may have prognostic significance, and measurement of distance from the lens or ciliary body may be useful when considering placement of a cobalt plaque.

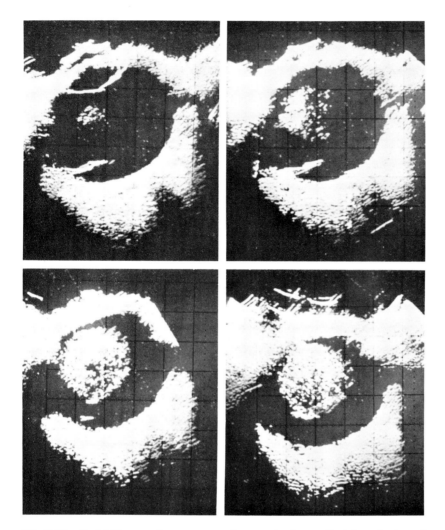

FIG. V-76. Serial B-scan ultrasonogram of an ocular tumor. Serial sectioning of tumors, particularly those of large size, is important for two aspects: (1) it demonstrates the total size of the lesion, and (2) it is useful in tracing the area of contact of the tumor to the ocular wall. Serial scanning, as these B-scans demonstrate, differentiates a mid-vitreal hemorrhage from a tumor extending into the vitreous from the ocular wall.

Evidence of Spread. It is possible with ultrasound to preoperatively suggest subclinical extension of a melanoma beyond the globe. In the case shown in Figure V-77, extension of the tumor into the optic nerve was suggested ultrasonically and was confirmed pathologically. This feature is not one of high confidence and must be carefully evaluated by using the clinical data. Massive orbital extension, however, can be easily shown, as demonstrated by Figure V-78, with a flat intraocular choroidal melanoma.

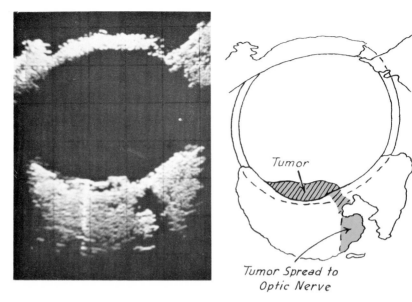

Tumor

Tumor Spread to
Optic Nerve

FIG. V-77. A B-scan ultrasonogram of a malignant melanoma near the optic nerve. Echoes are seen within the nerve, forming a pyramid-shaped abnormality. Histologic evaluation confirmed extension of the tumor to the nerve. In three cases to date with this finding, all have been confirmed histologically.

Change with Time. Repeating ultrasonic evaluation at various time intervals has been valuable to document the progressive growth (Fig. V-79) or regression of a mass lesion. Variation in scan plane is unavoidable in scans performed at different times, but scans through the area of maximum elevation with maximization of the A-scan vitreoretinal echo height will reduce measurement error. Ultrasonography has also been usefully employed to follow the response of tumors to local radiotherapy (cobalt 60 plaques). Hemangiomas have been followed after photocoagulation to document regression.

Metastatic carcinoma usually grows more rapidly than malignant melanoma, but we have not had the opportunity to follow a patient with such a lesion ultrasonically.

ACOUSTIC PROFILE. The acoustic profile of an ocular tumor includes the height of the echo from the leading boundary of the tumor (reflection coefficient), the loss of energy from the sound beam as it is transmitted through the tumor (absorption coefficient or decay slope), the presence, spacing and height of reflecting surfaces within the tumor (the internal tissue texture) and the variation of absorption and texture with changes of frequency of the transducer. Kinetic variations in both those projections can also be important. These acoustic parameters will be discussed individually but it must be kept in mind that they are interrelated.

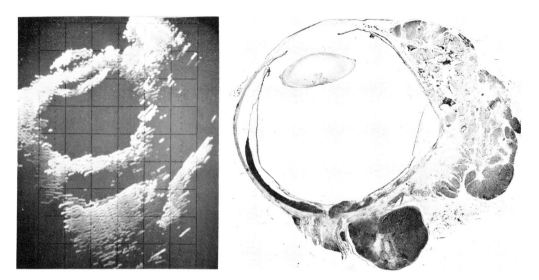

FIG. V-78. B-scan ultrasonogram (*left*) showing a flat posterior pole abnormality not identified as an ocular tumor. The retrobulbar changes are massive and consistent with extraocular extension of the homogeneous melanoma. The pathology section (*right*) of the exenterated orbital contents graphically shows the origin of the B-scan pattern.

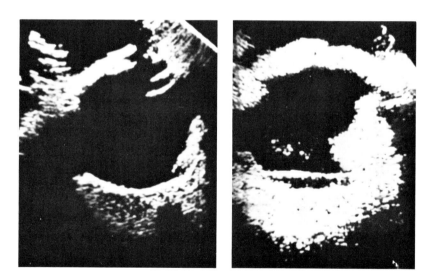

FIG. V-79. Repeat evaluation of an ocular tumor for measurement of growth allows accurate comparison of both the height and breadth of the tumor. The tumor seen in the B-scan on the left lies along the globe wall with an elevation of approximately 3 mm. The scan to the right, taken 9 months later, demonstrates the growth of the mass to a height of approximately 8 mm, which has caused secondary changes of retinal detachment and vitreous hemorrhage.

Boundary Properties. Echo amplitude is directly related to the change in impedance between the different tissue layers traversed by the examining ultrasound beam. High-amplitude echoes are produced at boundaries where there is great variation in tissue sound velocities or tissue densities (e.g., at fluid-tissue boundaries or at boundaries between highly disparate tissues such as lens and vitreous).

The leading edges of choroidal tumors produce high-amplitude echoes when the sound beam is perpendicular to the mass. It is essential for A-scan evaluation that this boundary echo be maximized in order to obtain proper values for the internal tissue echoes. The height of this leading edge is the high-amplitude echo from the vitreoretinal interface (Fig. V-80). The boundary properties of malignant melanomas, metastatic carcinomas, hemangiomas and subretinal hemorrhages thus are similar and have not aided in differentiation. Identification of this feature, however, separates tumor masses from intravitreal hemorrhages which, lacking regular boundaries, reflect only low-amplitude echoes from their anterior surfaces.

Absorption Coefficient. The absorption coefficient is a measure of the rate of energy loss from the ultrasound beam as it passes through tissue, i.e., the inverse of the ability of the tissue to transmit sound. The tissue absorbs ultrasound, and thus the height or strength of the echoes returned to the transducer diminishes. The amount of ultrasound energy absorbed is dependent on such factors as the molecular mobility and structural configuration of the tissue. Ultrasound is also attenuated by reflection and scatter from tissue elements. In a heterogeneous tissue both absorption and scattering losses combine to create a gradual falloff (decay slope) in echo height following the initial boundary spike. This decay slope is specific to each type of tissue. It is approximated for each tissue by a line connecting the peaks of echoes from within a tumor. The decay slope of a heterogeneous tumor which has internal reflecting surfaces produced by blood vessels or variations in tissue type is less easily approximated than the slope of a tumor with only one type of internal scattering element.

Ossoinig[10] has termed the decay slope as an "angle Kappa," referring to the angle between the echo peaks and a horizontal line parallel to the baseline. It should be noted that the decay slope in reality follows an exponential curve and appears as a line only when a logarithmic amplifier is used. Since the Kretz amplifier which Ossoinig uses (the S-shaped curve amplifier) approaches a logarithmic amplifier in character, the decay slope will be somewhat linear with this equipment. With linear amplifiers, which we use, the decay slope is exponential (see Chapter II). This curve is best discerned

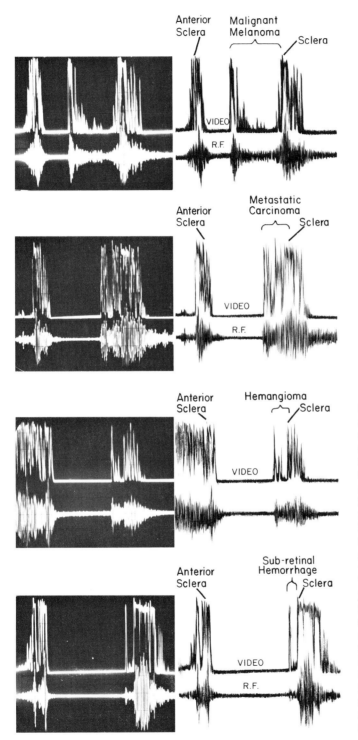

Anterior
Sclera

Malignant
Melanoma

Sclera

VIDEO

R.F.

Anterior
Sclera

Metastatic
Carcinoma

Sclera

VIDEO

R.F.

Anterior
Sclera

Hemangioma

Sclera

VIDEO

Anterior
Sclera

Sub-retinal
Hemorrhage

Sclera

VIDEO

R.F.

FIG. V-80. The A-scan through similar-sized ocular tumors demonstrates the differences between tissues that separate the high leading edge of the tumor, i.e., retina, and the scleral echo. Comparison of the relative echo amplitudes from within the tumor to the scleral echo can reliably identify the tissue present. Melanomas usually provide a high initial echo section followed by a rapid sloping off to echoes that are 10 to 40 per cent of the scleral echo. The percentage echo height is best judged from the radio-frequency trace. Metastatic tumors are usually sustained as 80 per cent of scleral echo and hemangiomas approximate the choroidal echo pattern at 60 to 70 per cent of the scleral echo on the radio frequency. Fluid or hemorrhage beneath retina is usually very low in amplitude, approximately 10 per cent of the scleral echo.

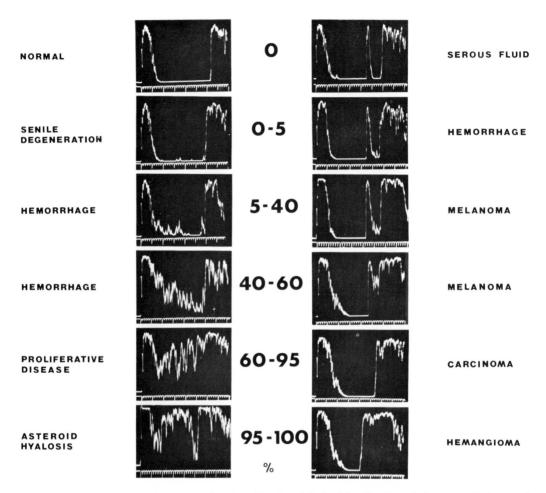

REFLECTIVITY
(% SPIKE HEIGHT)

VITREOUS		SUBRETINAL SPACE
NORMAL	0	SEROUS FLUID
SENILE DEGENERATION	0-5	HEMORRHAGE
HEMORRHAGE	5-40	MELANOMA
HEMORRHAGE	40-60	MELANOMA
PROLIFERATIVE DISEASE	60-95	CARCINOMA
ASTEROID HYALOSIS	95-100 %	HEMANGIOMA

FIG. V-81. A-scan diagnostic schema developed by Ossoinig for identification of vitreous pathology and ocular lesions. With the exception of the A-scan of serous fluid, the A-scans illustrate Type I quantitative echography used to evaluate internally heterogeneous structures. In this type of examination, the system is set at tissue sensitivity which is calibrated once for any instrument/probe combination with echoes obtained from citrated blood serving as biological tissue model. Echo patterns are classified according to their amplitude as a percentage of maximum display height; i.e., echoes from lesions such as melanomas lie below the 60 per cent level as opposed to tumors such as metastatic carcinoma and chorodial hemangioma which lie above the 60 per cent level. The slope of the returned signals (angle Kappa) is also used as an indication of ultrasonic attenuation within lesions.

Type II quantitative echography is used in evaluations of single surfaces within the eye such as those exhibited by foreign bodies and retinal detachments. Echo amplitudes are measured with reference to scleral echoes with the aid of a calibrated sensitivity control. This evaluation is an active process on the part of the observer who must ensure that the ultrasonic beam is normal to the surfaces being examined. (Photograph courtesy of Dr. Ossoinig.)

with the radio-frequency display, which is one reason we present radio-frequency as well as video A-scan signals. The other major reasons for observing the radio-frequency signal are (1) the radio frequency has minimal electronic processing and thus is less susceptible to amplifier overload or reject and is a more realistic, faithful, display of tissue reflections than is the "envelope" or video trace, and (2) tissue texture is better visualized with the radio-frequency than with the video display.

The decay slope is essential in differentiating tumor types. Malignant melanomas show a high-amplitude leading portion with a steep decay (or "angle Kappa"), often reaching baseline as the tumor adjoins the sclera (Fig. V-80). Hemangiomas generally exhibit a relatively mild, uniform decay slope, lacking the final low-amplitude section seen with malignant melanoma (Fig. V-80). The average amplitude of the tumor is usually about 70 per cent of the scleral echo height with our system, but is normally about 95 to 100 per cent of scleral echo height with the Kretz system utilized by Ossoinig (Fig. V-81).

Metastatic carcinomas, like hemangiomas, have relatively flat decay slopes but have higher initial amplitudes, usually about 80 per cent of the scleral height (Figs. V-80–V-82). Subretinal hemorrhages and cysts show low-amplitude internal reflections which are only 10 per cent to 20 per cent of the scleral height (Figs. V-80–V-82). The sclera is used as a reference for the height of choroidal tumor reflectance since it follows the tumor. Thus, absorption within the tumor by structures anterior to the tumor is subtracted from the scleral echo and relative absorption differences between tumor and sclera are thereby maintained.

Internal Tissue Texture. Echoes occurring within a tumor following the boundary spike delineate tissue "texture" by their spacing and height. Internal echoes are the result of inhomogeneities in the tissue such as blood vessels or poolings of fluid. These relatively small interfaces, known as scatterers, generally do not contribute significantly to absorption, but their presence and position are useful in differentiation between tumors.

Melanomas often have high-amplitude discontinuities, usually large blood vessels, that produce echoes rising above the decay slope (Fig. V-83). These echoes may show time variations in amplitude and position within the tumor. Ossoinig[10] has described these variations as "spontaneous movements." The rest of the radio-frequency echo complex in malignant melanoma appears as clustered, relatively coarse, widely spaced echoes mixed with closely spaced echoes. Hemangioma generally appears as fine-textured, closely

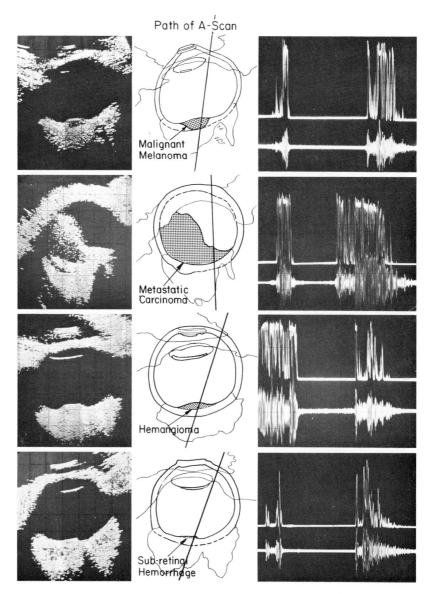

Path of A-Scan

Malignant
Melanoma

Metastatic
Carcinoma

Hemangioma

Sub-retinal
Hemorrhage

FIG. V-82. Comparisons of the B- and A-scan patterns through the four main tumor classes for ocular differential diagnosis are shown. The A-scan should be aligned as nearly perpendicular to the tumor as possible. Differentiation of tumors is afforded by studying the internal acoustic characteristics of the tumor. Variations in the frequency of transducer, orientation of the transducer, kinesis of the tissue and amplitude of echoes are all studied from the A-scan.

spaced echoes and metastatic carcinoma appears as coarse-textured echoes (Figs. V-80–V-82).

Work in progress evaluating the frequency spectra of tumor echoes indicates that these texture features will be increasingly important clues to tissue identification.

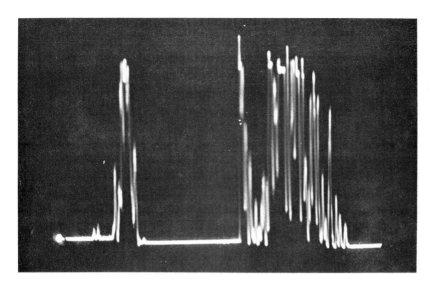

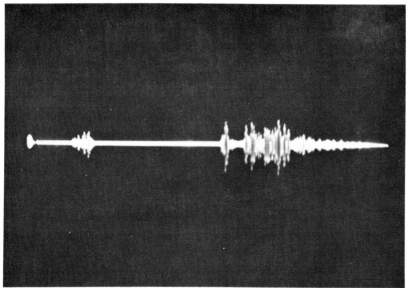

FIG. V-83. A-scan ultrasonograms of an eye with an intraocular malignant melanoma to demonstrate the high leading edge present in choroidal tumors. This high echo, most easily appreciated on the A-scan, is produced by overlying retina, and should be maximized to indicate that the examining beam is perpendicular to the mass. The slope and amplitude of echoes that follow this initial echo are then analyzed for differential diagnosis.

Frequency Variation. In discussing the above internal tissue characteristics, we have assumed that only a single transducer with a given frequency is used. When the ultrasound frequency is changed (by using a different transducer), each of the above internal tissue texture properties (i.e., echo amplitude, echo spacing, and

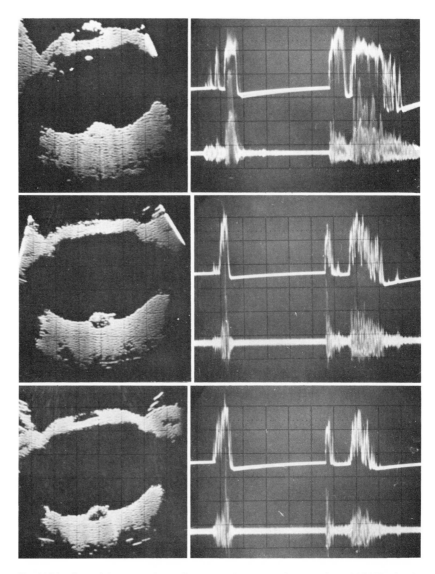

FIG. V-84. B- and A-scans of a malignant melanoma at frequencies of 10 MHz (*top*), 15 MHz (*middle*) and 20 MHz (*bottom*) demonstrating comparative frequency effects of tissue homogeneity. The A-scans demonstrate how the mass shows lower amplitude echoes in the deeper portion of the tissue due to acoustic absorption and relatively anechoic homogeneous tissue. The decay slope and tissue texture properties can be compared at the different frequencies. Melanomas show increasingly evident decay with higher frequencies; hemangiomas show little change with increased frequency, and metastatic carcinomas also show little change with frequency variation.

acoustic absorption) may vary (Fig. V-84). We have found this variation in tumor "acoustic profile" between examining frequencies of 10, 15 and 20 MHz to be valuable in distinguishing melanomas from metastatic carcinomas, hemangiomas, and organized subretinal hemorrhages. Melanomas exhibit a sharper drop to baseline on

ACOUSTIC CHARACTERISTICS OF CHOROIDAL TUMORS

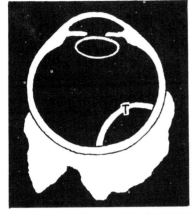

ACOUSTIC
"QUIET ZONE"
(OR "VACUOLE")

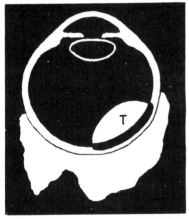

"CHOROIDAL
EXCAVATION"

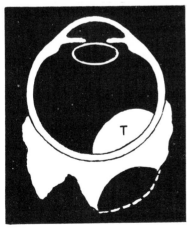

ACOUSTIC
"SHADOWING"
(OR "ABSORPTION DEFECT")

FIG. V-85. Three types of B-scan texture changes seen with ocular tumors that are useful in their identification. These morphologic changes are best seen on the two-dimensional B-scan, as they require comparison with adjacent tissues.

A-scan (increased hollowness on B-scan) with increased frequencies. Metastatic carcinomas are usually solid at all frequencies (i.e., maintain internal echoes on A-scan). Hemangiomas vary according to size, but are usually solid at all frequencies, and organized subretinal hemorrhages are usually hollow at all frequencies. Even the different cytological types of choroidal malignant melanoma may show different frequency-related variations, mixed cell or epithelioid tumors often showing greater hollowing with increased frequency than spindle cell tumors.[90]

Techniques for obtaining the frequency spectrum of tissue echoes are being developed that offer even greater tissue identification potential. Knowledge of frequency-tissue relationships as a means of augmenting the acoustic profiles of tumors will certainly grow even further as techniques are improved and experience is gained.

Kinetic Properties of Tumors. Ossoinig[10] has emphasized the value of using the A-scan probe as a means of ballotting tumors to stimulate changes in their acoustic patterns, as well as to permit observation of their compressibility. This test is obviously more useful in the orbit than in the globe, especially when dealing with cystic tumors. The detection of vascular echoes can be enhanced with this technique during ocular examination.

ACOUSTIC CHARACTERISTICS (B-SCAN). The acoustic profile of a tumor on A-scan translates into a B-scan display as variations in the appearance of a tissue texture. The phenomena of acoustic quiet zones, choroidal excavation, and acoustic shadowing (Fig. V-85) are major sources of B-scan tumor differentiation.

Acoustic "Quiet Zone." Malignant melanomas appear on B-scan as acoustically solid (white) areas protruding into the sonolucent vitreous cavity. Histologically, malignant melanomas are homogeneously cellular with varying degrees of vascularity (Fig. V-86). With increasing vascularity of the tumor tissue, there are many internal acoustic interfaces, so that more echoes are returned and the tumor appears more solid (white). This acoustic solidity in vascular tumors is apparent at transducer frequencies of 5, 10, 15 and 20 MHz. Polypoid-shaped melanomas almost always exhibit these characteristics of acoustic solidity. In relatively avascular melanomas (most often those with convex shape), the homogeneous cellularity of the tumor and lack of significant internal acoustic interfaces result in the appearance of an acoustic "quiet zone" or hollow within the tumor. This phenomenon is accentuated on the B-scan (Fig. V-87), although

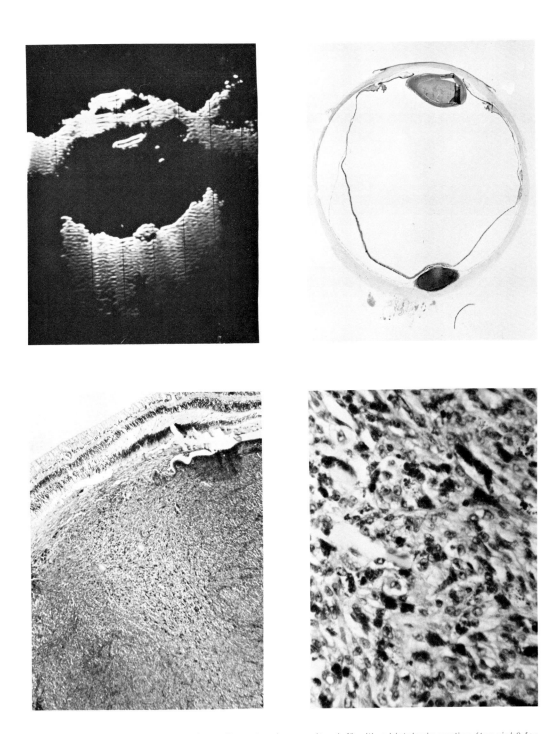

FIG. V-86. B-scan ultrasonogram of a malignant melanoma (*top left*) with a histologic section (*top right*) for comparison. Note that the tumor rests on the sclera and has replaced the normal choroid. The microscopic views (*bottom left and right*) of the tumor show it to be homogeneous tissue with large vascular channels indicating the cause for a steep decay slope (homogeneous) with interpersed ''spontaneous echoes'' (vascularity).

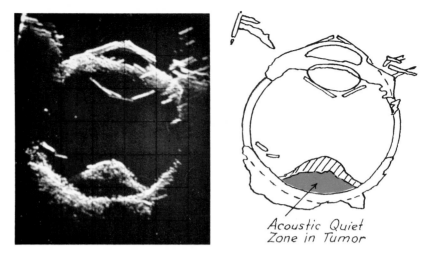

Acoustic Quiet
Zone in Tumor

Fɪɢ. V-87. An acoustic quiet zone shown in a solid tumor found to be so homogeneous that the mass appeared hollow. A-scan comparisons are essential with this type of
lesion to show that the tumor is actually solid, and not fluid filled.

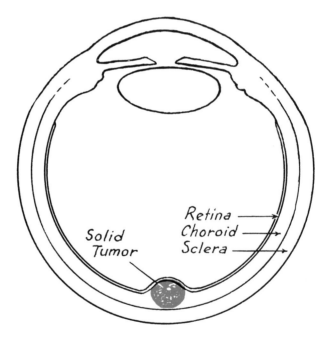

Retina
Choroid
Sclera

Solid
Tumor

Fɪɢ. V-88. Schematic drawing of an eye with a tumor of the
choroid to emphasize the manner in which tumor tissue can
replace the normal choroid, which is often .6 to .8 mm thick in
vivo. As demonstrated in the histologic section presented in
Figure V-86, the anterior edge of the choroid attaches high on
the tumor, indicating the marked difference in thickness of the
choroid in histologic sections compared to the in vivo state
portrayed during ultrasonography.

the A-scan tracing registers echoes of moderate though declining amplitude throughout the tumor. If the tumor were actually physically hollow and fluid filled, the A-scan would show absence of echoes after the initial leading echo (as seen in a retinal detachment). This phenomenon of acoustic hollowing in relatively avascular melanomas is most prominent at examining frequencies of 15 and 20 MHz. At 5 and 10 MHz, the tumors usually appear acoustically solid.

Choroidal Excavation. Involvement of the choroid by a melanoma can be shown dramatically by the presence of the "excavation" phenomenon. The area of tumor that has replaced the surrounding choroid is thereby demonstrated by a dish- or bowl-shaped indentation into the normally smooth concave choroidal outline. It must be remembered that the choroid in the living eye is an erectile tissue which may be as much as 1 mm thick (Fig. V-88). Excavation has been frequently noted in malignant melanoma (Fig. V-89), though not all melanomas exhibit this feature.

The incidence of choroidal excavation in a series of 110 intraocular tumors was computed.[87] Choroidal excavation was absent in all cases of metastatic carcinoma and hemangioma and was noted only in malignant melanoma. Of the 89 malignant melanomas, 42 per cent exhibited this characteristic and 58 per cent did not. Choroidal excavation was not seen in any melanoma lying anterior to the equator. The histologic similarity of metastatic carcinoma to certain melanomas, however, should perhaps lead us to expect a similar pattern. Subretinal hemorrhage and disciform macular degeneration, in our experience, do not show choroidal excavation.

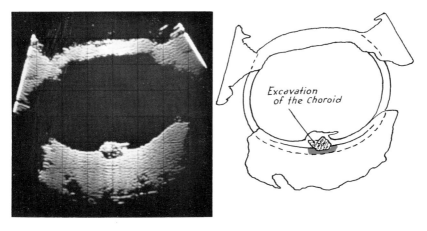

FIG. V-89. B-scan of a malignant melanoma demonstrating choroidal excavation. This feature is a reliable indication of melanoma, though only about 45 per cent of all melanomas demonstrate it.

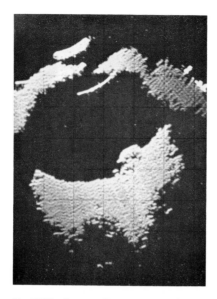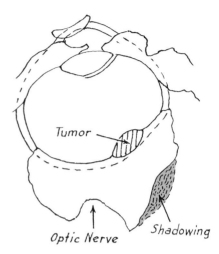

Fig. V-90. B-scan ultrasonogram of a tumor mass demonstrating that acoustic absorption in the tumor can cause "shadowing" or loss of definition of orbital structures immediately behind the tumor. This feature may also be useful in localizing the mass between the defect and the sound source, i.e. transducer.

Absorption Defect or "Shadowing." Absorption of sound by one tissue mass can cause an acoustic absorption defect or shadowing to appear in structures behind the mass. A solid mass will sometimes attenuate sound to such an extent that the area of retrobulbar fat behind it will seem fainter than the rest of the orbit, or the sound

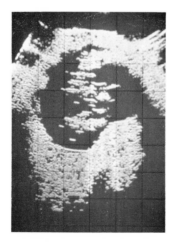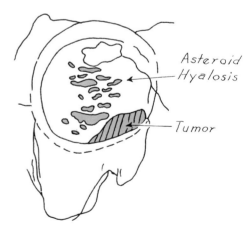

Fig. V-91. B-scan ultrasonogram of a solid elevated lesion at the posterior pole consistent with tumor mass. A nonassociated asteroid hyalosis pattern is present in mid-vitreous. Vitreous hemorrhage on B-scan could show a similar pattern, but the B-scan pattern would aid in differentiation of these entities since hyalosis usually has a distinct stalk connecting the vitreous to the optic nerve head and is of higher amplitude.

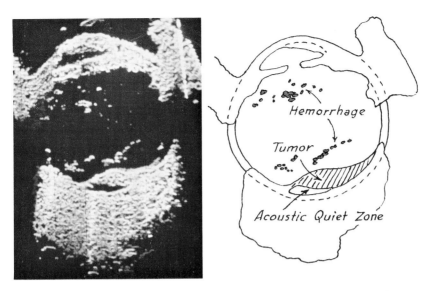

FIG. V-92. B-scan ultrasonogram of a posterior malignant melanoma, showing an acoustic quiet zone. Vitreous hemorrhage anteriorly has obscured the visual detection and evaluation of this tumor.

beam will not penetrate far into the orbit directly behind the tumor, causing a hollowed-out appearance (Fig. V-90). This absorption defect will not occur if the mass has good sound transmission properties. There is apparently no significant variation in the shadowing produced by melanoma and metastatic tumors with our techniques. Hemangiomas show little evidence of shadowing, probably as a result of their lesser density.

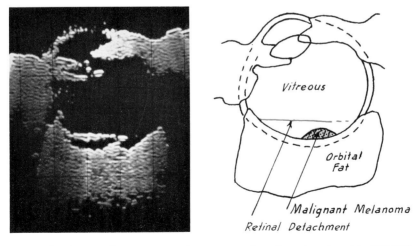

FIG. V-93. B-scan ultrasonogram of a very small malignant melanoma detected behind a retinal detachment. A tumor of this size may be exceedingly difficult to identify with A-scan alone.

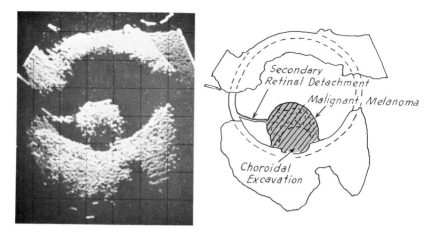

FIG. V-94. B-scan ultrasonogram of a malignant melanoma at the posterior pole with choroidal excavation and a secondary retinal detachment. The choroidal excavation here demonstrates the value of the two-dimensional portrayal of acoustic absorption as an aid in tumor identification, since no visual characterization is possible.

ASSOCIATED OCULAR CHANGES. Changes in the globe associated with intraocular tumors are also ultrasonically demonstrable. Asteroid hyalosis may mask the presence of a tumor (Fig. V-91). Vitreous hemorrhages occur infrequently with melanomas of the choroid, but one can be shown ultrasonically (Fig. V-92). Retinal detachments secondary to intraocular melanomas or metastatic carcinoma are of clinical importance (Figs. V-93, V-94 and V-95). They appear on B-scan ultrasonograms as bullous retinal elevations with a sharp, high-amplitude leading edge. Serous retinal detachments can also be associated with choroidal hemangioma (Fig. V-96).

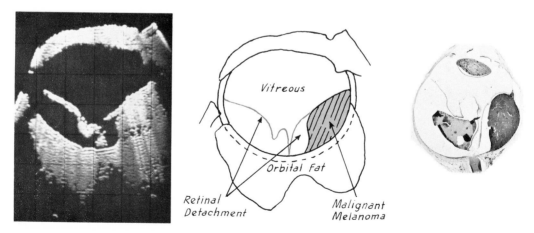

FIG. V-95. *Left:* B-scan ultrasonogram of a solid posterior tumor, underlying a retinal detachment, again showing a choroidal replacement and emphasizing the difference between a solid subretinal mass and subretinal fluid. *Right:* Histologic section of the enucleated globe, demonstrating the tissue basis for the ultrasonic appearance.

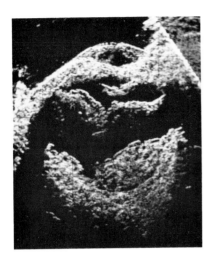
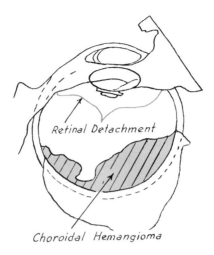

Retinal Detachment

Choroidal Hemangioma

FIG. V-96. A retinal detachment obscured this large hemangioma over the entire posterior pole. The sustained type of A-scan pattern seen with hemangioma is confirmed here on the B-scan. No choroidal replacement is seen as hemangioma and choroid are essentially similar tissue.

Conditions Simulating Choroidal Tumors

RETINAL LESIONS. In retinal detachment or retinoschisis, the ultrasonic pattern may show an elevated vitreoretinal interface echo, but since the subretinal space is acoustically sonolucent then the elevation is readily distinguishable from a tumor. Disciform macular degeneration also shows an elevated vitreoretinal interface. These hemorrhagic lesions show low-amplitude internal echoes on A-scan, but will appear hollow at 15 and 20 MHz (or with reduced gain at 10 MHz).

In chorioretinitis, an area of elevated retina may be seen, but the subretinal space is acoustically clear. RPE lesions (such as congenital hypertrophy of the pigment epithelium) that appear flat and highly pigmented ophthalmoscopically do not have sufficient elevation to be detected ultrasonically.

CHOROIDAL LESIONS. Most benign choroidal nevi fail to show significant elevation and thus cannot be demonstrated on B-scan ultrasonograms. Choroidal detachments present a typical B-scan convex circumferential elevation straddling the ora serrata with a sonolucent area between the retina and sclera. Organized choroidal hemorrhage may be difficult to distinguish acoustically from a tumor, but the internal echoes are of lower amplitude. Lymphoid hyperplasia of the choroid (Fig. V-97) may be ultrasonically indistinguishable from an "en plaque" melanoma but may be suspected due to greater sound absorption by inflammatory tissue.

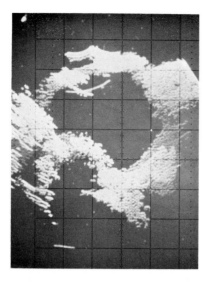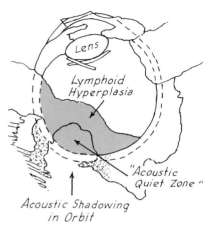

Lens

Lymphoid
Hyperplasia

"Acoustic
Quiet Zone"

Acoustic Shadowing
in Orbit

FIG. V-97. This B-scan shows the acoustic cross section of a globe enucleated for melanoma that was found to have lymphoid hyperplasia. Note that the scleral echo is absent behind the tumor, suggesting a marked absorption quality to the acoustic transmission properties of these tumors.

VITREOUS LESIONS. Vitreous hemorrhages that have undergone organization may appear as acoustically dense (white) masses. In contrast to collar-button melanomas, however, no connecting stalk can be found on serial sectioning, and the internal echo amplitudes are usually lower than those seen in melanoma. The presence of a vitreoretinal interface appearing smoothly curved and in normal position may help in differentiating these hemorrhages. Repeated ultrasonic evaluations may be necessary to distinguish a tumor which lies within a dense vitreous hemorrhage, a situation which arises more often with retinoblastoma than with choroidal tumors. The extremely difficult diagnostic problem of organized hemorrhage in conjunction with retinal detachment occurs rarely. The use of varying transducer frequencies, M-mode and quantitative scan methods may be required to establish the correct diagnosis.

Reliability and Limitations of Ultrasonic Differentiation

The reliability of ultrasonic diagnosis of ocular tumors in our laboratory has been reported[91] as better than 96 per cent for differentiation of neoplastic choroidal tumors from benign subretinal hemorrhages, vitreous hemorrhages and retinal detachments. Ossoinig[10] has reported a similar figure using his techniques.

We have to date examined nearly 1,000 patients with ocular tumors, both neoplastic and benign. It has not always been possible to identify the tissue present on one examination. Serial examinations are often requested to permit growth documentation as well as to repeat the evaluation. The methods described here, even when absolute differentiation cannot be made, can direct the course of treatment, small solid tumors can be followed, larger tumors can benefit from a search for metastatic lesions and ^{32}P tests can be indicated to the appropriate area.

In addition to the problems in identifying discrete lesions as discussed above, other difficulties in ultrasonic diagnosis of choroidal tumors exist that are related to size or position.

First, very small lesions cannot be demonstrated ultrasonically. In general, lesions causing more than 1 mm of elevation of the retina can be demonstrated, and when the tumor can be visualized and the ultrasonogram is performed under optimal conditions, tumors causing only 0.5 mm of elevation can be depicted. Smaller lesions can certainly be missed with ultrasonography. This is a problem of equivocal significance since there is a growing body of opinion that eyes with small lesions should not be enucleated immediately, but rather be followed or treated. It is customary clinically to follow a very small lesion in order to document a visual growth change. By the time such changes can be documented, the tumor should be demonstrable ultrasonically.

Second, very large lesions filling the vitreous are often confusing in that they may resemble vitreous hemorrhages. In our experience, these tumors have not exhibited choroidal excavation and their A-scan pattern can resemble hemorrhage. This is a particular problem with massive necrotic melanomas and it also occurs with retinoblastoma.

Finally, difficulties persist with optimal B-scan visualization of the ora serrata and pars plana regions. Even with the immersion technique, structures which lie perpendicular to the examining beam are well portrayed but structures lying parallel to the beam, such as the ocular walls at the ora, are not well outlined. Also, structures preceding a tumor will tend to mask some of its acoustic profile. Malignant melanomas seen in this area have not demonstrated choroidal excavation, which makes differentiation more difficult.

Ciliary Body Abnormalities

Ciliary body tumors occur less frequently than tumors of the choroid, representing approximately 10 per cent of all ocular melanomas.[92] Tumors of the ciliary body are often difficult to diagnose clinically, for they arise in an area of the eye not routinely examined and usually are not amenable to fluorescein angiography. They precipitate cataracts or secondary retinal detachments which will cause difficulty in clinical diagnosis. In addition, ophthalmoscopically visible masses may be difficult to distinguish from cystic lesions of the ciliary body, with elevation of the pigmented epithelium of the ciliary body in this area. Thus, ultrasonography is of great value in the diagnosis of such tumors.

Attention to certain technical features will improve ultrasonic portrayal of ciliary body tumors. First, it is important to rotate the eye as much as possible, bringing the mass perpendicular (in either an anterior or posterior position) to the transducer for best resolution. Second, small tumors in this region may be missed, particularly at the 6:00 and 12:00 meridians with horizontal scans, so vertical scans are thus required. Third, a range of transducer frequencies should be used to optimize differentiation. Fourth, serial examinations at a later date are necessary in equivocal cases.

CILIARY BODY TUMORS. The ultrasonographic characteristics of ciliary body tumors will be discussed as in choroidal tumors, in terms of both morphologic and acoustic characteristics.

The location and size of ciliary body tumors can be well demonstrated by B-scan ultrasound (Fig. V-98). Secondary changes such as retinal detachment, hemorrhage in the vitreous and cataractous lens changes can also be shown, as previously discussed.

As in tumors of the choroid, acoustic quiet zones at the posterior part of a ciliary body tumor can be appreciated. We have not had experience with sufficient ciliary body melanomas to establish the

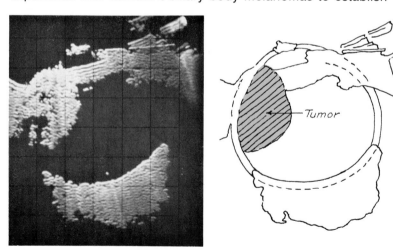

FIG. V-98. B-scan ultrasonogram at 10 MHz of a malignant melanoma of the ciliary muscle. Small tumors underlying the ciliary muscle are often more difficult to evaluate since the preceding normal tissue may obscure their outline and acoustic characteristics.

significance of frequency-related variation; however, the quiet zone phenomenon is best seen at high transducer frequencies. Choroidal excavation has not been seen with ciliary body tumors, and thus this useful differential sign is not available.

Lesions Simulating Ciliary Body Tumors. B-scan ultrasonography provides the differential diagnosis between ciliary body cysts and ciliary body tumors. The interior of the cysts is sonolucent and the A-scan trace remains at baseline throughout the cyst. A B-scan ultrasonogram of a patient with a ciliary body cyst is shown in Figure V-99, demonstrating the obviously anechoic cystic structure of the lesion.

Choroidal detachments or effusions can simulate a ring melanoma of the ciliary body, but ultrasonography can demonstrate their cystic or solid natures.

Clinical Usefulness of Ultrasound. Ciliary body tumors are often misdiagnosed. In one series, 40 per cent of misdiagnoses were due to obscuration by retinal or choroidal detachment and 5 per cent were misinterpreted as cystic lesions.[93] Ultrasonography can improve the differential diagnosis, even in patients with clear media. The size and the posterior extent of these tumors, as determined by serial acoustic tomography, influence a decision regarding corneoscleral iridocyclectomy. The clinician can often fail to appreciate the position of the posterior edge of the tumor with ophthalmoscopic or slit-lamp examination techniques, even in the presence of clear media, while ultrasonography can show this variable.

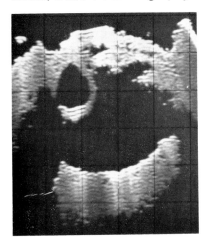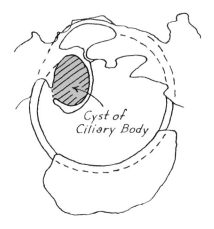

FIG. V-99. B-scan ultrasonogram of a ciliary body cyst appearing as a clearly hollow outlined structure. A small tumor at the base of the cyst may be difficult to identify, and scans in both horizontal and vertical planes with variations in sensitivity settings and frequencies are advised.

We do not presently have enough experience to differentiate melanomas from metastatic tumors in this area using quantitative A-scan ultrasonography. Metastatic tumors, however, are quite unusual in a postion anterior to the ora serrata. Ordinarily, the diagnosis of a metastatic tumor can be made clinically on the basis of multiple tumors, known primary tumor, and relatively rapid growth.

Choroidal Effusions

Choroidal effusions (detachments) occur commonly following intraocular surgery. In some patients, these cannot be diagnosed clinically because of a cloudy cornea, hazy aqueous or vitreous, or miotic pupil. Since ultrasound is not subject to the limitations of optical techniques, it is uniquely useful in this postoperative complication.

A choroidal effusion appears ultrasonographically as a convex line of echoes extending into the vitreous compartment from the globe wall in any quandrant. In a fully developed choroidal effusion, the echo lines may extend into the central vitreous from each side of the eye and may even appear to touch (Fig. V-100, courtesy of Dr. R. Dallow). The choroidal effusion is always seen to straddle the ora

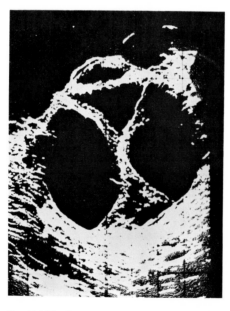
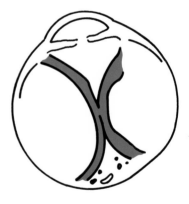

Choroidal Detachment

FIG. V-100. B-scan ultrasonogram of a choroidal effusion in a patient with a shallow anterior chamber, following a filtering procedure. The characteristic pattern of a choroidal effusion is the rounded bullous outline extending into mid-vitreous with a relatively obtuse angle noted at the posterior pole. The anterior attachment point of the effusion precedes the ora, and aids in differentiating these effusions from retinal detachment. (Courtesy of Dr. R. Dallow.)

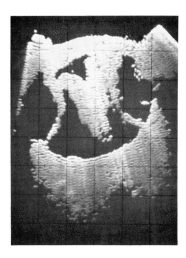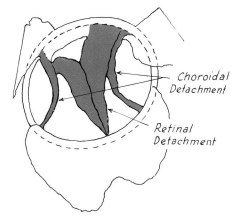

Choroidal
Detachment

Retinal
Detachment

FIG. V-101. B-scan ultrasonogram of a choroidal effusion and a retinal detachment. The choroidal detachments have obtuse angles at the posterior pole and the retinal detachment can be traced back to attachment at the optic nerve head. The point of attachment of the retina to the ora serrata and the optic nerve head can be discerned even in the presence of choroidal effusion, and the anterior attachment of the effusion is again emphasized.

serrata, and at its juncture with the posterior wall echo there is an acute angle anteriorly. The space peripheral to the line of echoes is acoustically clear, and an A-scan through the choroidal space shows no echoes. This characteristic differentiates a choroidal detachment from a choroidal hemorrhage, which shows low-amplitude echoes in the choroidal space, similar in amplitude to echoes obtained in vitreous hemorrhage. Infrequently, however, large choroidal detachments will show scattered low-amplitude echoes in the subchoroidal space, indicative of organized exudate. Other ocular abnormalities such as retinal detachment (Fig. V-101) may coexist with choroidal effusion.

A flat or shallow chamber is most commonly encountered as a postoperative condition. It may also appear in other situations such as penetrating injury, pupillary block, dislocated lens, swollen lens, choroidal hemorrhage or intraocular tumors. Most flat chambers are associated with a serous choroidal detachment (effusion). Examination of the posterior segment may therefore provide information vital for the diagnosis and management of each individual case. In a majority of cases, the cause of the flat chamber is discernible and treatment may be initiated.

There does exist, however, a small subgroup in which the posterior segment cannot be visualized and the proper approach to management is not apparent. In such cases, B-scan ultrasonography has proven to be extremely helpful.

In evaluating an eye with a flat or shallow anterior chamber, it is essential to detect relevant abnormalities in the anterior segment, to search carefully for evidence of external fistulization, to measure the intraocular pressure and to determine the presence or absence of a choroidal detachment in the posterior segment, as discussed by Forbes and Coleman.[94] Unfortunately, one or more factors such as corneal edema, hyphema, cataract, miosis and vitreous hemorrhage may intercede to prevent adequate visualization of the posterior segment. Clinical experience suggests that such problems are likely to be encountered in the more complex cases where information regarding the posterior segment is most needed.

In persistent postoperative flat chamber syndrome where the posterior segment cannot be visualized, data from B-scan ultrasonography can be essential prior to surgical intervention. First, demonstration that a serous choroidal detachment is, in fact, present confirms the diagnosis and establishes the need for posterior sclerotomy as part of the operative procedure. Second, localization of the choroidal detachment enables the surgeon to place the posterior sclerotomy at the site of maximum choroidal elevation.

An eye with a flat chamber following a filtering procedure for angle-closure glaucoma always raises the possibility of malignant glaucoma. In this condition, aqueous humor is trapped within the vitreous compartment despite a patent iridectomy, and the lens is anteriorly displaced. Malignant glaucoma is readily distinguished from postoperative pupillary block glaucoma, which is characterized by lack of a patent iris coloboma and aqueous humor trapped in the posterior chamber causing iris bombé without anterior displacement of the lens. In malignant glaucoma, the intraocular pressure is usually quite high, but it may fall within the normal range during the early phase. The tension in the flat chamber syndrome is generally quite soft, but may transiently rise to a normal level in some cases despite the continued presence of a choroidal detachment. Hence, a differential diagnosis between malignant glaucoma and the flat chamber syndrome cannot always be made by tonometry alone. In equivocal cases, the presence of a choroidal detachment would be diagnostic of the flat chamber syndrome, whereas the absence of such a finding would strongly suggest incipient malignant glaucoma. Thus, when visualization of the posterior segment is not possible, and the intraocular pressure is not elevated, ultrasonography should be employed.

In a case of flat chamber with elevated pressure after surgery for angle-closure glaucoma, a diagnosis of malignant glaucoma would appear to be firmly established, providing there is no choroidal elevation representing either serous detachment or hemorrhage.

When the fundus cannot be seen in this type of situation, Chandler et al.[95] and Simmons[96] recommended preliminary sclerotomies in both lower quadrants to determine whether or not a ciliochoroidal detachment or hemorrhage is present before proceeding with their effective surgical procedure for malignant glaucoma, i.e., pars plana vitreous aspiration and anterior chamber air injection. In all probability this matter could be settled by B-scan ultrasonography, not only prior to surgery but as soon as the possibility of malignant glaucoma is considered.

Abnormalities of the Optic Nerve Head

Papilledema, papillitis, pseudopapilledema, drusen and melanocytoma can be appreciated ultrasonically as a protrusion of the intrascleral portion of the optic nerve into the vitreous, and an increased reflectivity of this region for anatomic reasons. Papilledema and papillitis usually cannot be separated by the ultrasonic appearance of the scleral portion of the nerve alone, although a clear subretinal fluid level may occasionally be seen with papilledema (Fig. V-102). The appearance of the orbital portion of the nerve may indicate the correct diagnosis ophthalmoscopically in cases of both visible and nonvisible elevations of the optic nerve head. In cases of pseudopapilledema due to drusen, the orbital echoes are normal, corresponding to the histologic findings that drusen in the nerve are not found posterior to the lamina cribrosa.

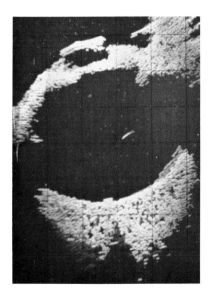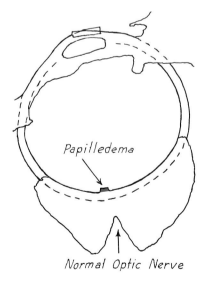

FIG. V-102. B-scan ultrasonogram demonstrating prominence of the optic nerve head.

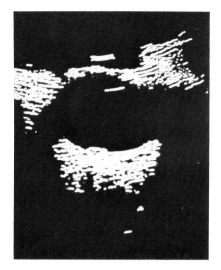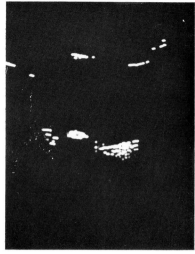

Fig. V-103. B-scan ultrasonograms of optic nerve head drusen taken at varying sensitivity settings. The mass seen on the higher gain setting (*left*) persists even when the sensitivity is lowered to a threshold point (*right*), demonstrating the internal solidity of the drusen.

Drusen may be so large that shadowing or internal echoes can cause apparent enlargement or internal reflections in the anterior nerve segment (Fig. V-103). In cases of optic neuritis, echoes from the nerve wall may produce a contiguous line appearing to separate the nerve and the sheath. When optic neuritis is seen in association with enlarged, inflamed rectus muscles, this doubling of the wall sign may permit the diagnosis of class VI Graves' disease to be made ultrasonically. When optic neuritis is associated with pseudo-

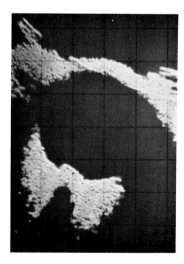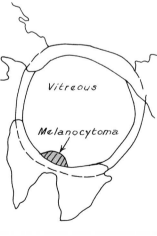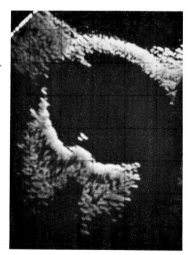

Fig. V-104. Melanocytoma.

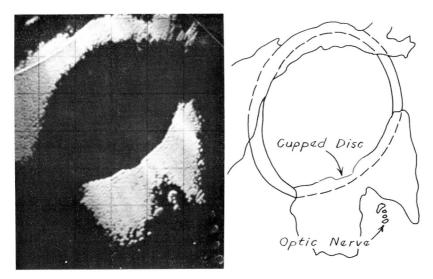

FIG. V-105. B-scan ultrasonogram taken with a narrow beamwidth transducer to demonstrate an indentation or cupping of the optic nerve head. This pathologic condition cannot usually be detected with standard examining transducers.

tumor of the orbit, the inflammatory character of these mass lesions can be suspected by the nerve changes as well as edema of normal structures such as Tenon's capsule.

Shrinkage of the optic nerve cannot be appreciated with B-scan ultrasound. Thus ultrasonography usually cannot differentiate an atrophied from a normal optic nerve. However, when the optic nerve is invaded by tissue which is acoustically dissimilar to that of the normal optic nerve tissue, acoustic interfaces occur and abnormal echoes are returned from within the nerve. As an example, when a juxtapapillary melanocytoma (Fig. V-104) extends into the nerve, many abnormal intraneural echoes can be identified. Melanocytomas are composed of polyhedral cells with large amounts of pigment and are histologically and ultrasonically very unlike normal nerve tissue.

Optic nerve cupping is not usually demonstrable ultrasonically since the beamwidth utilized in ocular evaluation is too wide to permit resolution of such a small depression. The standard beamwidth causes the nasal and temporal cup edges to merge, and the beamwidth artifact causes merging of echoes from the floor of the optic cup with echoes from adjoining tissue. Studies utilizing precisely focused, very narrow beamwidth transducers can demonstrate cupping of the optic nerve head (Fig. V-105).

Elevation of the optic nerve head may also be seen with intrinsic tumors of the optic nerve such as melanocytoma which may resemble drusen ultrasonically.

Ocular Trauma

The preceding sections of ocular diagnosis have been presented in a manner based on the anatomic landmarks of the eye. Changes produced in these structures by trauma have been alluded to; however, the importance of ultrasound in the evaluation of a traumatized globe merits a separate discussion so that specific changes, examining techniques and approaches to clinical management may be more adequately summarized.

Ocular trauma may be classified into three categories: contusion or concussion injuries, penetrating or lacerating wounds, and foreign body injuries. Eyes subjected to any of these forms of trauma often exhibit cloudy media due to corneal or lens damage, hyphema or vitreous hemorrhage. In these situations, ultrasonography becomes essential for complete evaluation of the globe prior to primary repair. Effective medical and surgical therapy of the traumatized eye is thereby enhanced with ultrasonic evaluation. Table V-4 summarizes some of the conditions evaluable with ultrasound and the modes of treatment that may be initiated or expedited.

Careful visual inspection and radiographic examination for ocular foreign bodies should be performed first, so that the ultrasonographer may direct the examination to the most pertinent clinical questions. Identification of an ocular foreign body by X-ray enables the examiner more rapidly to localize the foreign body in relation to ocular structures, shortening the total time required for the examination, which is desirable in traumatized eyes.

In patients with recent ocular trauma, every attempt is made to maintain sterile technique. We do not sterilize our transducer, but it can be immersed in Zephiran prior to scanning or a rubber glove tip can be placed over the end of the transducer. In addition, an antibiotic solution can be instilled in the sterile water bath. With a severely

TABLE V-4.   Improvements in Management Aided by Ultrasound

Conditions	Treatment
Vitreous hemorrhage	Vitrectomy
Retinal perforation	Prophylactic cryopexy
Retinal detachment	Encircling band
Lens dislocation	Observation or removal
Lens rupture	Aspiration
Choroidal hemorrhage	Drainage
Scleral rupture	Repair
Foreign body localization	Extraction
Foreign body magnetic properties	Extraction

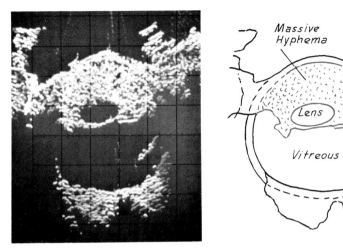

FIG. V-106. B-scan ultrasonogram of a traumatized globe showing dense hyphema, posterior displacement of the lens and hemorrhage into the vitreous compartment. There is no acoustic evidence of retinal detachment.

traumatized globe, clinical judgment would determine whether immersion B-scan or contact A- or B-scan is indicated.

Contusion and Concussion Injuries

HYPHEMA. The presence of hyphema can be noted ultrasonically, but usually adds little information in and of itself to that already obtained visually. A moderately dense hyphema can be appreciated ultrasonically as echoes occurring within the anterior chamber,

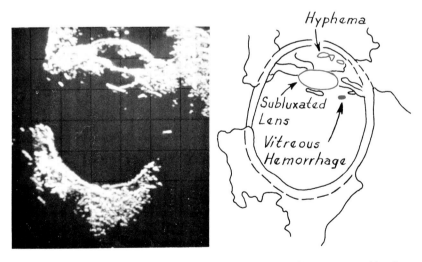

FIG. V-107. Following trauma, a deep anterior chamber with a concave iris plane indicates angle recession. This globe also demonstrates hyphema, a dislocated lens, and an anterior vitreous hemorrhage.

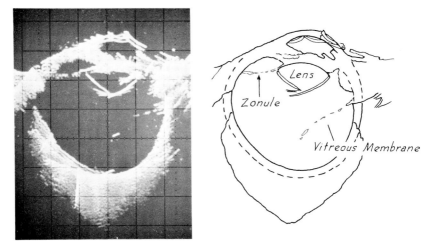

Fig. V-108. B-scan ultrasonogram demonstrating a deep anterior chamber. The possibility of angle recession exists in an eye of this type following trauma. The lens has been subluxated but the zonular attachment remains, seen as a separate line of echoes extending from the equator of the lens to the ora serrata.

whereas a relatively light, nonclotted hyphema may be sonolucent. Extension of the hyphema into the posterior chamber may be discerned. Figure V-106 demonstrates hemorrhage into the anterior chamber as well as deepening, probable angle recession and hemorrhage into the posterior chamber.

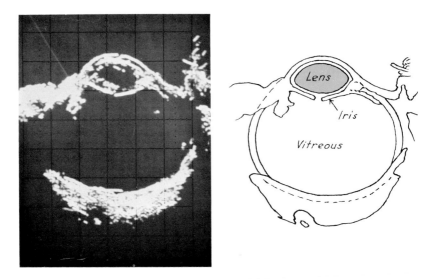

Fig. V-109. B-scan ultrasonogram demonstrating traumatic displacement of the lens into the anterior chamber. The vitreous is acoustically clear, except for possible vitreous hemorrhage along the nasal aspect of the ciliary muscle.

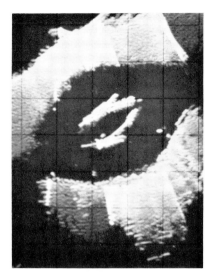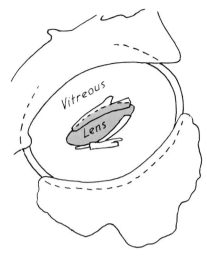

FIG. V-110. B-scan ultrasonogram of a traumatized globe with the lens displaced into the mid-vitreous.

ANGLE RECESSION. Ultrasound is not able to depict actual cleavage of the angle, but can demonstrate an abnormal deepening of the anterior chamber and widening of the angle as seen in recession. These findings, as seen in Figures V-107 and V-108, indicate the severity of the trauma to the anterior segment.

DISLOCATED LENS. In any form of severe concussion, the lens may become subluxated or totally dislocated from its usual position. Even minor variations in position may be portrayed with the B-scan ultrasound display. Figure V-109 shows an anterior displacement of the lens and Figure V-110 shows dislocation of the lens into the vitreous body. In contusion injuries, the lens is usually not ruptured, and maintains its normal configuration.

VITREOUS HEMORRHAGE. Vitreous hemorrhage occurs frequently following ocular trauma, and has been discussed previously. To reiterate, light diffuse vitreous hemorrhage is usually sonolucent, although coagulation and clotting accompanying more massive hemorrhage will appear as reflective aggregates. As mentioned, the density, location, and extent of hemorrhage can be well demarcated with the B-scan display. In younger patients with formed vitreous, this demarcation orients the examiner to sites of stress and thus possible retinal tears.

RETINAL DETACHMENT. We have previously dealt with the ultrasonographic appearance of retinal detachment. To summarize, the vitreoretinal interface produces a high-amplitude echo from the

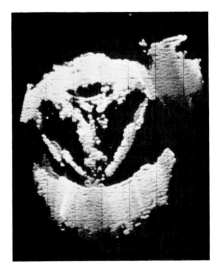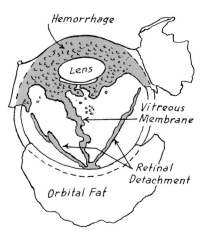

FIG. V-111. B-scan ultrasonogram of a retinal detachment with central vitreous hemorrhage, demonstrating the flat, cord-like appearance seen with old fibrotic retina.

retinal surface, usually allowing identification of this surface in retinal detachment, distinguishing it from hemorrhage along the posterior vitreous membrane caused by trauma. On rapid motion of the eye in kinetic scanning, a retinal detachment will usually move freely but maintain its points of attachment at the ora and the disk. In most situations, lower-amplitude echoes characterize a vitreous veil versus a retinal detachment, but this feature becomes less reliable in long-standing vitreal membranes, where the echo heights may approximate those from the vitreoretinal interface, and absolute differentiation may no longer be possible (Fig. V-111).

SCLERAL INJURY. Ultrasound cannot detect a scleral rupture, but by demonstrating the presence of a hemorrhage in the vitreous and the areas of contiguity between hemorrhage and sclera, such injury may be deduced.[97,98] If rupture at the equator is suspected, the globe should be fully rotated to permit perpendicular examination of this region.

Perforating or Lacerating Wounds

ANTERIOR SEGMENT. As in blunt trauma, hyphema or complete absence of anterior chamber often follows a perforating injury, and can be delineated acoustically.

LENS INJURIES. The interior of the lens is normally sonolucent. Intralenticular echoes can therefore indicate early cataract formation

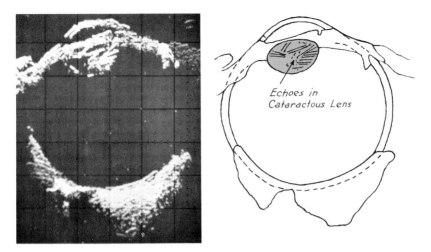

FIG. V-112. B-scan ultrasonogram of a traumatic cataract, demonstrating the acoustic discontinuities from within the lens capsule.

secondary to perforation (Fig. V-112). Knowledge of rupture of the posterior lens capsule with dispersion of lens material into the anterior vitreous (Fig. V-113) can indicate the need for early lens extraction with anterior vitrectomy.

VITREOUS HEMORRHAGE. Perforating injuries into the vitreous nearly always produce vitreous changes visible acoustically. In young individuals, who suffer the majority of traumatized eyes, the solid vitreous permits a track of hemorrhage to be traced through the

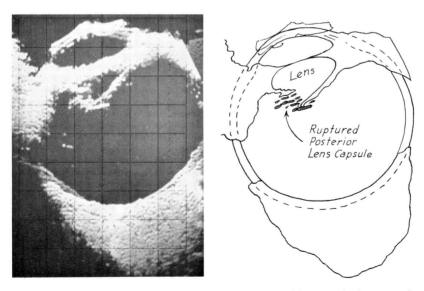

FIG. V-113. B-scan ultrasonogram demonstrating rupture of the posterior lens capsule with evidence of lens material in the anterior vitreous.

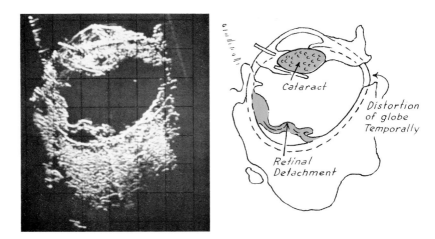

FIG. V-114. B-scan ultrasonogram of a traumatized globe demonstrating a localized retinal detachment and distortion of the globe indicative of possible scleral rupture.

entire vitreous compartment. If this path leads to the posterior globe wall, perforation may be assumed. Surgery can then be directed to the correct quadrant, minimizing unnecessary exploration and reducing the possibility of extrusion of ocular contents through an unidentified posterior laceration. A posterior perforation site can be localized with reference to its distance from the limbus as well as the correct meridian, so that during surgical exploration the wound can be examined and appropriate therapy, such as cryopexy and scleral buckling, can be instituted.

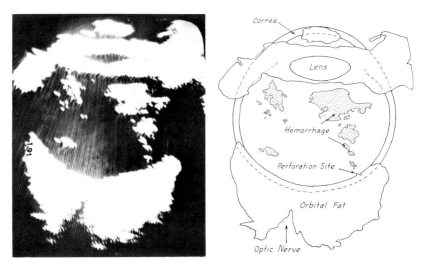

FIG. V-115. A posterior perforation site exemplified by the track of vitreous hemorrhage back to the globe wall. The retina is in place. This ultrasonic finding is useful in orienting the surgeon not only to the quadrant but to the distance back from the limbus, when applying prophylactic retinal surgery to these areas.

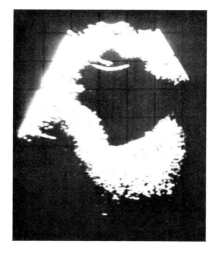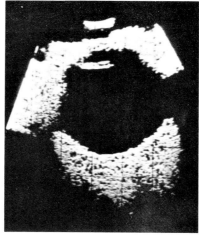

FIG. V-116. *Left:* B-scan ultrasonogram taken one hour following an incision for cataract extraction. The suspected ocular changes (i.e., shallow anterior chamber and choroidal hemorrhage) are confirmed by the ultrasonogram. *Right:* The following day, the ultrasonogram was repeated and demonstrated a settling of the choroidal bulge.

SCLERAL PERFORATION. As noted previously, the presence of scleral rupture may not be ultrasonically noted, but distortion of the globe contour, as seen in Figure V-114, or a path of blood through the vitreous as seen in Figure V-115, can be used to identify the site of perforation.

Surgical perforation of the sclera, which is only rarely complicated by choroidal hemorrhage and anterior dislocation of the vitreous, may necessitate ultrasonic evaluation. Figure V-116 shows an ultrasonogram performed one hour following an incision for cataract extraction. After the initial incision, the lens was noted to bulge anteriorly and an increased vitreous pressure was suspected. The wound was closed without removal of the lens. An ultrasonogram taken shortly thereafter showed a shallow anterior chamber with the lens in place and a marked choroidal bulge at the posterior pole, indicating hyperemia and possible local hemorrhage of the choroid. Ultrasonography was repeated 24 hours later and showed a normal anterior chamber and vitreous compartment. This patient underwent satisfactory intracapsular cataract extraction at a later date.

Foreign Bodies

A major use of ultrasound in ophthalmology has been the localization of intraocular foreign bodies and the determination of their magnetic properties. Bronson[99] has published extensively on the use

INTRAOCULAR FOREIGN BODY
LOCALIZATION
RADIOGRAPHIC-ULTRASONIC

RADIOGRAPHIC LOCALIZATION   RIGHT EYE ☐   LEFT EYE ☐

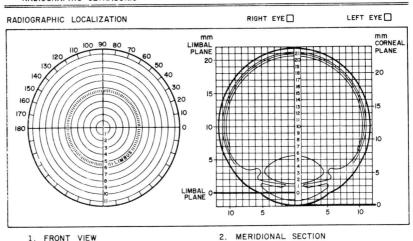

1. FRONT VIEW   2. MERIDIONAL SECTION

ULTRASONIC LOCALIZATION

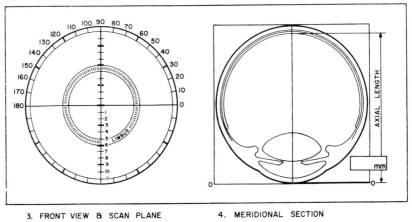

3. FRONT VIEW & SCAN PLANE   4. MERIDIONAL SECTION

Fig. V-117. *A:* Chart used for reporting combined radiographic and ultrasonic localization of foreign bodies. Radiographic localization of a metallic foreign body is advised prior to any attempt at ultrasonic evaluation. The axial length, as determined by ultrasound, combined with radiographic localization will determine whether the foreign body lies in the globe or in the orbit.

of ultrasound for the localization of intraocular foreign bodies and has described an intraocular forceps directed by ultrasound.[9]

RADIOPAQUE FOREIGN BODIES. In evaluating radiopaque foreign bodies, it is essential that the X-ray report be available to the ultrasonographer prior to doing the scan. The number and position of foreign bodies as determined by radiography can be of inestimable help in directing and shortening the ultrasonic evaluation. Figure

RADIOGRAPHIC LOCALIZATION   RIGHT EYE ☐   LEFT EYE ☒

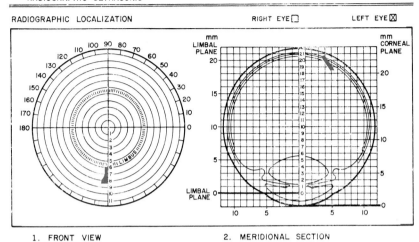

1. FRONT VIEW   2. MERIDIONAL SECTION

ULTRASONIC LOCALIZATION

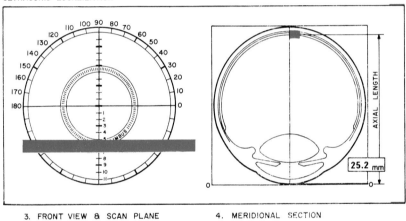
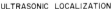

3. FRONT VIEW & SCAN PLANE   4. MERIDIONAL SECTION

FIG. V-117. *B:* Data on a combined foreign body localization entered on the chart. The ultrasonic examination and globe measurement confirmed the intraocular location of the foreign body in an elongated globe.

V-117 shows a report form devised at the E. S. Harkness Eye Institute by Drs. Trokel and Coleman for combined radiographic and ultrasonic localization.[100] The radiographic localization using the Comberg-Pfeiffer technique is presented in the upper portion of the chart. The radiographic position of the foreign body relative to the cornea is enhanced by the ultrasonographic determination of the axial length. The ultrasonic localization in the lower portion of the chart, in addition to confirming the radiography findings, will indicate the position of the foreign body relative to other struc-

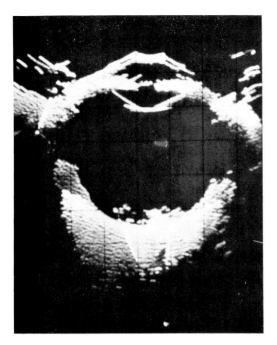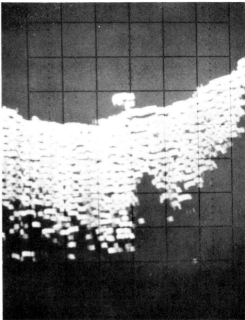

FIG. V-118. *Left:* B-scan ultrasonogram demonstrating a metallic fragment at the back of the eye surrounded by hemorrhage. *Right:* Electronic magnification at a lower sensitivity setting shows the metallic fragment to lie anterior to the retina. Acoustic absorption from the fragment produces shadowing in the orbit, a feature useful in localizing the foreign body.

tures, such as the lens, retina or optic nerve. The magnetic properties of the foreign body may be noted at the bottom of the chart.

Because of the random size and material of foreign bodies, absolute criteria for their identification cannot be supplied. Their distance from the transducer, orientation and acoustic impedance variation from surrounding tissue all affect the reflected echoes. A rigorous, meticulous search for foreign bodies is thus indicated in all cases where they are suspected. Careful B-scan serial sectioning of the globe and increased attention to the amplitude of echoes on the A-scan are essential. The localization of a foreign body and determination of its magnetic properties are therefore far more time consuming than routine ocular diagnosis.

Several acoustic features of metallic foreign bodies are demonstrated by Figure V-118. In this ultrasonogram, a metallic foreign body is located on the retinal surface at the posterior pole. In the left section, which was taken at an increased sensitivity setting, hemorrhage obscures the position of the foreign body. At the right, this same posterior portion of the eye has been electronically expanded and the sensitivity has been reduced so that hemorrhage surrounding the foreign body is not seen. This technique of repeating the serial sectioning at varying sensitivity settings is useful in foreign body localization as it permits distinction of the high-amplitude echoes produced by the foreign body from lower-amplitude echoes produced by the surrounding hemorrhage. This particular ultrasonogram demonstrates two other important acoustic characteristics of metallic foreign bodies:

1. The foreign body tends to absorb sound energy, so that the region posterior to it will appear shadowed, or anechoic. In this photograph, the retrobulbar fat has a wedge-shaped shadow resembling an optic nerve shadow in the region directly posterior to the foreign body.
2. Sound travels faster through metal than through surrounding vitreous. Consequently, the region posterior to the foreign body shows slight prominence of the retina, an artifactual result of the increased transmission velocity of sound through metal. This mound posterior to a foreign body on the retina can be aligned with a shadowed area posteriorly to direct attention to a foreign body.

These features, and additional acoustic characteristics, are of assistance in identifying the position of a foreign body. Figure V-119 shows a foreign body that has penetrated the sclera. Because of the high-amplitude echoes in the surrounding sclera, the foreign body itself cannot be seen here even at lower gain. However, a path of hemorrhage through the vitreous leads to the presumed site of foreign body penetration. A trail of reduplication echoes posterior to mid-vitreal (Fig. V-120) or intrascleral (Fig. V-121) foreign bodies will allow the examiner to trace back to the position of the foreign body. In all cases, the foreign body will produce a high-amplitude spike on

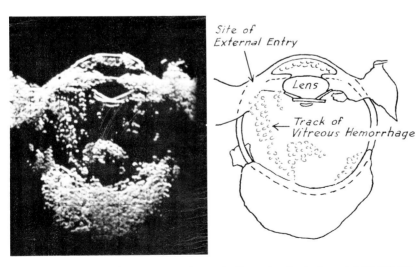

FIG. V-119. B-scan ultrasonogram demonstrating a track of vitreous hemorrhage leading to the presumed site of a posterior perforating injury.

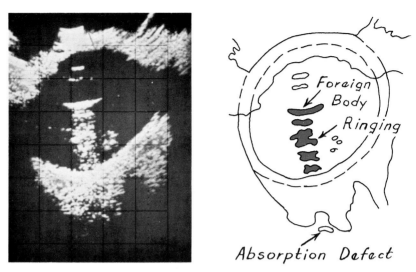

FIG. V-120. B-scan ultrasonogram of an eye containing an intraocular metallic foreign body. The foreign body, indicated by a bright, high-amplitude echo in mid-vitreous, is followed by a dense trail of echoes which are artifactual reduplications.

the A-scan which will maintain its height even at reduced gain (Fig. V-122).

Isometric viewing may be implemented to demonstrate graphically the acoustic characteristics of a foreign body. The color plates show a three-dimensional view of the ultrasonogram of a retrobulbar foreign body. A cursor line, superimposed on this three-dimensional display, indicates the amplitude of echoes in its path, and an isolated high-amplitude spike posterior to the sclera identifies the position of the foreign body.

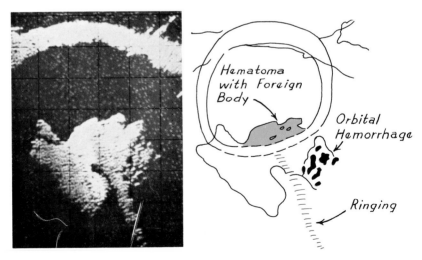

FIG. V-121. The ultrasonic artifact of multiple reduplication echoes or "ringing" helps to localize a metallic foreign body obscured by hemorrhage.

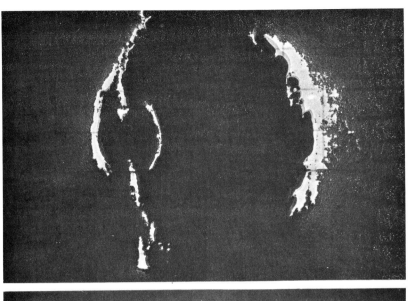

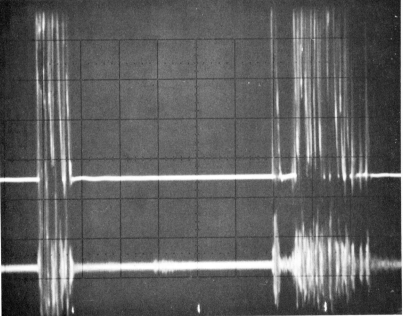

FIG. V-122. B- and A-scans demonstrating a foreign body at the back of the eye. The A-scan pattern shows the characteristic high-amplitude echoes returned from metallic or glass foreign bodies which may approach or exceed the echo amplitude of the vitreoretinal interface.

MAGNETIC FOREIGN BODIES. The magnet test during ultrasonic examination is one of the most useful preoperative studies in the evaluation of foreign bodies. The test was initially described independently by Purnell[25] and by Penner and Passmore,[21] and utilizes ultrasonic display of the motion of the foreign body induced by a

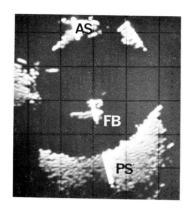

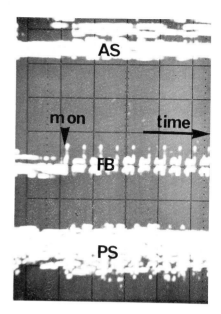

Fig. V-123. B- and M-scans of an intraocular foreign body surrounded by blood. The response of the foreign body to a pulsating magnetic field is demonstrated by the aberrations on the M-scan. (M = magnet, AS = anterior segment, PS = posterior segment, FB = foreign body.)

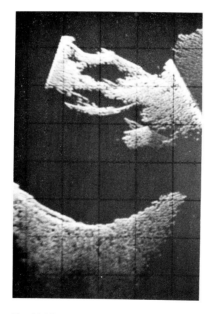

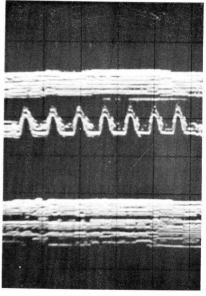

Fig. V-124. M-scans of an intraocular foreign body showing the velocity and rate of motion as well as the rate of recoil to the initial position. The magnet should be positioned relatively far from the globe at the initiation of the test, so that introduction of the magnetic field will not pull the foreign body unexpectedly into the ocular wall or into the lens.

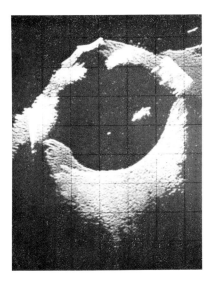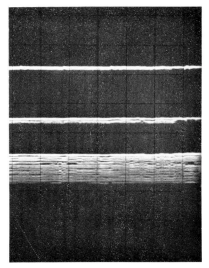

Fig. V-125. M-scan ultrasonogram of an intraocular foreign body of nonmagnetic composition. Upon introduction of a magnetic field, no motion of the foreign body is seen.

magnet; it is usually performed with the A-scan as a simple visual correlation. We prefer the use of the M-scan as it provides the most graphic way of demonstrating movement of foreign bodies.

We use a Bronson-Magnion pulsed magnet, so that the easily recognized pulsating movement of the foreign body can be related to the lack of response from the surrounding tissue structures (Fig. V-123). The magnet should be placed in position over the pars plana so that any induced motion of the foreign body will not displace it into the lens or other delicate ocular structures. The magnet should be turned on while positioned well away from the eye, so that there is minimum excursion. It is drawn closer to the eye until motion of the foreign body is seen on the M-scan or the A-scan. The M-scan can demonstrate the velocity of movement, the amount of excursion and the recoil of the foreign body to its original position (Fig. V-124). A nonmagnetic foreign body will not produce any motion on the M-scan (Fig. V-125). These graphs, in conjunction with the suspected mass of the foreign body as determined by X-ray, can indicate the likelihood of successful magnetic extraction as well as direct the optimum position for surgical incision, whether at the pars plana or directly over the foreign body.

RADIOLUCENT FOREIGN BODIES. Suspected foreign bodies of glass, plastic, wood and other nonradiopaque materials require careful serial sectioning for ultrasonic localization. Glass or plastics, particularly when discrete surfaces are present, can be well visualized

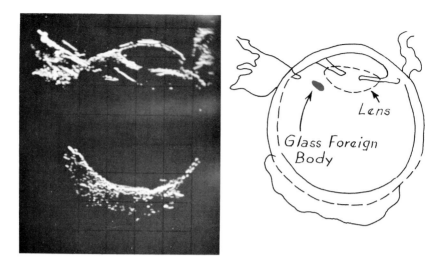

Fig. V-126. A radiolucent glass foreign body seen behind the lens. The relation of the foreign body to lens and globe wall was uniquely portrayed with ultrasound as blood had obscured this foreign body to visual evaluation.

ultrasonically. Figure V-126 shows a piece of glass posterior to the lens, underlying the ciliary body. In general, glass, plastics or wood material do not have the mass and velocity to penetrate deeply into the eye and are usually seen in the anterior chamber, the lens or anterior vitreous. We have found it difficult or impossible to localize small pieces of glass in the sclera, angle or cataractous lens. Occasionally, when previous radiographic localization has been performed, a foreign body can be located within the lens but, because of the layered structure of the lens, traumatic separation of planes may make it difficult to absolutely distinguish tissue planes from intralenticular foreign bodies. Except for wood, these materials are usually inert and the reduced efficacy of ultrasound in these situations is less critical than it would be in the identification of metallic materials.

The uses of ultrasound in foreign body managment are summarized in Table V-5.

TABLE V-5   Uses of Ultrasound in Intraocular Foreign Body Management

Foreign body localization
Axial length measurements to augment X-ray localization
Assessment of associated globe damage
Determination of magnetic properties using pulsed magnet
Extraction of nonmagnetic foreign bodies using ultrasonic data

1. Mundt, G. H., and Hughes, W.: Ultrasonics in ocular diagnosis. Am. J. Oph-thalmol., 41:488–498, 1956.
2. Oksala, A., and Lehtinen, A.: Diagnostic value of ultrasonics in ophthalmology. Ophthalmologica, 134:387–395, 1957
3. Jansson, F.: Measurement of intraocular distances by ultrasound and compari-son between optical and ultrasonic determinations of the depth of the anterior chamber. Acta Ophthalmol., 41:25–61, 1963.
4. Jansson, F.: Measurements of intraocular distances by ultrasound. Acta Oph-thalmol. (Suppl.), 74:1–51, 1963.
5. Oksala, A., and Lehtinen, A.: Measurement of the velocity of sound in some parts of the eye. Acta Ophthalmol., 36:633–639, 1958.
6. Baum, G., and Greenwood, I.: The application of ultrasonic locating techniques to ophthalmology. Part I. Reflective properties. Am. J. Ophthalmol., 46:319–329, 1958.
7. Coleman, D. J., and Weininger, R.: Ultrasonic M-mode technique in ophthalmol-ogy. Arch. Ophthalmol., 82:475–479, 1969.
8. Oksala, A.: The echogram in the diagnosis of eye diseases. Klin. Monatsbl. Augenheilkd., 137:72–87, 1960.
9. Bronson, N. R.: Techniques of ultrasonic localization and extraction of intra-ocular and extraocular foreign bodies. Am. J. Ophthalmal., 60:596–603, 1965.
10. Ossoinig, K.: Clinical echo-ophthalmology, In: Current Concepts of Ophthalmol-ogy, Vol. III, St. Louis, C. V. Mosby Co., 1972, pp. 101–130.
11. Ossoinig, K.: The evaluation of kinetic properties of echo signals. In: Ultrasonics in Ophthalmology. Edited by A. Oksala, and H. Gernet. Basel, S. Karger, 1967, pp. 88–96.
12. Buschmann, W., and Staudt, J.: Fundamentals of echographic differential diagnosis. In: Ultrasonographia Medica (SIDUO III). Edited by J. Bock and K. Ossoinig. Vienna, Verlag der Weiner Med. Akad., 1971, pp. 395–409.
13. Gernet, H., and Franceschetti, A.: Ultrasound biometry of the eye (review). In: Ultrasonics in Ophthalmology. Edited by A. Oksala and H. Gernet, Basel, S. Karger, 1967, pp. 175–200.
14. Massin, M., and Poujol, J.: Clinical value of time-amplitude ultrasonography in 1,000 patients. In: Ophthalmic Ultrasound. Edited by K. Gitter et al. St. Louis, C. V. Mosby Co., 1969, pp. 306–310.
15. Francois, J., Goes, F., and Yobbagyi, P.: Ultrasonic echography in ophthalmol-ogy. Ann. Ocul., 201:609–645, 1968.
16. Vanysek, J., Preisova, J., and Obraz, J.: Ultrasonography in Ophthalmology. London, Butterworths, 1969.
17. Bertenyi, A., Betko, J., and Greguss, P.: Comparison between ultrasound and isotope diagnosis of intraocular tumors. In: Ultrasonographia Medica (SIDUO III). Edited by J. Bock and K. Ossoinig, Vienna, Verlag der Weiner Med. Akad., 1971, pp. 291–297.
18. Gallenga, R.: The role of diagnostic ultrasound after nine years of routine clinic. In: Ultrasonographia Medica, (SIDUO III). Edited by J. Bock and K. Ossoinig. Vienna, Verlag der Weiner Med. Akad.. 1971, pp. 313–320.
19. Sarin, L. K., Meyer, D., Gitter, K., and White, R.: The clinical evaluation of the use of ultrasound (A-scan) in 500 patients. In: Diagnostica Ultrasonica in Ophthalmologia (SIDUO II). Edited by J. Vanysek. Brno, University of Brno, 1968, pp. 297–300.
20. Keeney. A. H.: Ultrasound in clinical ophthalmological diagnosis. Trans. Pac. Coast Otoophthalmol. Soc., 48:89, 1967.
21. Penner, R., and Passmore, J. W.: Magnetic vs. nonmagnetic intraocular foreign bodies. An ultrasonic determination. Arch. Ophthalmol., 76:676–677, 1966.
22. Cowden, J. W., and Runyan, T. E.: Localization of intraocular foreign bodies.

Further experiences in ultrasonic vs. radiologic methods. Arch. Ophthalmol., 3:299–301, 1969.

23. Baum, G., and Greenwood, I.: Ultrasonography—an aid in orbital tumor diagnosis. Arch. Ophthalmol., 64:180–194, 1960.

24. Baum, G.: Use of ultrasonography in the differential diagnosis of ocular tumors. *In:* Ocular and Adnexal Tumors. Edited by M. Boniuk. St. Louis, C. V. Mosby Co., 1964, pp. 308–321.

25. Purnell, E. W.: Ultrasound in ophthalmological diagnosis. *In:* Diagnostic Ultrasound. Edited by C. Grossman, et al. New York, Plenum Press, 1966, pp. 95–109.

26. Purnell, E.: Ultrasonic interpretation of orbital disease. *In:* Ophthalmic Ultrasound. Edited by K. Gitter, et al. St. Louis, C. V. Mosby Co., 1969, pp. 249–255.

27. Purnell, E. W., et al.: The production of focal chorioretinitis by ultrasound. A preliminary report. Am. J. Ophthalmol., 58:953–957, 1964.

28. Purnell, E.: Therapeutic use of ultrasound. *In:* Ultrasonics in Ophthalmology. Edited by R. Goldberg and L. Sarin. Philadelphia, W. B. Saunders, 1967, pp. 145–149.

29. Holasek, E., and Sokollu, A.: Direct contact, hand held, diagnostic B-scanner. Proceedings IEEE Ultrasonics Symposium, 1972.

30. Coleman, D. J., Konig, W. F., and Katz, L.: A hand operated ultrasound scan system for ophthalmic evaluation. Am. J. Ophthalmol., 68:256–263, 1969.

31. Coleman, D. J.: Reliability of ocular and orbital diagnosis with B-scan ultrasound. Part 1: Ocular diagnosis. Am. J. Ophthalmol., 73:501–516, 1972.

32. Coleman, D. J.: Reliability of ocular and orbital diagnosis with B-scan ultrasound. Part II: Orbital diagnosis. Am. J. Ophthalmol., 74:708–718, 1972.

33. Coleman, D. J., and Katz, L.: Color-coding of B-scan ultrasonograms. Arch. Ophthalmol., 91:429–431, 1974.

34. Coleman, D. J., Katz, L., and Lizzi, F.: Isometric, three-dimensional viewing of ultrasonograms. Arch. Ophthalmol., 93:1362–1367, 1976.

35. Kossoff, G., and Robinson, D. E.: The C.A.L. ultrasonic echoscope for ophthalmological investigations. J. Coll. Radiol. Aust., 9:168–173, 1965.

36. Bronson, N. R.: Development of a simple B-scan ultrasonoscope. Trans. Am. Ophthalmol. Soc., 70:365–408, 1972.

37. Coleman, D. J., Jack, R. L., and Franzen, L. A.: Ultrasonography in ocular trauma. Am. J. Ophthalmol., 75:279–288, 1973.

38. Coleman, D. J.: Measurement of choroidal pulsation with M-scan ultrasound. Am. J. Ophthalmol., 71:363–365, 1971.

39. Baum, G., and Greenwood, I.: The application of ultrasonic locating techniques in ophthalmology, Part II. Ultrasonic slit lamp in the ultrasonic visualization of soft tissues. Arch. Ophthalmol., 60:263–279, 1958.

40. Oksala, A., and Varonen, E.-R.: The influence of the eyeball on the ultrasonic field of the transducer and its diagnostic significance. Acta Ophthalmol., 43:268–271, 1965.

41. Kossoff, G.: Ultrasonic visualization system. *In:* Ophthalmic Ultrasound. Edited by K. Gitter, et al. St. Louis, C. V. Mosby Co., 1969, pp. 27–37.

42. Baum, G.: An evaluation of ultrasonic techniques. Am. J. Ophthalmol., 64:926–936, 1967.

43. Coleman, D. J., Jack, R. L., and Cardona, H.: Ultrasonic evaluation of eyes with keratoprosthesis. Am. J. Ophthalmol., 74:543–554, 1972.

44. Oksala, A.: Acoustic structure of the opaque and of the transparent lens. Klin. Monatsbl. Augenheilkd., 138:374–380, 1961.

45. Metz, G., and Bronson, N.: Ultrasound appearance of senile lens changes. *In:* Ophthalmic Ultrasound. Edited by K. Gitter, et al. St. Louis, C. V. Mosby Co., 1969, pp. 218–223.

46. Cibis, P.: Vitreoretinal Pathology and Surgery in Retinal Detachment. St. Louis, C. V. Mosby Co., 1965.

47. Cibis, P. A., and Yamashita, T.: Experimental aspects of ocular siderosis and hemosiderosis. Am. J. Ophthalmol., 48:465–480, 1958.

48. Regnault, F. R.: Vitreous hemorrhage: An experimental study. Arch. Ophthalmol., 83:458–465, 1970.

49. Oksala, A., and Lehtinen, A.: Investigation on the structure of the vitreous body by ultrasound., Am. J. Ophthalmol., 46:361–366, 1958.

50. Coleman, D. J., and Franzen, L. A.: Vitreous surgery- pre-operative evaluation and prognostic value of ultrasonic display of vitreous hemorrhage. Arch. Ophthalmol., 92:375–381, 1974.

51. Goldberg, R. E., et al.: Application of ultrasonography in ophthalmology. Trans. Am. Acad. Ophthalmol. Otolaryngol., 71:880–888, 1967.

52. Jaffe, N.: The Vitreous in Clinical Ophthalmology. St. Louis, C. V. Mosby Co., 1969.

53. Oksala, A.: The echogram in vitreous opacities. Am. J. Ophthalmol., 49:1301–1307, 1960.

54. Coleman, D. J.: Ultrasound in vitreous surgery. Trans. Am. Acad. Ophthalmol. Otolaryngol., 76:467–479, 1972.

55. Jack, R. L., Hutton, W. L., and Machemer, R.: Ultrasonography and vitrectomy. Am. J. Ophthalmol., 78:265–274, 1974.

56. Oksala, A., and Lehtinen, A.: Diagnostics of detachment of the retina by means of ultrasound. Acta Ophthalmol., 35:461–467, 1957.

57. Baum, G.: Problems in ultrasonographic diagnosis of retinal disease. Am. J. Ophthalmol., 71:723–739, 1971.

58. Coleman, D. J., and Jack, R. L.: B-scan ultrasonography in the diagnosis and management of retinal detachments. Arch. Ophthalmol., 90:29–34, 1973.

59. Boniuk, M., and Zimmerman, L. E.: Problems in differentiating idiopathic serous detachments from solid retinal detachments. Int. Ophthalmol. Clin., 2:411, 1962.

60. Norton, E. W.: Differential diagnosis of retinal detachment. *In:* Symposium on Retina and Retinal Surgery. Edited by W. Cockerham, et al. St. Louis, C. V. Mosby Co., 1969, p. 56.

61. Boniuk, M., and Zimmerman, L. E.: Occurrence and behavior of choroidal melanomas in eyes subjected to operations for retinal detachment. Trans. Am. Acad. Ophthalmol. Otolaryngol., 66:642, 1962.

62. Deneuville, J. P.: Diagnosis of melanoma of the choroid—is it always easy? Ann. Ocul., 201:45, 1968.

63. Reese, A. B.: Pigment freckles of the iris (benign melanomas): Their significance in relation to malignant melanoma of the uvea. Am. J. Ophthalmol., 27:217, 1944.

64. Reese, A. B.: Tumors of the Eye, 2nd ed. New York, Harper and Row, 1963, pp. 84–161.

65. Howard, G. M.: Erroneous clinical diagnosis of retinoblastoma and uveal melanoma. Trans. Am. Acad. Ophthalmol. Otolaryngol., 73:199, 1969.

66. Stafford, W. R., Yanoff, M., and Parnell, B. L.: Retinoblastoma initially mis-diagnosed as primary ocular inflammation. Arch. Ophthalmol., 82:771, 1969.

67. Howard, G. M., and Ellsworth, R. M.: Differential diagnosis of retinoblastoma. A statistical survey of 500 children. Am. J. Opthalmol., 60:610, 1965.

68. Oksala, A.: The echogram in retinoblastoma. Acta Ophthalmol., 37:132–137, 1959.

69. Fridman, F. E., and Khvatova, A. V.: The use of ultrasonic echography in the diagnosis of retinoblastoma. Vestn. Oftalmol., 82:73, 1969.

70. Sezer, N., and Barishak, R.: The diagnosis of retinoblastomas. Ophthalmologica, 151:184–195, 1966.

71. Bellone, G., and Gallenga, P. E.: Diagnostic echography of retinoblastoma. Arch. Rass. Ital. Ottal., 4:241–248, 1970–71.

72. Till, P., and Ossoinig, K.: Echography of retinoblastoma. Ber. Dtsch. Ophthalmol. Ges., 69:203–209, 1969.

73. Sterns, G. K., Coleman, D. J., and Ellsworth, R. M.: The ultrasonographic characteristics of retinoblastoma. Am. J. Ophthalmol., 78:606–611, 1974.

74. Schepens, C. L.: Discussion. *In:* Controversial Aspects of the Management of Retinal Detachment. Edited by C. Schepens and C. Regan. Boston, Little, Brown and Co., 1965, p. 315.

75. Reese, A.: Tumors of the Eye, 2nd ed., New York, Harper and Row, 1963, p. 269.

76. Norton, E. W., and Gutman, F.: Fluorescein angiography and hemangiomas of the choroid. Arch. Ophthalmol., 78:121–125, 1967.

77. Shields, J. A., and Font, R. L.: Melanocytoma of the choroid clinically simulating a malignant melanoma. Arch. Ophthalmol., 87:396–400, 1972.

78. Naumann, G., Zimmerman, L. E., and Yanoff, M.: Visual field defect associated with choroidal nevus. Am. J. Ophthalmol., 62:914–917, 1966.

79. Tamler, E., and Maumenee, A. E.: Clinical study of choroidal nevi. Arch. Ophthalmol., 62:196–202, 1959.

80. Terner, I. S., Leopold, I. H., and Eisenberg, I. J.: The radioactive phosphorus (P32) uptake test in opththalmology: A review of the literature and analysis of results in 262 cases of ocular and adnexal pathology. Arch. Ophthalmol., 55:52–53, 1956.

81. Dunn, A., and McTigue, J. W.: The radioactive phosphorus uptake test for malignant melanoma of the eye: A study of 40 consecutive cases of suspected intraocular malignant melanoma. Arch. Ophthalmol., 57:668–671, 1957.

82. Oksala, A.: Echogram in melanoma of the choroid. Br. J. Ophthalmol., 43:408–414, 1959.

83. Oksala, A.: Ultrasound diagnosis in intraocular melanoma. Ann. N.Y. Acad. Sci., 100:18–27, 1963.

84. Ossoinig, K., and Till, P.: Methods and results of ultrasonography in diagnosing intraocular tumors. *In:* Ophthalmic Ultrasound. Edited by K. Gitter, et al. St. Louis, C. V. Mosby Co., 1969, pp. 294–300.

85. Poujol, J.: Clinical echography in intraocular tumors. *In:* Ultrasonographia Medica (SIDUO III). Edited by J. Bock and K. Ossoinig. Vienna, Verlag der Weiner Med. Akad., 1971, pp. 275–290.

86. Baum, G.: Ultrasonic characteristics of malignant melanoma. Arch. Ophthalmol., 78:12–15, 1967.

87. Coleman, D. J., Abramson, D. H., Jack, R. L., and Franzen, L. A.: Ultrasonic diagnosis of tumors of the choroid. Arch. Ophthalmol., 91:344–354, 1974.

88. Mackley T. A., and Teed, R. W.: Unsuspected intraocular malignant melanomas. Arch. Ophthalmol., 60:475–478, 1958.

89. Ferry, A. P.: Lesions mistaken for malignant melanoma of the posterior uvea: A clinico-pathologic analysis of 100 cases with ophthalmoscopically visible lesions. Arch. Ophthalmol., 72:463–469, 1964.

90. Coleman, D. J., and Abramson, D. H.: Correlation of ultrasonic characteristics and tissue morphology of malignant melanoma. *In:* Diagnostica Ultrasonica in Ophthalmologia. Edited by M. Massin and J. Poujol. Paris, Centre National d'Ophtalmologie des Quinze-Vingts, 1973, pp. 215–218.

91. Coleman, D. J.: Reliability of ocular tumor diagnosis with ultrasound. Trans. Am. Acad. Ophthalmol. Otolaryngol., 77:677–683, 1973.

92. Reese, A.: Tumors of the Eye, 2nd ed. New York, Harper and Row, 1963, p. 292.

93. Ferry, A. P.: Lesions mistaken for malignant melanoma of the posterior uvea: A clinico-pathologic analysis of 100 cases with ophthalmoscopically visible lesions. Arch. Ophthalmol., 72:463–469, 1964.

94. Forbes, M., and Coleman, D. J.: Ultrasonography in management of the postoperative flat chamber. Presented at the American Medical Association, Section on Ophthalmology, June 1973.

95. Chandler, P., and Grant, M.: Lectures on Glaucoma. Philadelphia, Lea and Febiger, 1965.

96. Simmons, R. J.: Malignant glaucoma. Br. J. Ophthalmol., 56:263–272, 1972.

97. Oksala, A., and Lehtinen, A.: Diagnostics of rupture of the sclera by means of ultrasound. Acta Ophthalmol., 36:37–42, 1958.
98. Freyler, H.: Ultrasonic studies in experimental scleral rupture. *In:* Ultrasonographia Medica (SIDUO III). Edited by J. Bock and K. Ossoinig. Vienna, Verlag der Weiner Med. Akad., 1971, pp. 167–178.
99. Bronson, N. R.: Management of foreign bodies. Am. J. Ophthalmol., 66:279–284, 1968.
100. Coleman, D. J., and Trokel, S.: Improved foreign body localization with combined radiographic and ultrasound methods. *In:* Ultrasonographia Medica (SIDUO III). Edited by J. Bock and K. Ossoinig. Vienna, Verlag der Weiner Med. Akad., 1971, pp. 265–269.

Additional References

Lens

Gernet, H., and Schneller, E.: The question of absorption and refraction of ultrasonic waves by the lens. *In:* Ultrasonics in Ophthalmology. Edited by A. Oksala and H. Gernet. Basel, S. Karger, 1967, pp. 110–115.
Lavine, O., and Langerstrass, K. H.: Ultrasound in cataract research. Br. J. Phys. Med., 16:159–162, 1953.
Leverè, P., and Cazalis, R.: Ultrasonics in failure of simple discission for congenital cataract. J. Radiol. Electrol. Med. Nucl., 35:502–503, 1954.
Macoul, K. L.: Dislocated lens simulating retinal detachment by ultrasonography. Arch. Ophthalmol., 80:724–726, 1968.
Minix, M. B.: Dislocation of lens—Diagnosis by ultrasonography. J.A.M.A., 207:1354, 1969.
Oguchi, Y., and van Marle, G.: Study of the ultrasonic characteristics of the lens. *In:* Ultrasonography in Ophthalmology. Edited by J. Francois and F. Goes. Basel, S. Karger, 1975, pp. 252–258.
Oksala, A., and Varonen, E.-R.: The effect of the lens on the ultrasonic field in diagnosis of the eye by ultrasound. Acta Ophthalmol., 43:260–267, 1965.
Oksala, A., and Varonen, E.-R.: The echogram of the normal and opaque lens. Acta Ophthalmol., 43:273–280, 1965.
Ursin, K. V.: Ultrasonographic examination of the vitreous body before cataract extraction. Duodecim, 80:422–424, 1964.

Vitreous

Bellone, G., and Gallenga, P.: Congenital malformation of the vitreous body. Echographic and biomicroscope study. Arch. Rass. Ital. Ottal., 37:160, 1969.
Bellone, G., and Gallenga, P. E.: A new method of treatment by A-scan echography of the vitreous. Arch. Rass. Ital. Ottal., 1:169–177, 1970.
Bellone, G., and Gallenga, P.: Ultrasonic features of changes in the vitreous body caused by degenerative, inflammatory, vascular amd deforming disease of the eye. *In:* Ultrasonographia Medica (SIDUO III). Edited by J. Bock and K. Ossoinig. Vienna, Verlag der Weiner Med. Akad., 1971, pp. 229–246.
Czerek-Jaguczanska, H., and Czerek, K.: An analysis of vitreous hemorrhage with the use of ultrasound. Klin. Oczna, 36:343–344, 1966.
Freeman, H. M.: The lens and the vitreous. Arch. Ophthalmol., 82:551, 1969.
Gallenga, P.: Echographic classification of diseases of the vitreous body. *In:* Diagnostica Ultrasonica in Ophthalmologia (SIDUO IV). Edited by M. Massin and J. Poujol. Paris, Centre National d'Ophtalmologie des Quinze-Vingts, 1973, pp. 163–168.

Gartner, J., et al.: On changes in the vitreous body during aging. Studies using ultrasonics Graefe. Arch. Klin. Exp. Ophthalmol., 173:282–292, 1967.

Gartner, J., and Lopping, B.: Vitreous body in systemic connective tissue changes. Studies using ultrasonics. Ber. Dtsch. Ophthalmol. Ges., 68:40, 1968.

Gernet, H.: Discussion of the paper: Biology and surgery of the vitreous body. Bull. Mem. Soc. Fr. Ophtalmol., 81:44–48, 1968.

Jack, R., and Machemer, R.: Ultrasonic preoperative examination for vitrectomy. *In:* Diagnostica Ultrasonica in Ophthalmologia (SIDUO V). Basel, S. Karger, in press.

Lopping, B., Maratos, P., and Nover, A.: Echographic studies of the vitreous in primary chronic polyarthritis. *In:* Ultrasonographia Medica (SIDUO III). Edited by J. Bock and K. Ossoinig. Vienna, Verlag der Weiner Med. Akad. 1971, pp. 255–258.

Massin, M., and Poujol, J.: Ultrasonic examination of the vitreous body. Bull. Mem. Soc. Fr. Ophtalmol., 81:63–73, 1968.

Nover A., et al.: Ultrasonic studies of the vitreous body of healthy and diseased eyes. Klin. Monatsbl. Augenheilkd., 152:639–48, 1968.

Oksala, A., and Lehtinen, A.: Experimental researches on vitreous hemorrhages and on the echo gram emitted by them. Acta Ophthalmol., 37:17–25, 1959.

Oksala, A.: Experimental and clinical observations on the echograms in vitreous hemorrhages. Br. J. Ophthalmol., 47:65–70, 1963.

Oksala, A., and Mäntyjärvi, M.: Experimental researches on difficulties of pathological echograms due to vitreous haemorrhages. Acta Ophthalmol., 42:503–513, 1964.

Oksala, A., and Lunden, P.: Experimental researches on the significance of the interference field of the crystal in the ultrasonic diagnosis of vitreous opacities and of tumor. Acta Ophthalmol., 42:211–218, 1964.

Perez-Llorca, J.: The appearance of the echoes in the anterior vitreous of the normal eye: their frequency and characteristics. *In:* Diagnostica Ultrasonica in Ophthalmologia (SIDUO IV). Edited by M. Massin and J. Poujol. Paris, Centre National de'Ophtalmalogie des Quinze-Vingts, 1973, pp. 173–174.

Ricci, A., and Itin, W.: Echographic studies of vitreo-retinal degenerations. Bull. Mem. Soc. Fr. Ophtalmol., 79:446–453, 1966.

Rossi, A., and Gallenga, P.: Ultrasonographic features of the senile vitreous body. *In:* Ultrasonographia Medica (SIDUO III). Edited by J. Bock and K. Ossoinig. Vienna, Verlag der Weiner Med. Akad., 1971, pp. 247–254.

Rousselie, F., Clay, C., and Karantinos, D.: Intra-vitreous hemorrhages and echography. Arch. Ophtalmol., 31:399–412, 1971.

Schum, U.: Ultrasonic diagnosis of the area of the vitreous body. Ophthalmologica, 159:239–245, 1969.

Schum, U., and Mueller-Jensen, K.: Ultrasonic results with artificial vitreous implants. *In:* Ophthalmic Ultrasound. Edited by K. Gitter, et al. St. Louis, C. V. Mosby Co., 1969, pp. 224–226.

Schum, U.: Ultrasonic diagnosis of the vitreous. *In:* Ultrasonographia Medica (SIDUO III). Edited by J. Bock and K. Ossoinig. Vienna, Verlag der Weiner Med. Akad., 1971, pp. 299–306.

Simbinova, R. M.: A study of echographic changes during hemorrhages into the vitreous body under experimental and clinical conditions. Vestn. Oftalmol., 1:59–62, 1971.

Tane, S., Funahashi, T., and Horiuchi, T.: Studies on an ultrasonic diagnosis in ophthalmology. Report 3. An ultrasound technique for the vitreous body of healthy and affected eyes. Folia Ophthalmol. Jap., 22:79–85, 1971.

Tane, S., and Horiuchi, T.: Ultrasonic diagnosis of vitreous body opacity. Ophthalmology (Tokyo), 13:511, 1971.

Tane, S.: The studies on the ultrasonic diagnosis in ophthalmology. The quantitative ultrasono-tomography in intravitreal hemorrhages. Acta Soc. Ophthalmol. Jap., 76:1318–1325, 1972.

Ursin, K. V.: Prognosis of intravitreal hemorrhages—ultrasound studies. *In:* Ultrasonics in Ophthalmology. Edited by A. Oksala and H. Gernet. Basel, S. Karger, 1967, pp. 161–166.

Ursin, K. V.: Ultrasound studies on changes in the vitreous body after contusion: a preliminary report. *In:* Ophthalmic Ultrasound. Edited by K. Gitter, et al. St. Louis, C. V. Mosby Co., 1969, pp. 227–230.

Yamamoto, Y., Kaburagi, H., Hikawa, T., and Sueno, M.: Echogram in the diagnosis of vitreous hemorrhage. Jap. J. Clin. Ophthalmol., 25:1385–1930, 1971.

Yamamoto, Y.: Ultrasono-tomography and treatment of vitreous hemorrhage. *In:* Diagnostica Ultrasonica in Ophthalmologia (SIDUO IV). Edited by M. Massin and J. Poujol. Paris, Centre National d'Ophtalmologie des Quinze-Vingts, 1973, pp. 175–178.

Retinal and Choroidal Detachments

Alajmo, A.: Usefulness of ultrasound in the diagnosis of retinal detachment. Atti Soc. Oftal. Ital., 20:335–336, 1962.

Alekseev, B. N.: Ultrasonic echography in surgery for retinal detachment. Vestn. Oftalmol., 2:15–19, 1973.

Araki, M.: Diagnosis of retinal detachment by ultrasonic examination. Acta Soc. Ophthalmol. Jap., 66:46–52, 1962.

Bertenyi, A.: Preparation for surgery for retinal detachment using ultrasound. Wiss. Z. Humboldt Univ. Berlin [Math. Naturwiss.], 14:199, 1965.

Carlin, D.: Ultrasound in retinal detachment surgery. J. Audio Eng. Soc., 19:20–23, 1971.

Dyszynska-Rosciszewska, B., and Szreterowa, M.: Ultrasonic studies in patients with retinal detachment. Klin Oczna, 42:37–44, 1972.

Freyler, H.: Echography of hemorrhagic choroidal detachment. *In:* Diagnostica Ultrasonica in Ophtalmalogia (SIDUO IV). Edited by M. Massin and J. Poujol. Paris, Centre National d'Ophtalmologie des Quinze-Vingts, 1973, pp. 189–194.

Gernet, H.: On relative and absolute frequency of retinal detachment in myopia. Klin. Monatsbl. Augenheilkd, 149:545–550, 1966.

Hillman, J. S.: An assessment of ultrasonography in retinal detachment and retinoschisis. *In:* Ultrasonography in Ophthalmology. Edited by J. Francois and F. Goes. Basel, S. Karger, 1975, pp. 63–67.

Jack, R. L., and Coleman, D. J.: Diagnosis of retinal detachments with B-scan ultrasound. Can. J. Ophthalmol., 8:10–18, 1973.

Lopping, B., and Nover, A.: Experimental ultrasonic studies in primary and secondary retinal detachment. Graefe. Arch. Ophthalmol., 165:585–594, 1963.

Nónay, T., Bertényi, A., and Greguss, P.: Choroidal detachments in cases of retinal detachment demonstrated by ultrasound. *In:* Ophthalmic Ultrasound. Edited by K. Gitter, et al. St. Louis, C. V. Mosby Co., 1969, pp. 256–259.

Offret, G., and Rousselie, F.: Diagnosis and surveillance of retinal detachment by means of time amplitude ultrasonography. *In:* Ophthalmic Ultrasound. Edited by K. Gitter, et al. St. Louis, C. V. Mosby Co., 1969, pp. 260–268.

Oksala, A.: Observations on choroidal detachment by means of ultrasound Acta Ophthalmol., 36:651–657, 1958.

Oksala, A.: The echogram in detachment of the retina. Ophthalmologica, 138:350–361, 1959.

Oksala, A.: The echogram in exudative retinitis in Coats' disease. Acta Ophthalmol., 38:364–371, 1960.

Oksala, A.: The echogram in postoperative choroidal detachment. Acta Ophthalmol., 40:475–479, 1962.

Oksala, A.: Ultrasonography in the diagnosis of retinal detachment. Bibl. Ophthalmol., 72:218, 1967.

Oksala, A., and Koponen, J.: Choroidal detachment associated with scleritis—A case report with echograms. Ultrasound Med. Biol., 1:283–285, 1974.

Ossoinig, K. C.: Clinical value of echography in traumatic retinal detachment. Mod. Probl. Ophthalmol., 10:437–42, 1972.

Sanna, G., and Rivara, A.: Differential diagnosis of idiopathic retinal detachment and secondary retinal detachment with the aid of ultrasonics. Ann. Ottal., 89:572–580, 1963.

Schupbach, M.: Ultrasonic diagnosis of retinal detachment. Mod. Probl. Ophthalmol., 10:443–448, 1972.

Till, P., and Ossoinig, K.: Echographic findings in proliferative retinopathy. Klin. Monatsbl. Augenheilkd., 161:297–301, 1972.

Ulrich, C.: Reliability of ultrasonic diagnosis of retinal and choroidal detachment. Wiss. Z. Humboldt Univ. Berlin [Math. Naturwiss.], 14:175–178, 1965.

Intraocular Tumors

Araki, M., Takano, Y., and Honmura, S.: Diagnosis of ocular tumors by ultrasonic examination. Acta Soc. Ophthalmol. Jap., 69:2043–2051, 1965.

Baum, G.: Ultrasonic characteristics of malignant melanoma. In: Ultrasonics in Ophthalmology. Edited by A. Oksala and H. Gernet, Basel, S. Karger, 1967, 22–26.

Bertenyi, A.: Ultrasonography of Intra-ocular tumours. Arch. Rass. Ital. Ottal., 1:81–89, 1970.

Bigar, F., Kaefring, S., and Ossoinig, K. C.: Malignant melanoma of the choroid and ciliary body. A differential diagnosis in clinical echography. In: Ultrasonography in Ophthalmology. Edited by J. Francois and F. Goes. Basel, S. Karger, 1975, pp. 141–154.

Bock, J., and Ossoinig, K.: The correlation between histological structure and the echogram as the basis of non-operative tissue differentiation. Klin. Monatsbl. Augenheilkd., 155:687–695, 1969.

Buschmann, W.: Ultrasonic diagnosis of intraocular tumors. Wiss. Z. Humboldt Univ. Berlin [Math. Naturwiss.], 14:163–167, 1965.

Buschmann, W.: Clinical results and methodological advances in echographic diagnosis of intraocular tumors. Klin. Monatsbl. Augenheilkd., 148:625–641, 1966.

Buschmann, W., Lommatzech, P., Goder, G., and Brausewetter, K.: New examination methods in diagnosis of intraocular tumors. Klin. Monatsbl. Augenheilkd., 152:73–79, 1968.

Czerek-Jaguczanska, H.: Clinical application of echogram in retinal detachment and intrabulbar tumors. Wiss. Z. Humboldt Univ. Berlin [Math. Naturwiss.], 14:151–153, 1965.

Dadd, M. J., Hughes, H. L., and Kossoff, G.: Ultrasonic characteristics of choroidal melanoma. In: Ultrasonography in Ophthalmology. Edited by J. Francois and F. Goes. Basel, S. Karger, 1975, pp. 155–162.

Desvignes, P., Haut, J., and Legras, M.: Pseudo-melanosarcoma of the choroid. Bull. Soc. Ophtalmol. Fr., 68:545–550, 1968.

Dyszynska-Rosciszewska, B., and Szreterowa, M.: Diagnosis of intraocular tumors by means of ultrasound (system A). Klin. Oczna, 42:709–15, 1972.

Gitter, K. A., and Annesley, W. H.: Recognition of a case of choroidal melanoma by ultrasound. Arch. Ophthalmol., 78:358–359, 1967.

Gitter, K. A., Meyer, D., and Sarin, L. K.: Fluorescein and ultrasound in diagnosis of intraocular tumors. Am. J. Ophthalmol., 66:719, 1968.

Hildebrandt, I.: Ultrasonic diagnosis of the course of light coagulated intraocular tumors. Wiss. Z. Humboldt Univ. Berlin [Math. Naturwiss.], 14:141–144, 1965.

Jack, R. L., and Coleman, D. J.: Detection of retinal detachments secondary to choroidal malignant melanoma. Am. J. Ophthalmol., 74:1057–1065, 1972.

Kaneko, A.: Differential diagnosis of the retinoblastoma using ultrasonography. Acta Soc. Ophthamol. Jap., 75:2147–2157, 1971.

Karlin, D. B.: Ultrasound in the diagnosis of intraocular and retrobulbar tumors. Int. Ophthalmol. Clin., 1:121–143, 1972.

Massin, M.: The causes of errors of A-scan echography in the diagnosis of uveal tumors. Arch. Ophtalmol., 28:857–860, 1968.

Meyer, D., et al.: Ultrasonic diagnosis of malignant melanoma. *In:* Diagnostica Ultra-sonica in Ophthalmologia (SIDUO II). Edited by J. Vanysek. Brno, University of Brno, 1968, pp. 309–311.

Mozherenkov, V. P.: The diagnostic value of unidimensional echography in intraocular tumors. Vestn. Oftalmol., 84:45–48, 1971.

Nover, A., and Gerbaulet, K.: Tumor diagnosis by means of ultrasonics and radioactive isotopes in the eye. Fortschr. Med., 78:285–287, 1960.

Nover, A.: Clinical studies with ultrasonics in retinal detachment and intraocular tumors. Klin. Monatsbl. Augenheilkd., 142:176–194, 1963.

Oksala, A.: Melanoma of the choroid examined with an acoustic biomicroscope. Br. J. Ophthalmol., 45:218–222, 1961.

Oksala, A., and Lehtinen, A.: Acoustic biomicroscopy of intraocular tumors. Am. J. Ophthalmol., 51:1203–1211, 1961.

Oksala, A. et al.: Haemangioma of the ciliary body. Br. J. Ophthalmol., 48:669–672, 1964.

Oksala, A., and Varonen, E.-R.: Experimental researches on the influence of various tumors on the ultrasonic field. Acta Ophthalmol., 44:253–260, 1966.

Oksala, A., and Kause, E.: On the differential diagnosis of retinitis proliferans-intraocular tumor, by ultrasound. *In:* Ultrasonics in Ophthalmology. Edited by A. Oksala and H. Gernet. Basel, S. Karger, 1967, pp. 143–149.

Oksala, A., and Salminen, L.: Investigations of the effects of blood and tumor tissue on the height of the rear eye wall echoes. *In:* Ultrasonics in Ophthalmology. Edited by A. Oksala and H. Gernet. Basel, S. Karger, 1967, pp. 154–160.

Ossoinig, K.: On the ultrasonic diagnosis of eye tumors. Clinical and experimental studies with saw-tooth recorders. Klin. Monatsbl. Augenheilkd., 146:321–337, 1965.

Ossoinig, K.: The problem of acoustic diagnosis of tumors of the eye and orbit. Experimental studies and clinical studies with time-amplitude methods. Wiss. Z. Humboldt Univ. Berlin [Math. Naturwiss.], 14:185–191, 1965.

Ossoinig, K., and Steiner, H.: The problem of standardization in ultrasonic diagnosis; a test object for the diagnosis of intraocular tumors. Wiss. A. Humboldt Univ. Berlin [Math. Naturwiss.], 14:129–133, 1965.

Poujol, J., and Bonnin, P.: Diagnosis of intraocular retroequatorial tumors by ultra-sonography and fluorescein angiography. *In:* Ophthalmic Ultrasound. Edited by K. Gitter, et al. St. Louis, C. V. Mosby Co., 1969, pp. 273–281.

Poujol, J., and Bonnin, P.: Diagnosis of intraocular tumors by ultrasonography associated with fluoroscein angiography. Report of 60 cases confirmed histolog-ically. Ann. Ocul., 202:305–324, 1969.

Poujol, J., Iris, L., and Armand, M. J.: Correlations between the reflectivity and ultrasound attenuation of intraocular tumors and their histologic structure. *In:* Ultrasonography in Ophthalmology. Edited by J. Francois and F. Goes. Basel, S. Karger, 1975, pp. 172–177.

Preisová, J.: Ultrasonic image of intraocular tumors. *In:* Ophthalmic Ultrasound. Edited by K. Gitter, et al. St. Louis, C. V. Mosby Co., 1969, pp. 269–272.

Ricci, A., Psilis, K., and Soriano, H.: Diagnosis of intraocular and orbital tumors by echography and gammagraphy. Ophthalmologica, 161:132–138, 1970.

Rousselie, F.: Ultrasonography in choroid tumors. Arch. Ophtalmol., 28:851, 1968.

Sommer, P., and Kunze, P.: Pseudo-uveitis in retinoblastoma. Klin. Monatsbl. Augen-heilkd., 6:844–850, 1969.

Sonoda, Y., Kizima, M., and Uchida, H.: Melanoma of the choroid. Folia Ophthalmol. Jap., 8:828–831, 1968.

Thomas, C. L., and Purnell, E. W.: Ocular melanocytoma. Am. J. Ophthalmol., 1:79–86, 1969.

Ulrich, C., Lommatzsch, P., Buschmann, W., and Ulrich, W.: Results of a combination of ultrasonography and radiophosphor test for diagnosis of intraocular tumors. *In:* Diagnostica Ultrasonica in Ophthalmologia (SIDUO II). Edited by J. Vanysek. Brno, University of Brno, 1968, pp. 313–316.

Ulrich, C., Lommatzch. P., and Ulrich, W. P.: Combined method for diagnosis of intra-ocular tumors. Klin. Monatsbl. Augenheilkd., 155:425, 1969.

Ursin, K. V.: A case of intrabulbar melanoma confirmed by ultrasound. Acta Ophthalmol., 44:708, 1966.

Vannini, A., and Bellone, G.: Diagnostic possibilities of ultrasound in intraocular tumors. Consideration of a case of melanocytoma with malignant degeneration. Arch. Rass. Ital. Ottal., 31:81–92, 1962.

Intraocular Foreign Bodies and Trauma

Alajmo, A., and De Concillis, N.: On the application of ultrasonics-ophthalmology diagnosis. III. Possibilities of ultrasonics in the detection of endo-ocular foreign bodies. Riv. Inofort Mal. Prof. Fasc., 6:956–961, 1960.

Baum, G.: Problems in ultrasographic localization and attempts at their solution. In: Ophthalmic Ultrasound. Edited by K. Gitter et al. St. Louis, C. V. Mosby Co., 1969, pp. 231–236.

Bellone, G., and Gallenga, P. E.: Diagnostic echography of ophthalmic foreign bodies. Part I. Foreign bodies located in the anterior segment. Arch. Rass. Ital. Ottal., 37:296, 1969.

Bellone, G., and Gallenga, P. E.: Diagnostic ultrasonography for ophthalmic foreign bodies. Part II. Foreign bodies located in the posterior segment. Arch. Rass. Ital. Ottal., 37:317, 1969.

Bronson, N. R.: Localization and extraction of foreign bodies by ultrasound. In: Diagnostic Ultrasound. Edited by C. Grossman, et al. New York, Plenum Press, 1966, pp. 72–78.

Bronson, N.: Localization and extraction of intraocular foreign bodies. In: Ultrasonics in Ophthalmology. Edited by R. Goldberg and L. Sarin. Philadelphia, W B. Saunders, 1967, pp. 160–182.

Bronson, N.: Ultrasonic localization (of F. B.). Int. Ophthalmol. Clin., 8:199–203, 1968.

Bronson, N.: Foreign body management. In: Ultrasonographia Medica, (SIDUO III). Edited by J. Bock and K. Ossoinig. Vienna, Verlag der Weiner Med. Akad., 1971, pp. 259–264.

Coleman, D. J.: Ultrasound in ocular trauma. Rev. Soc. Colombiana Oftalmol., 3:105–110, 1972.

Cowden, J., and Runyan, T.: Further experiences in ultrasonic versus radiologic localization of intraocular foreign bodies. In: Ultrasonographia Medica (SIDUO III). Edited by J. Bock and K. Ossoinig. Vienna, Verlag der Weiner Med. Akad., 1971, pp. 271–274.

Czerek-Jaguczanska, H.: The possibilities of ultrasonic localization as a diagnostic aid in ophthalmology. Ophthalmologica, 148:151–159, 1964.

Dallow, R.: Ultrasonography in ocular and orbital trauma. Int. Ophthalmol. Clin., 14:23–56, 1974.

Franceschetti, A.: Foreign body localization with ultrasound. Ber. Dtsch. Ophthalmol. Ges., 67:294, 1966.

Francois, P., Asseman, R., and Constantinides, G.: Non-magnetic intraocular foreign bodies. Bull. Mem. Soc. Fr. Ophtalmol., 79:307–318, 1966.

Fridman, F. E.: Ultrasonic biolocalization in the eye under experimental and clinical conditions. Wiss. Z. Humboldt Univ. Berlin [Math. Naturwiss.], 14:147–149, 1965.

Gernet, H., and Hennewig, J.: Clinical, biometric and roentgenologic results in traumatic intraocular foreign bodies. Ber. Dtsch. Ophthalmol. Ges., 67:280–283, 1969.

Kutshera, E., and Kosmath, B.: Eye injuries in hunting accidents. Klin. Monatsbl. Augenheilkd., 153:808, 1968.

Liubarskii, S. A.: The value of ultrasonic biometry in locating foreign bodies in the eye. Oftalmol. Zh., 23:115, 1968.

Nover, A., and Stallkamp, H.: Experimental studies with ultrasonics on eye with intraocular foreign bodies. Graefe. Arch. Ophthalmol., 164:517–523, 1962.

Oksala, A.: A wooden splinter in the eye, diagnosed by ultrasound. Klin. Monatsbl. Augenheilkd., 134:88–93, 1959.

Oksala, A., and Lehtinen, A.: Use of the echogram in the location and diagnosis of intraocular foreign bodies. Br. J. Ophthalmol., 43:744, 1959.

Oksala, A.: Copper splinters in the anterior chamber and in the vitreous body diagnosed by ultrasound. Klin. Monatsbl. Augenheilkd., 136:81–88, 1960.

Oksala, A., and Mela, M. J.: Experimental researches on the significance of the interference phenomenon within the near field in the diagnosis of the eye by ultrasound, particularly with regard to the search for a foreign body. Acta Ophthalmol., 42:179–187, 1964.

Oksala, A., and Salminen, L.: Some aspects dealing with the ultrasonic diagnosis of intraocular foreign bodies. *In:* Diagnostic Ultrasound. Edited by C. Grossman, et al. New York, Plenum Press, 1966, pp. 79–94.

Ossoinig, K., and Seher, K.: Ultrasonic diagnosis of intraocular foreign bodies. *In:* Ophthalmic Ultrasound. Edited by K. Gitter, et al. St. Louis, C. V. Mosby Co., 1969, pp. 311–320.

Preisova, J., and Paul, M.: Contribution to the localization of intraocular foreign bodies by means of ultrasound. Wiss. Z. Humboldt Univ. Berlin, 14:221, 1965.

Sanna, G., and Quilici, G.: Experimental research in the use of ultrasound in diagnosis and localization of intraocular foreign bodies. Ann. Ottal., 89:877–884, 1963.

Schum, U.: A combination of magnet and ultrasound for localization and extraction of intraocular foreign bodies. Klin. Monatsbl. Augenheilkd., 157:256–258, 1970.

Ustimenko, L.: Diagnostic application of ultrasound in intraocular foreign bodies. Vestn. Oftalmol., 4:68–74, 1965.

Vanysek, J.: Contribution to the localization of intraocular foreign bodies by means of ultrasound. Wiss. Z. Humboldt. Univ. Berlin [Math. Naturwiss.], 14:221–222, 1965.

Wainstock, M. A.: Combined use of ultrasonic biometry and a new silicone lens for ophthalmic foreign body localizations. Ultrasonography in Ophthalmology. Edited by J. Francois and F. Goes. Basel, S. Karger, 1975, pp. 102–108.

General Ophthalmic Ultrasound

Alajmo, A.: Application of ultrasound in ophthalmologic diagnosis I. General part: experimental research, use of ultrasound in ocular diagnosis and treatment. G. Ital. Oftalmol., 11:241–251, 1958.

Alajmo, A.: The use of ultrasonic energy in ophthalmological diagnosis II. Further experimental and clinical data (A review of the literature). G. Ital. Oftalmol., 13:41–50, 1960.

Aldridge, E. E.: Preliminary investigation of the use of ultrasonic holography in ophthalmology. Br. J. Radiol., 44:126–130, 1971.

Aldridge, E. E., et al.: Scanned ultrasonic holography for ophthalmic diagnosis. Ultrasonics, 12:155–160, 1974.

Barkhash, A. S.: Role of ultra-acoustic studies in the diagnosis of initial sub-atrophy of the eye in children. Oftalmol. Zh., 28:500–503, 1973.

Baum, G.: An evaluation of techniques used in the radiation of the eye with ultrasonic energy. Am. J. Phys. Med., 36:212–220, 1957.

Baum, G., and Greenwood, I.: Ultrasonic visualization of the eye. *In:* 12th Annual Conference on Electrical Techniques in Medicine and Biology: Digest of Technical Papers. New York, Lewis Winger, 1959, pp. 66–69.

Baum, G., and Greenwood, I.: Ultrasound in ophthalmology. Am. J. Ophthalmol., 49:249–261, 1960.

Baum, G., and Greenwood, I.: Ultrasonic techniques in ophthalmology (abstract). J. Acoust. Soc. Am., 33:84, 1961.

Baum, G., and Greenwood, I.: A critique of time-amplitude ultrasonography. Arch. Ophthalmol., 65:353–365, 1961.

Baum, G., and Greenwood, I.: High resolution ultrasonography and its application to clinical ophthalmology. *In:* Proceedings Third International Conference Medicine and Electronics. Springfield, Charles C Thomas, 1961, pp. 412–421.

Baum, G.: Ultrasonography in clinical ophthalmology. Trans. Am. Acad. Ophthalmol. Otolaryngol., 68:265–276, 1964.

Baum, G.: Ophthalmic ultrasonography. *In:* Ultrasound as a Diagnostic and Surgical Tool. Edited by D. Gordon. Baltimore, Williams and Wilkins, 1964, pp. 176–184.

Baum, G.: A synopsis of ophthalmic ultrasonography. Wiss. Z. Humboldt Univ. Berlin [Math. Naturwiss.], 14:51–62, 1965.

Baum, G.: A discussion of acoustic artifacts in ophthalmic ultrasonography Am. J. Ophthalmol., 60:493–498, 1965.

Baum, G., and Greenwood, I.: Current status of ophthalmic ultrasonography. *In:* Ultrasonic Energy. Edited by E. Kelly. Urbana, Univ. of Illinois Press, 1965, pp. 260–277.

Baum, G.: A comparison of the merits of scanned intensity modulated ultrasonography vs. unscanned A-scope ultrasonography. *In:* Diagnostic Ultrasound. Edited by C. Grossman, et al. New York, Plenum Press, 1966, pp. 59–71.

Baum, G.: Instrumentation problems in ophthalmic ultrasonography. Ultrasonics, 6:43, 1968.

Baum, G.: Quantized ultrasonography. Ultrasonics, 10:14–15, 1972.

Baum, G.: Ultrasonics and ophthalmology. Eye Ear Nose Throat Mon., 51:430–435, 1972.

Baum, G.: The use of isodensitometric processing in ophthalmic ultrasonography. *In:* Ultrasonography in Ophthalmology. Edited by J. Francois and F. Goes. Basel, S. Karger, 1975, pp. 9–10.

Bellone, G., and Gallenga, P. E.: Idiopathic retinoschisis in the young subject to sexlinked recessive transmission. Arch. Rass. Ital. Ottal., 37:8, 1969.

Belz, B.: Ultrasound in ophthalmology. Ann. Ocul., 184:673–678, 1951.

Bronson, N. R.: Quantitative ultrasonography. Arch. Ophthalmol., 81:460–472, 1969.

Bronson, N. R.: Quantitative ultrasonography. *In:* Ophthalmic Ultrasound. Edited by K. Gitter, et al. St. Louis, C. V. Mosby Co., 1969, pp. 69–75.

Bronson, N. R.: Quantitative ultrasonography. Arch. Rass. Ital. Ottal., 1:201–210, 1970.

Bronson, N. R.: Ultrasonic examination in keratoplasty. Int. Ophthalmol. Clin., 10:253–260, 1970.

Bronson, N. R.: Contact B-scan ultrasonography. Am. J. Ophthalmol., 77:181–191, 1974.

Bruckner, H. L.: The role of A-scan ultrasonics in ophthalmology. Ann. Ophthalmol., 3:1014–1024, 1971.

Buschmann, W.: The present status of diagnostic ultrasound in the eye. Rehabilitation, 15:137, 1962.

Buschmann. W.: Investigation of a new optical-acoustic device. Klin. Monatsbl. Augenheilkd. 142:170–176, 1963.

Buschmann, W.: The present status of ultrasonic diagnosis in the eye. Therapiewoche, 13:261–262, 1963.

Buschmann, W.: Acoustic illusions in ophthalmologic ultrasonography. Am. J. Ophthalmol., 57:461–466, 1964.

Buschmann, W.: A new apparatus for ultrasound diagnosis. Wiss Z. Humboldt Univ. Berlin [Math. Naturwiss.], 14:31–35, 1965.

Buschmann, W.: Problems and progress in the ultrasonic diagnosis of the eye. Klin. Monatsbl. Augenheilkd., 144:321–347, 1964.

Buschmann, W.: New equipment and transducers for ophthalmic diagnosis. Ultrasonics, 3:18–21, 1965.

Buschmann, W.: Some measuring procedures for the evaluation of examination devices used in ultrasonic diagnosis (instrument and transducers). Wiss. Z. Humboldt Univ. Berlin [Math. Naturwiss.], 14:115–119, 1965.

Buschmann, W.: Bases, methods and reliability of ultrasonic diagnosis on the eye (review). *In:* Ultrasonics in Ophthalmology. Edited by A. Oksala and H. Gernet.

Basel, S. Karger, 1967, pp. 54–75.

Buschmann, W.: Special transducer probes for diagnostic ultrasonography of the eyeball. *In:* Ultrasonics in Ophthalmology. Edited by R. Goldberg and L. Sarin. Philadelphia, W. B. Saunders, 1967, pp. 87–101.

Buschmann, W., and Hauff, D.: Results of diagnostic ultrasonography in ophthalmology. Am. J. Ophthalmol., 63:926–933, 1967.

Buschmann, W., Linnert, D., Bluth, K., and Staudt, J.: Results and problems in the use of B-scanning equipment ophthalmologic ultrasonics diagnosis. Schweiz. Med. Wochenschr., 99:1025–1033, 1969.

Buschmann, W., Vogel, A., and Hermann, G.: Frequency changes and results in diagnostic ultrasonography depending on amplifier characteristics of ultrasonoscopes. Proceedings of the Conference of Ultrasonics in Biology and Medicine UBIOMED-70, Warsaw, 1970.

Buschmann, W., Klopp, R., and Seefeld, B.: Selection of superior scanning methods of A- and B-scan ultrasonography of the eye and orbit. Ophthalmol. Res., 2:149–164, 1971.

Cascio, G. Ultrasonics in ophthalmology. I. General physical, biological technical aspects of ultrasonics; clinico-experimental uses. Boll. Ocul., 33:675–688, 1954.

Chivers, R. C.: B-scanning and holography in ophthalmic diagnosis. Ultrasonics, 12:209–213, 1974.

Coleman, D. J., and English, F.: The role of ultrasonography in ophthalmology. Med. J. Aust., 2:570–573, 1971.

Coleman, D. J., Jack, R. L., and Franzen, L. A.: Ultrasonography in pediatric ophthalmology. J. Pediatr. Ophthalmol., 9:111–119, 1972.

Cowden, J.: Ultrasonic gross pathologic correlation. *In:* Ultrasonographia Medica (SIDUO III). Edited by J. Bock and K. Ossoinig. Vienna, Verlag der Weiner Med. Akad., 1971, pp. 351–355.

Czerek-Jaguczanska, H.: Ultrasonic diagnosis in ophthalmology. Klin. Oczna, 33:73–76, 1963.

Czerek-Jaguczanska, H.: Detection of intraocular changes by means of ultrasound. Klin. Oczna, 35:373–376, 1965.

Czerwinska, W.: Ultrasonics in ophthalmology. Klin. Oczna, 28:261–267, 1958.

Damascelli, B., Palmia, C., and Milani, F.: Diagnostic value of bidimensional echography. Minerva Radiol., 13:581, 1968.

Decker, D., Epple, E., Leiss, W., and Nagel, M.: Digital computer analysis of time-amplitude ultrasonograms from the human eye. II. Data processing. J. Clin. Ultrasound, 1:156–160, 1973.

Dysznska-Rosciszewska, B., and Lypacewicz, G.: First clinical experiences with ultrasonograph B. Klin. Oczna, 42:27–30, 1972.

Ernyei, A.: Experiences with ultrasonic diagnosis in ophthalmology. Wiss. Z. Humboldt Univ. Berlin [Math. Naturwiss.], 14:171–174, 1965.

Ferreira, L. E.: Ultrasonic recording in ophthalmology. Arq. Bras. Oftalmol., 30:311, 1967.

Filipczynski, L.: Compound and rapid scan ultrasonic imaging of eye structures. *In:* Ophthalmic Ultrasound. Edited by K. Gitter, et al. St. Louis, C. V. Mosby Co., 1969, pp. 207–212.

Filipczynski, L.: Present day state and prospects of developments of ultrasonic techniques for diagnostic purposes in ophthalmology. Klin. Oczna, 42:21–26, 1972.

Flament, J.: Echographic findings in scleral pockets. Experimental study. Bull. Soc. Ophtalmol. Fr., 70:165–168, 1970.

Fodor, F.: Application of ultrasound in ophthalmology. Oftalmologia, 9:1–4, 1965.

Franceschetti, A., and Luyckx, J.: The use of ultrasound in ophthalmology. Med. Hyg., 24:36–37, 1966.

Francois, J., and Goes, F.: Ultrasonography in the diagnosis of ocular affections. Possibilities and limitations of the method. Bull. Soc. Belge Ophtalmol., 150:600–614, 1968.

Francois, J., and Goes, F.: Ultrasonography in pediatric ophthalmology. J. Pediatr.

Ophthalmol., 8:221–233, 1971.

Freeman, M. H.: Ultrasonic pulse-echo techniques in ophthalmic examination and diagnosis. Ultrasonics, 1:152–160, 1963.

Fridman, F. E., and Dainlkova, A. J.: Modern views on the use of ultrasound in ophthalmology. Vestn. Oftalmol., 6:51–54, 1960.

Fridman, F. E.: Ultrasound echography in diagnosing certain eye diseases. Vestn. Oftalmol., 4:62–68, 1965.

Gallenga, R.: Diagnostic ultrasonography in ophthalmology. Arch. Rass. Ital. Ottal., 1:9–36, 1970.

Gernet, H.: Open questions on ultrasonic methodology for the eye. Wiss. Z. Humboldt Univ. Berlin [Math. Naturwiss.], 14:135–140, 1965.

Gernet, H.: On microphthalmia, macular changes and refraction in the case of mandibulofacialis dystrophy. Klin. Monatsbl. Augenheilkd., 144:887–899, 1964.

Gernet, H: In: Echography: An Advanced Course, Vols. I–IV. Edited by H. Merte. Munich, Urban and Schwarzenberg, 1972.

Gerstner, R.: A comparison between section-picture representation and peak-type recording in ultrasonic diagnosis. Wiss Z. Humboldt Univ. Berlin [Math. Naturwiss.], 14:37–38, 1965.

Gerstner, R.: Sound output of impulse echo equipment for ophthalmological examinations. Wiss. Z. Humboldt Univ. Berlin [Math. Naturwiss.], 14:95–97, 1965.

Gitter, K., Meyer, D., and White, R.: Ultrasonic aid in the evaluation of leukocoria. Am. J. Ophthalmol., 65:190–195, 1968.

Gitter, K. A., et al.: The role of ultrasound in evaluation of eyes with opaque media. In: Diagnostica Ultrasonica in Ophthalmologia (SIDUO II). Edited by J. Vanysek. Brno, University of Brno, 1968, pp. 287–291.

Gitter, K., Meyer, D., and Sarin, L.: Limitations and misinterpretations of time-amplitude ultrasonography. In: Ophthalmic Ultrasound. Edited by K. Gitter, et al., St. Louis, C. V. Mosby Co., 1969, pp. 237–248.

Gitter, K.: The use of diagnostic ultrasonography in pediatric ophthalmology. In: Ultrasonographia Medica (SIDUO III). Edited by J. Bock and K. Ossoinig, Vienna, Verlag der Weiner Med. Akad., 1971, pp. 321–332.

Goldberg, R. E., and Sarin, L. K.: Experience with ultrasonography. Part 1. The posterior segment of the globe. Am. J. Ophthalmol., 61:1497–1502, 1966.

Goldberg, R., and Sarin, L.: Time-amplitude (A-mode) ultrasonography. In: Ultrasonics in Ophthalmology. Philadelphia, W. B. Saunders, 1967, pp. 45–75.

Gordon, D.: Ultrasonic rays in diagnosis and surgery. Trans. Med. Soc. Lond., 79:173–180, 1963.

Gordon, D.: A suitable ultrasonic section-picture apparatus for ophthalmology. Wiss. Z. Humboldt Univ. Berlin [Math. Naturwiss.], 14:29–30, 1965.

Gordon, D.: Ultrasonic stereotaxic surgery. Wiss. Z. Humboldt Univ. Berlin [Math. Naturwiss.], 14:45–49, 1965.

Gordon, D. Transducer design for ultrasonic ophthalmology. In: Ophthalmic Ultrasound. Edited by K. Gitter, et al. C. V. Mosby, Co., St. Louis, 1969, pp. 65–68.

Greguss, P., and Bertenyi, A.: Ultrasonic holography in ophthalmology. In: Ophthalmic Ultrasound. Edited by K. Gitter, et al.: St. Louis, C. V. Mosby Co., 1969, pp. 81–87.

Greguss, P., and Galin, M.: Holography. Ann. Ophthalmol., X:817–820, 1972.

Groder, G.: The anatomical basis for ultrasonic diagnosis of the eye. Wiss. Z. Humboldt Univ. Berlin [Math. Naturwiss.], 14:11–16 1965.

Hamard, H.: Intra-ocular exploration by means of B ultrasonography. Bull. Soc. Ophtalmol. Fr., 68:1013–1018, 1968.

Hamard, H., and Rietzler, F. X.: Use of the B-echography in the exploration of the eyeball. Arch. Ophthalmol., 29:673, 1969.

Hapten, K.: Ultrasonics and the eye. Sven Lakartidn., 49:2714–2727, 1962.

Hauff, D., and Buschmann, W.: Results of ultrasound examinations in 1,000 patients. In: Diagnostica Ultrasonica in Ophthalmologia (SIDUO II). Edited by J. Vanysek. Brno, University of Brno, 1968, pp. 301–308.

Herrmann, G., and Buschmann, W.: Methods for measuring the HF oscillation frequency in ultrasound pulses of equipment for diagnostic ultrasonography. Ophthalmol. Res., 3:274–282, 1972.

Hess, S.: The physical basis for ultrasonic diagnosis. Wiss. Z. Humboldt Univ. Berlin [Math. Naturwiss.], 14:7-10, 1965.

Holasek, A., Sokollu, A., and Purnell, E. W.: A digitized, direct contact B-scanner for ophthalmic application. J. Clin. Ultrasound, 1:36–41, 1973.

Howry, D. H.: Techniques used in ultrasonic visualization of soft tissues. *In:* Ultrasound in Biology and Medicine. Edited by E. Kelly. Washington, American Institute of Biological Sciences, 1957, pp. 49–65.

Hudelo, A., et al.: Ultrasound in ophthalmology. Ann. Ocul., 190:684–697, 1957.

Hughes, H., and Dadd, M. J.: The application of ultrasonography to the examination of the eye. Med. J. Aust., 2:848, 1969.

Jack, R. L., and Coleman, D. J.: B-scan ultrasonographic diagnosis of ocular and orbital disease. Can. J. Ophthalmol., 7:257–267, 1972.

Katz, L. L., and Konig, W. F.: Signal processing in ultrasonic tomography. *In:* Ophthalmic Ultrasound. Edited by K. Gitter, et al. St. Louis, C. V. Mosby Co., 1969, pp. 110–115.

Kennerdell, J-S.: Evaluation of eyes with opaque anterior segments, using both ultrasonography and electroretinography. Am. J. Ophthalmol., 5:853–860, 1973.

Kossoff, G., and Liu, C. N.: The C.A.L. ophthalmological echoscope. Wiss. Z. Humboldt Univ. Berlin [Math. Naturwiss.], 14:39–43, 1965.

Kossoff, G.: Improved techniques in cross sectional echography. Ultrasonics, 10:221–228, 1972.

Lamer, L.: Diagnostic ultrasonography in ophthalmology. Union Med. Can., 96:841, 1967.

Linnert, D., Bluth, K., Engler, M., and Buschmann, W.: Comparison of examination conditions in ophthalmic diagnostic ultrasound. *In:* Ultrasonographia Medica (SIDUO III). Edited by J. Bock and K. Ossoinig. Vienna, Verlag der Weiner Med. Akad., 1969, pp. 71–81.

Marek, P.: Use of ultrasonics in ophthalmology. Szemeszet, 95:104–108, 1958.

Marmur, R. K.: Echographic criteria for the diagnosis of pathological changes in the anterior chamber of the eye. Oftalmol. Zh., 27:486–489, 1972.

Massin, M.: Generalities on ocular echography. Clin. Ophthalmol., 1:17–24, 1968.

Massin, M., and Poujol, J.: Indication and diagnostic value of A ultrasonography in ophthalmology. Arch. Ophthalmol., 29:613–624, 1969.

McDicken, W. N., et al.: 3-D images using a fibreoptic ultrasonic scanner. Br. J. Radiol., 45:70–71, 1972.

Mitkokh, D. I., and Mozherenkov, V. P.: Use of the EKHO-21 echoophthalmograph for ophthalmologic ultrasonic studies. Nov. Med. Priborostr., 1:103, 1970.

Nakajima, A.: Ophthalmology congress in America. Ophthalmology, 10:681, 1968.

Nover, A., and Nuding, J.: Diagnostic ultrasound examination in normal and pathological tissues. Graefe. Arch. Ophthalmol., 168:290–303, 1965.

Nover, A., and Grote, W.: Investigations on the reflection of ultrasound on the retina, the choroid and sclera—so-called back-wall echo. Graefe. Arch. Ophthalmol., 168:388–404, 1965.

Nulikov, I. A., et al.: Ultrasonic biolocator for the diagnosis of some eye diseases on the basis of the UDM-IM defectoscope. Med. Prom. SSSR, 10:52–55, 1965.

Obraz, J.: A few measurements to determine the characteristics of ultrasonic equipment. *In:* Diagnostica Ultrasonica in Ophthalmologia (SIDUO II). Edited by J. Vanysek. Brno, University of Brno, 1968, p. 55.

Obraz, J.: Ultrasonic transducers and their properties. Wiss. Z. Humboldt Univ. Berlin [Math. Naturwiss.], 14:121–127, 1965.

Offret, G., and Rousselie, F.: Ocular echography. Bull. Soc. Ophtalmol. Fr., 70:1009–1014, 1970.

Oksala, A.: Ultrasonic apparatus in examination of the eye and its diseases. Nord. Med., 59:721–725, 1958.

Oksala, A.: A case of glaucoma absolutum diagnosed by echography. Duodecim, 75:77–84, 1959.

Oksala, A., and Lehtinen, A.: Magnification of the echogram of the eye by a high-frequency oscilloscope. Acta Ophthalmol., 38:19–24, 1960.

Oksala, A.: Analysis of echoes from the posterior bulbar wall. Acta Ophthalmol., 38:25–31, 1960.

Oksala, A., and Lehtinen, A.: Experimental observations on acoustic biomicroscopy of various parts of the eye. Acta Ophthalmol., 38:599–605, 1960.

Oksala, A.: About selective echography in some eye diseases. Acta Ophthalmol., 40:466–472, 1962.

Oksala, A.: Observations on the depth resolution in ultrasonic examination of the eye. Acta Ophthalmol., 40:575–579, 1962.

Oksala, A., and Varonen, E.-R.: Analysis of echoes from the rear eye wall with the aid of experimental research. I. The sound beam directed to the rear wall past the lens. Acta Ophthalmol., 42:616–628, 1964.

Oksala, A., and Varonen, E-R.: Analysis of echoes from the rear eye wall with the aid of experimental and clinical research. II. Effect of the absorption of the lens and of amplification. Acta Ophthalmol., 42:782–793, 1964.

Oksala, A.: Earlier experiences on the diagnosis of eye disease with ultrasonics. Klin. Monatsbl. Augenheilkd., 144:347–360, 1964.

Oksala, A.: On ultrasonic diagnosis of intraocular diseases. Rehabilitation, 17:82–83, 1964.

Oksala, A.: The clinical value of time amplitude ultrasonography. Am. J. Ophthalmol., 57:453–460, 1964.

Oksala, A.: Diagnostics by ultrasound in ophthalmology. Eye Ear Nose Throat Mon., 26:45–58, 1964.

Oksala, A.: On the increased understanding of ultrasonics in the diagnosis of intra-ocular diseases. Ophthalmologica, 149:467–480, 1965.

Oksala, A.: Development and significance of ultrasonic diagnosis in ophthalmology. In: Ultrasonics in Ophthalmology. Edited by A. Oksala and H. Gernet. Basel, S. Karger, 1967, pp. 1–21.

Oksala, A., and Hakkinen, L.: An experimental comparison between A- and B-scan ultrasonography. Acta Ophthalmol., 45:773, 1967.

Oksala, A.: Basic problems in A-mode ultrasonography. In: Ultrasonics in Ophthal-mology. Edited by R. Goldberg and L. Sarin. Philadelphia, W. B. Saunders, 1967, pp. 76–86.

Oksala, A.: The pathology of ultrasound in the eye and its clinical aspects. Klin. Monatsbl. Augenheilkd., 150:408, 1967.

Oksala, A., and Hakkinen, L.: Experimental studies of the behavior of ultrasound in the sclera and cornea. In: Ophthalmic Ultrasound. Edited by K. Gitter, et al. St. Louis, C. V. Mosby Co., 1969, pp. 59–64.

Oksala, A.: General problems in ophthalmic ultrasonography techniques. In: Ophthal-mic Ultrasound. Edited by K. Gitter, et al. St. Louis, C. V. Mosby Co., 1969, pp. 205–206.

Oksala, A.: Ultrasonics in ophthalmology. Duodecim, 85:854, 1969.

Oksala, A.: The clinical use of ultrasonic methods of diagnosis in ophthalmiatrics. Lakartidningen, 68:993, 1971.

Oksala, A.: On the use of ultrasonic diagnosis in ophthalmology and medicine. Ann. Clin. Res., 3:5–8, 1971.

Orso, G. P.: Ultrasonics in scleroderma. Radiobiol. Radioter. Fis. Med., 11:437–445, 1956.

Ossoinig, K. C.: Ultrasonic diagnosis on the eye: An aid for the clinic. In: Ultrasonics in Ophthalmology. Edited by A. Oksala and H. Gernet. Basel, S. Karger, 1967, pp. 116–133.

Ossoinig, K., and Till, P.: Echo-ophthalmography. Ber. Dtsch. Ophthalmol. Ges., 70:605–613, 1969.

Preisova, J., and Vanysek, J.: The present state of diagnostic ultrasonography in ophthalmology. Wiss. Z. Humboldt Univ. Berlin [Math. Naturwiss.], 14:157–162, 1965.

Preisova, J., and Vanysek, J.: Our experiences with ultrasound diagnosis of eye diseases. Cesk. Oftalmol., 21:361–369, 1965.

Preisova, J. and Vanysek, J.: Current status of ultrasonic diagnosis in ophthalmology. Cesk. Oftalmol., 25:297, 1969.

Preisova, J., Anton, M., and Vanysek, J.: Comparison of ultrasonic diagnosis with findings on enucleated bulbs. *In:* Ultrasonographia Medica (SIDUO III). Edited by J. Bock, and K. Ossoinig. Vienna, Verlag der Weiner Med. Akad., 1971, pp. 357–365.

Psilas, K., and Itin, W.: On the utility of ultrasonics in ophthalmology. Ultrasonography or echography. Rev. Med. Suisse Romande, 90:873, 1970.

Purnell, E. W., and Sokollu, A.: An evaluation of time-amplitude sonography in ocular diagnosis. Am. J. Ophthalmol., 54:1103–1109, 1962.

Purnell, E.: Intensity modulated B-scan ultrasonography. *In:* Ultrasonics in Ophthalmology. Edited by R. Goldberg and L. Sarin. Philadelphia, W. B. Saunders, 1967, pp. 102–123.

Purnell, E. W.: Diagnostic and therapeutic ultrasonics. *In:* Centennial Symposium of Manhattan Eye, Ear, and Throat Hospital, New York. 1968 Proceedings, Vol. I, Ophthalmology. Edited by A. Turtz. Philadelphia, W. B. Saunders, 1969, pp. 206–212.

Ricklefs, G.: The avoidance of erroneous diagnoses by means of echography. Klin. Monatsbl. Augenheilkd., 149:79–83, 1966.

Rivara, A., and Sanna, G.: Observations on the technique of use of ultrasonics in ophthalmological diagnosis. Minerva Oftalmol., 6:33–36, 1964.

Robinson, D., Dadd, M., and Kossoff, G.: Two-dimensional ultrasonography in the eye. *In:* Ophthalmic Ultrasound. Edited by K. Gitter, et al. St. Louis, C. V. Mosby Co., 1969, pp. 75–80.

Rousselie, F.: Ultrasonography in ophthalmology. Presse Med., 76:1523–1524, 1968.

Rousselie R., Clay, C., Bernard, J., and Offret, G.: A-scan echography and electro-retinography in uveitis. *In:* Diagnostica Ultrasonica in Ophthalmologia (SIDUO IV). Edited by M. Massin and J. Poujol. Paris, Centre National d'Ophtalmologie des Quinze-Vingts, 1973, pp. 179–183.

Sander, E.: Ultrasound echography in the clinic. Klin. Monatsbl. Augenheilkd., 146:728–737, 1965.

Shereshevskaya, L. Y., and Fridman, F. E.: Use of ultrasonics in some diseases of the eye. Vestn. Oftalmol., 6:61–67, 1963.

Sokollu, A.: The use of diagnostic ultrasound in eye research. *In:* Diagnostic Ultrasound. Edited by C. Grossman, et al. New York, Plenum Press, 1966, pp. 46–58.

Sokollu, A.: A critical evaluation of ultrasonic images of the eye obtained by various echoscopic scan modes. *In:* Diagnostica Ultrasonica in Ophthalmologia. Edited by J. Vanysek. Brno, University of Brno, 1968, pp. 35–50.

Sokollu, A.: Surgical and therapeutic use of ultrasound in ophthalmology. *In:* Ophthalmic Ultrasound. Edited by K. Gitter, et al. St. Louis, C. V. Mosby Co., 1969, pp. 323–332.

Stallkamp, H., and Nover, A.: Diagnostic studies with ultrasonics on the healthy eye. Graefe. Arch. Ophthalmol., 164:399–410, 1962.

Sundmark, E.: Diagnostic use of ultrasound in ophthalmology. Nord. Med., 63:826, 1960.

Susal, A. L.: An ophthalmic ultrasound scanning system. Ultrasonics, 12:36–39, 1974.

Sverdlov, D. G.: Uses of ultrasonics in ophthalmology for diagnostic purposes. Oftalmol. Zh., 16:373–378, 1961.

Szczypinski, J., and Smogulecka, E.: Ultrasonography in the diagnosis of eye disease (method B). Klin. Oczna, 42:31–36, 1972.

Till, P., and Ossoinig, K.: A ten year study of clinical echography in intraocular disease. *In:* Ultrasonography in Ophthalmology. Edited by J. Francois and F. Goes. Basel, S. Karger, 1975, pp. 49–62.

Trier, H. G., and Bohm, H. W.: B-scan in posterior staphyloma. *In:* Diagnostica Ultrasonica in Ophthalmologia (SIDUO II). Edited by J. Vanysek. Brno, University of Brno, 1968, pp. 263–267.

Trier, H. G., and Reuter, R.: Digital computer analysis of time-amplitude ultrasonograms from the human eye. I. Signal acquisition. J. Clin. Ultrasound, 1:150–156, 1973.

Ursin, K. V.: The filming of echograms (a new method of recording ultrasonograms of the eye). Acta Ophthalmol., 42:794–799, 1964.

Ustimenko, I. L.: Use of ultrasound in ophthalmology for diagnostic purposes. Oftalmol. Zh., 22:37, 1967.

von Ardenne, M. H., Gossman, R., and Millner, R.: An analysis of the ultrasound Focoscan method. Wiss. Z. Humboldt Univ. Berlin [Math. Naturwiss.], 14:71–72, 1965.

Vanysek, J., Obraz, J., and Preisova, J.: On the possibilities of an ultrasonic examination in ophthalmology. Ophthalmologica, 144:20–28, 1962.

Vanysek, J., and Preisova, J.: Diagnostic evaluation of ultrasound in ophthalmology. Rev. Czech. Med., 10:73–85, 1964.

Vanysek, J., and Preisova, J.: On the possibilities of ultrasonic diagnosis in ophthalmology. Cas. Lek. Cesk., 103:193–198, 1964.

Vanysek, J., Preisova, J., and Paul, M.: Ultrasonic image of the anterior eye segment by TAU and SIMU. *In:* Ophthalmic Ultrasound. Edited by K. Gitter, et al. St. Louis, C. V. Mosby Co., 1969, pp. 213–217.

Wainstock, F. L.: Use of ultrasound in ophthalmology: report of 6 cases. Ohio State Med. J., 69:674–678, 1973.

Wainstock, M. (Editor): Ultrasonography in ophthalmology. Int. Ophthalmol. Clin., 9:523–847, 1969.

Ziskin, M. C.: Contrast agents for diagnostic ultrasound. Invest. Radiol., 7:500–505, 1972.

Acoustic Characteristics of Tissues and Effects of Ultrasound on Tissue

Amar, L.: On the generation of elastic waves in the eye irradiated by a laser beam. Bibl. Ophthalmol., 72:414, 1967.

Badtke, G.: The effect of ultrasonic waves on the eye. Arch. Phys. Ther., 2:119–122, 1950.

Begui, Z. E.: Acoustic properties of the refractive media of the eye. J. Acoust. Soc. Am., 26:365–368, 1954.

Buschmann, W.: Use of the frequency filtering effect of tissues in diagnostic ultrasonography. Ophthalmol. Res., 4:122–127, 1973.

Cleary, S. F., and Pasternack, B. S.: Lenticular changes in microwave workers. A statistical study. Arch. Environ. Health, 12:23–29, 1966.

Darabos, G., and Gombos, K.: The effect of ultrasound on the blind spot. Szemeszet, 98:101–106, 1961.

Fry, W.: Mechanism of acoustic absoption in tissue. J. Acoust. Soc. Am., 24:412–415, 1952.

Fry, W., and Dunn, F.: Ultrasound: Analysis and experimental methods in biological research. *In:* Physical Techniques in Biological Research, Vol. 4. New York, Academic Press, 1962, pp. 261–394.

Greguss, P.: Ultrasonic propagation in the hetero-dispersive media of the eye. Ultrasonics, 2:134–136, 1964.

Greguss, P.: Ultrasonic pathways and fields in hetero-dispersive rheologic media. Wiss. Z. Humboldt Univ. Berlin [Math. Naturwiss.], 14:83–85, 1965.

Grün, F., et al.: On the action of ultrasound on the vitreous and the lens. Klin. Monatsbl. Augenheilkd., 116:358–367, 1950.

Hallerman, W., et al.: Effects of ultrasonics on the eye of the animal. Klin. Monatsbl. Augenheilkd., 119:401–411, 1951.

Hapten, K., and Palm, E.: The effect of ultrasonic vibrations on the living rabbit eye. Acta Ophthalmol., 32:227–234, 1954.

Jankowiak, J., and Majewski, C.: Effect of exposure of one eyeball to ultrasound on the cerebral vision centers of the rabbit. Am. J. Phys. Med., 44:109–112, 1965.

Kawamoto, I.: Experimental studies on the effect of ultrasonic waves on the eyeball. Soc. Ophthalmol. Jap. Acta, 51:21–16, 1947.

Koch, S. A., and Rubin, L. F.: Diagnostic ultrasonography of the dog eye. J. Small Anim. Pract., 10:357, 1969.

Kossoff, G., and Robinson, D.: Basic physics of diagnostic ultrasound. In: Ultrasonics in Ophthalmology. Edited by R. Goldberg and L. Sarin. Philadelphia, W. B. Saunders, 1967, pp. 23–44.

Krasnow, M. M., Subbotina, I. N., and Boguslavskania, E. S.: Experimental ultrasonic retinopathy. Vestn. Oftalmol., 1:34–38, 1972.

Larsen, J. S., et al.: Experimental ultrasonic examinations of intraocular, intrascleral and retrobulbar foreign bodies. Acta Ophthalmol., 51:499–511, 1973.

Lavine, O., et al.: Effects of ultrasonic waves on the refractive media of the eye. Arch. Ophthalmol., 47:204–219, 1952.

Lazuk, V. A.: Effect of ultrasound on the healthy eye of the rabbit and on hemorrhage in rabbit eyes. Vopr. Kurortol. Fizioter. Lech. Fiz. Kult., 30:139–143, 1965.

Levchenko, O. G.: Ultrasound in the treatment of various eye diseases. Oftalmol. Zh., 26:207–210, 1971.

Lizzi, F., Burt, W. J., and Coleman, D. J.: Effects of ocular structures on propagation of ultrasound in the eye. Arch. Ophthalmol., 84:635–640, 1970.

Lutz, H., and Lutz-Ostertag, Y.: Effect of ultrasonics on the epithelium of the crystalline lens. C. R. Acad. Sci., 249:2122–2124, 1959.

Marmur, R. K.: Influence of ultrasound on the permeability of the blood-eye barrier and of the refractive media of the eye. Bull. Exp. Biol. USSR, 57:578–580, 1964.

Marmur, R. K., and Bushmitch, D. G.: Influence of ultrasound on retrocorneal membranes developed after keratoplasty. Oftalmol. Zh., 19:362–365, 1964.

Marmur, R. K.: The effect of ultrasonics on reparative regeneration of the cornea. Oftalmol. Zh., 22:450, 1967.

Marmur, R. K., and Skorodinskaia, V. V.: Ultrasonics in the complex therapy of pigmented degeneration of the retina. Oftalmol. Zh., 22:207, 1967.

Marmur, R. K., et al.: Sub-microscopic and cytochemical changes of retinal photoreceptors under the action of ultrasound. Oftalmol. Zh., 28:589–592, 1973.

Nowak, A.: Investigations on the influence of acoustic and ultra-acoustic fields on biochemical processes. VIII. Influence on miotic activity in the corneal epithelium in guinea pigs. Acta Physiol. Pol., 12:901–904, 1961.

Oksala, A.: The influence of the eye globe on the ultrasonic intensity. Eye Ear Nose Throat Mon., 52:332–335, 1973.

Oksala, A.: Experimental investigations of the effect of various parts of the eye on the sound field in the ultrasonic method. Acta Ophthalmol., 48:1157–1165, 1970.

Oksala, A.: Experimental studies on the effect of the eye globe on the ultrasonic field. Acta Ophthalmol., 49:308–316, 1971.

Oksala, A., and Blok, P.: Influence of lenses on the sonic field. Experimental studies using swine lenses. Acta Ophthalmol., 47:295, 1969.

Oksala, A., and Hakkinen, L.: Influence of the eye tunic on the sonic field. Experimental studies on swine eyes. Acta Ophthalmol., 47:295, 1969.

Oksala, A., and Jaaslahti, S. L.: Experimental observations on the acoustic shadows caused by some pathological conditions on the echogram of the sclera. Acta Ophthalmol., 50:116, 1972.

Oksala, A., and Jaaslahti, S.: Experimental observations on the acoustic shadow in B-scan examination of the eye. Acta Ophthalmol., 49:151–158, 1971.

Oksala, A., and Lehtinen, A.: Additional experimental observations of acoustic section of the eye. Acta Ophthalmol., 39:302–307, 1961.

Oksala, A., and Lehtinen, A.: Absorption of ultrasound in the aqueous humor, lens and vitreous humor. Acta Ophthalmol., 36:761–768, 1958.

Oksala, A., and Piiroinen, L.: Experimental researches on the ultrasonic field and the point of departure of the echo from the scleral calotte, using the sclera as a test piece. Acta Ophthalmol., 44:549–557, 1966.

Oxilia, E.: Action of ultrasonic waves on the cornea of rabbits. G. Ital. Oftalmol., 3:350–365, 1950.

Patetta-Queirolo, M. A., and Glaussiuss Olivera, J. A.: Action of ultrasonic waves on the lens. Arch. Soc. Biol. Montevideo, 19:32–36, 1952.

Quintieri, C., and Falcinelli, M.: Effects of ultrasonics in ophthalmology: experimental study. Boll. Ocul., 33:702–712, 1954.

Raue, H.: The use of microwaves in ophthalmology, Klin. Monatsbl. Augenheilkd, 142:563–567, 1963.

Schwab, F., et al.: On the action of ultrasound on the anterior section of the living rabbit eye. Klin. Monatsbl. Augenheilkd., 116:367–376, 1950.

Schwab, F.: Experiments with ultrasonic impulses on the eye. Experiments on the lens. Graefe. Arch. Ophthalmol., 155:97–114, 1954.

Sokollu, A., and Holasek, E.: Model study of propagation of ultrasonic waves in ocular media. *In:* Ophthalmic Ultrasound. Edited by K. Gitter, et al. St. Louis, C. V. Mosby Co., 1969, pp. 88–99.

Torikai, T., and Sato, G.: Ultrasonic waves. Naika, 14:804–810, 1964.

Tsok, R. M.: The action of ultrasound on normal eye tissues in the course of experimental hemophthalmos. Vestn. Oftalmol., 4:65–71, 1963.

Yamamoto, Y., et al.: Diffusion of colimycin into the aqueous humor and the effect of ultrasonic waves. Rimsho Ganka, 17:875–877, 1963.

Ziskin, M. C., Romayananda, N., and Harris, K.: Ophthalmologic effect of ultrasound at diagnostic intensities. J. Clin. Ultrasound, 2:119–123, 1974.

CHAPTER VI

Orbital Diagnosis

VI

Orbital
Diagnosis

Ultrasound aids greatly in the diagnosis of orbital abnormalities by providing information often not obtainable by any other examination technique. As discussed in Chapter V, we prefer to use combined A-, B- and M-scan ultrasonic techniques for evaluation of both the globe and orbit. In orbital diagnosis, the topographic outlining capabilities of the B-scan are ideally suited to localizing and delineating abnormalities. Orientation difficulties (due to the lack of distinctive anatomic landmarks in the orbit) preclude total reliance on an A-scan method. In our combined technique we depend upon the A-scan for specific tissue characterization and upon the M-scan for determination of the vascular properties of tissues, once the initial localization with B-scan has been achieved.

We feel that the orbital penetration available through transducer variation denotes immersion B-scan as the technique of choice in orbital examination.[1] This method of B-scan ultrasonography provides a two-dimensional acoustic section of the orbit that quickly directs attention to specific areas where abnormalities may be suspected. Kinetic scanning and A-scan analysis of these areas are employed to add supplemental information to the overall pattern obtained from the B-scan.

When a lesion is palpable (e.g., a cyst or mass in the eyelid) it is useful to use contact A- or B-scan techniques, for in these cases there is definite clinical information as to the topography and the location of the mass. In addition, the contact A-scan can be used to identify a lesion which is concealed by the bony overhang of the superior orbital rim. These techniques are of particular use with lacrimal gland tumors. A contact probe to compress various orbital lesions has been described by Ossoinig[2] and is of use in characterizing the cystic or solid components of orbital masses.

Our ultrasonic orbital evaluation consists of serial tomographic sections utilizing both static and kinetic A- and B-scanning. In general, horizontal scans are made serially across the eye and orbit at 2-mm intervals. Dallow[3] has emphasized the importance of vertical as well as horizontal scanning of the orbit to portray structures partially obscured by the orbital rim. Lower-frequency transducers (such as 5 MHz) should be used to outline the posterior extent of the orbit and should be used if ocular disease prevents adequate penetration at the normal examining frequency of 10 MHz. Kinetic scanning, i.e., having the patient move his eye from side to side and up and down while fast sector scans are performed, is important in orbital diagnosis. Kinetic scanning indicates the degree of adherence of a mass to the mobile anatomic features of the orbit, such as the optic nerve, and to the fixed structures, such as the orbital wall.

Comparative evaluation of the patient's other orbit is usually not done, since variations from the normal orbital pattern are usually easily discerned. However, in patients with subtle pathologic changes, such as disease of the optic nerve, a comparative evaluation of the companion orbit may aid in differentiation.

Obviously, a thorough knowledge of orbital anatomy and of the pathologic situations likely to arise in the orbit greatly enhances the ability to interpret information that can be obtained from the ultrasonic evaluation. It is for these reasons that ultrasonic orbital examination is best performed by an ophthalmologist.

Diagnostic Parameters

Echoes are produced in the orbit at planes of acoustic impedance mismatch between adjacent tissues. Measuring acoustic characteristics of orbital tissues, Buschmann[4] reported sound velocities of 1,462 m/sec for fat compared with 1,615 m/sec for optic nerve and 1,631 m/sec for muscle. These velocity differences cause the acoustic discontinuities which sharply define the interfaces between fat and optic nerve or muscle and cause partial reflection of an ultrasonic wave as it meets interfaces between these structures.

Within a heterogeneous tissue such as retrobular fat are many smaller tissue elements, including vessels, nerves and fat globules with many fibrous septae. The multiple tissue interfaces produce echoes and result in a nearly uniform confluence of echoes representing the entire fat pad. The relatively uniform tissue structures of optic nerve and extraocular muscles have less marked impedance mismatches and produce only low-amplitude echoes within the tissue substance. In addition, they are organized in tissue planes parallel to the ultrasonic beam, thus failing to produce echoes that are detectable along the transmitter-receiver beam path. The same principle of reflections from internal structural elements of a tissue applies to tumors and other abnormalities as well, and is an important criterion for differentiation of tissue types.

Types of Diagnostic Information

We feel that ultrasonography should be the first test utilized for orbital evaluation in that it provides information on soft tissues not detectable with traditional radiologic methods. It is a highly sensitive test and rarely misses any significant orbital abnormality. This inherent sensitivity is occasionally misleading (in that inflammatory tissues can resemble neoplasms) so that further tests may be desirable if the ultrasonographic findings indicate a pathologic situation.

In the past, clinicians have relied upon radiographic techniques for orbital evaluation. Plain films and tomography depict bony abnormalities well—fractures, erosion, or hyperostosis. Vascular contrast studies demonstrate arteriovenous lesions and intracranial abnormalities causing exophthalmos. Some indications of orbital soft tissue lesions may be gained from these studies also, but the findings are often not definitive.[5] Direct injection of contrast material into the orbit (contrast orbitography) has fallen out of favor because of morbidity and diagnostic unreliability. Radioisotope scans of the orbit seem promising for differentiating orbital lesions, but more extensive studies are needed to validate the specificity of findings. Thermography,[6] likewise, is in early stages of development and may aid in diagnosis of some vascular problems. A revolutionary new neuroradiologic procedure, called computerized tomography, is capable of showing soft tissue lesions within the bony cranium and orbit. Tumors of sufficient size are shown well by this technique, although other orbital abnormalities are not.

Ultrasonography, in contrast, provides unique high-resolution information regarding tumors and inflammatory orbital changes that is not obtainable by any other diagnostic techniques. Bony changes and vascular abnormalities, however, are not well demonstrated, although soft tissue is generally well seen. Ultrasonography, thus, serves as an invaluable complement to the usual radiographic studies, and can often demonstrate an abnormality when all other tests are negative.

Medical and surgical therapies are aided considerably by ultrasonographic findings. For instance, the effect of steroid administration in presumed pseudotumors can be monitored by following the inflammatory signs ultrasonically. Surgical approaches to a tumor can be planned with full knowledge, ultrasonically, of the location, size, extent, tissue composition and circumscribed or invasive character of the tumor.

Indications for Orbital Ultrasound

The indications for orbital ultrasonography are summarized in Table VI-1. In addition, ultrasound is of specific use in documenting clinical evaluable pathologic states such as myositis, Graves' disease or optic neuropathy. In general, ultrasound is indicated when orbital disease is suspected, and the findings may aid in the management and treatment of these orbital pathologic conditions.

TABLE VI-1.   Indications for Orbital Ultrasound

Unilateral or bilateral exophthalmos
Retinal striae
Unexplained optic atrophy
Papilledema without evident cause
Suspected orbital foreign body

The Normal Orbit

A-scan

SCAN PLANE DIRECTED THROUGH THE OPTIC NERVE. In an A-scan oriented through the optic nerve, echoes of diminishing amplitude are seen posterior to the posterior globe wall complex. These echoes drop off to baseline because of attenuation of sound energy. The distance from the posterior wall of the globe to the posterior part of the retrobulbar complex depends upon the scan position (directly through the nerve, or tangential to it).

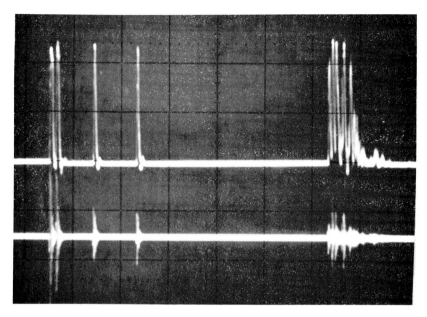

Fɪɢ. VI-1. An A-scan through normal retrobulbar structures shows an initial high-amplitude return from the vitreoretinal interface followed by a gradually decaying echo pattern from the retrobulbar fat.

SCAN PLANE ABOVE OR BELOW THE OPTIC NERVE. The A-scan oriented inferior or superior to the optic nerve also shows echoes from the retrobulbar fat, which gradually diminish until baseline is reached (Fig. VI-1).

B-scan

HORIZONTAL SCAN PLANE THROUGH THE OPTIC NERVE. With the ultrasonic scan plane passing through the optic nerve, the normal retrobulbar echo pattern is a W-shaped acoustically opaque (white) area (Fig. VI-2). This opaque W-shaped area is bounded anteriorly by the globe, and is indented posteriorly by an acoustically empty (black) notch that widens toward the orbital apex. This notch, or triangle, is formed by the optic nerve and associated structures.

The source of the echoes which give rise to the relatively uniform W-shaped retrobulbar echo pattern is not definitely known. Purnell[7] has postulated that the orbital fat provides the major source of these echoes, and his view is widely shared. Acoustic discontinuities presumably occur throughout this loculated tissue between intracellular lipids and cell membranes and between cell membranes and loose connective tissue septae. (Similar echo patterns can be produced experimentally in fine-mesh silicone sponge.) M-scans of the orbit have shown marked pulsatile vascular activity, and acoustic

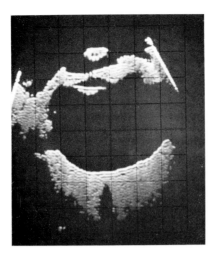 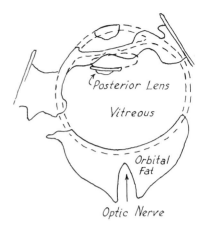

FIG. VI-2. A horizontal B-scan section through the optic nerve showing the characteristic crescentic pattern bisected by the sonolucent optic nerve shadow. The pattern is W-shaped with the apex of the nerve pattern forming a relatively acute angle of less than 90 degrees.

discontinuities in the blood vessel network in the muscle cone probably contribute to this echo pattern.

In all normal orbits we have examined, the optic nerve consistently appears as an acoustically empty triangular notch in the retrobulbar fat pattern. It is probable that the optic nerve appears acoustically sonolucent because of homogeneous tissue structure, and because the nerve fibers, septae and meninges lie parallel to the

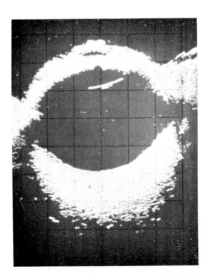 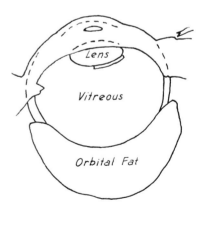

FIG. VI-3. A horizontal B-scan section taken inferior or superior to the optic nerve produces a crescentic pattern. Occasionally, a section of the orbital walls may be shown (most usually the temporal orbital wall) even in normal orbits.

examining ultrasonic beam, thus causing no reflections. The anterior angle of the optic nerve triangle or notch is usually less than 90 degrees (with a range of 40 degrees to 70 degrees normally). Widening or any rounding of this angle is an indication of pathologic enlargement of the optic nerve or its sheaths.

HORIZONTAL SCAN PLANE ABOVE OR BELOW THE OPTIC NERVE. When scans of the orbit are made inferior or superior to the optic nerve, the acoustically empty (black) optic nerve triangle is, of course, absent. The retrobulbar pattern appears as a uniform, acoustically opaque (white) crescent lying immediately posterior to the globe (Fig. VI-3). This crescent becomes progressively wider as the center of the orbit is approached.

VERTICAL SCAN PLANE. While horizontal scan planes are generally employed, it is important to perform vertical scans of the orbit, for in this way areas of pathology which might be missed in serial horizontal scans may be demonstrated more readily. The vertical scans (Fig. VI-4) resemble horizontal scans quite closely. On an axial scan, the

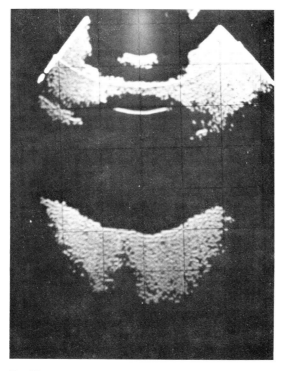

FIG. VI-4. A vertical B-scan through the nerve resembles horizontal sections through the nerve with the crescentic orbital fat pattern bisected by the sonolucent nerve shadow.

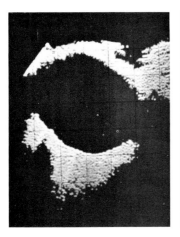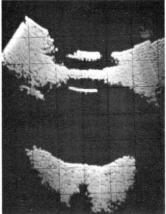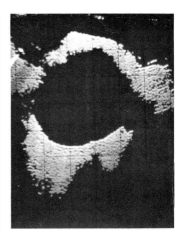

FIG. VI-5. B-scan ultrasonogram demonstrating the location of the optic nerve in different positions of gaze. In general, these different positions are observed during fast sector kinetic scanning.

optic nerve notch is demonstrable. On scans not intersecting the optic nerve, an acoustically opaque (white) crescent is demonstrated.

VARIATIONS WITH POSITIONS OF GAZE. The normal retrobulbar fat pattern has been described with the eye in a straight-ahead direction of gaze. Gaze to the far right or left results in a foreshortening of the retrobulbar pattern (decreasing its thickness) and in a bending of the optic nerve pattern toward the direction of gaze as shown in Figure VI-5. The movement of the optic nerve with changing positions is

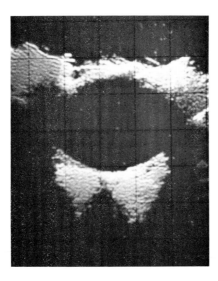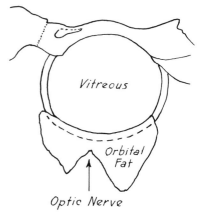

FIG. VI-6. B-scan ultrasonogram of a 1-month-old infant demonstrating that the orbital ultrasonic pattern closely resembles that seen in adults.

diagnostically important. If a mass lesion is found in the orbit, a fast sector scan should be performed as the patient moves his eye, in order that the relationship of the mass to the mobile optic nerve can be determined.

VARIATIONS WITH AGE. Age has relatively little effect on the B-scan ultrasonographic orbital pattern. The retrobulbar pattern in infants is, of course, smaller than in adults but is identical in outline (Fig. VI-6). It is our impression that the retrobulbar fat pattern in infants

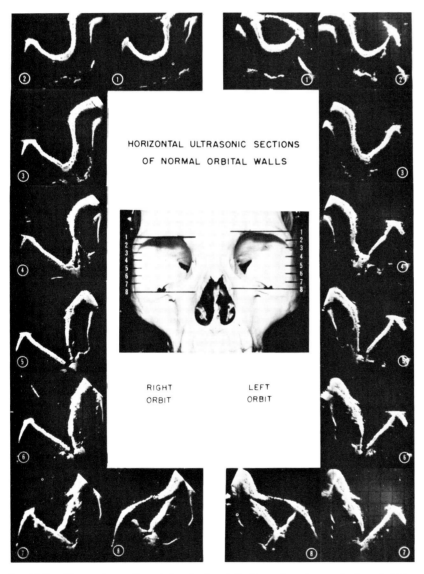

HORIZONTAL ULTRASONIC SECTIONS
OF NORMAL ORBITAL WALLS

RIGHT ORBIT

LEFT ORBIT

FIG. VI-7. Ultrasonic sections taken horizontally through a demonstration skull to illustrate the typical acoustic appearance of the orbital walls.

and children usually appears more "dense" and more uniformly white than in adults, possibly indicating fat distribution in smaller micelles.

EXTRAOCULAR MUSCLES AND ORBITAL WALL. The outer limit of the acoustically opaque (white) W-shaped retrobulbar pattern is formed by the rectus muscles and intermuscular septae. In B-scans made exactly in the horizontal meridian, a rectus muscle outline can often be seen and traced forward to the globe at its insertion.

The ultrasonic patterns formed by the normal orbital walls in different horizontal scan planes are shown for reference in Figure VI-7.

A small portion of one orbital wall (usually the lateral orbital wall) is often seen on our B-scan ultrasonograms (Fig. VI-8), but if a large portion of the orbital wall or if both medial and lateral walls are seen, edema or inflammation of the ocular muscles or periorbital tissue is indicated. The orbital apex is rarely seen in clinical ultrasonograms but can be approximated by tracing the optic nerve and the rectus muscle/orbital wall echoes to their juncture.

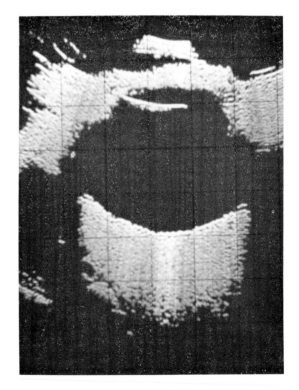

FIG. VI-8. B-scan ultrasonogram of a normal orbit taken at 10 MHz at an increased sensitivity setting to enhance the orbital wall.

Demonstration of the orbital wall is not a dependable ultra-sonographic finding, but is a feature dependent on the transducer frequency (more likely to be seen with the lower-frequency trans-ducers, i.e., 5 MHz), depth of ultrasonic beam penetration, and on receiver gain. It is imperative to obtain familiarity with the area of orbital wall seen in normal orbits with a given instrument, using a given transducer, and calibration of the receiver gain before conclu-sions can be made with regard to abnormal prominence of the orbital wall on one or both sides in a scan of an abnormal orbit.

FREQUENCY-RELATED VARIATION. The orbital ultrasonographic appearance varies according to the transducer frequency selected. Figure VI-9 demonstrates a comparison of the normal orbital pat-terns found using a 5- and 10-MHz transducer. As a rule, the lower the transducer frequency, the deeper the orbital penetration achieved.

EFFECT OF SCANNING MODE. Some variation in the normal orbital pattern results from the use of different scanning methods. Figure VI-10 demonstrates the difference between a compound scan and a sector scan of the normal orbit.

Artifacts Encountered in Orbital Ultrasonography

Numerous artifacts may occur during B-scan ultrasonography of the orbit, and knowledge of these possible artifacts will help avoid erroneous interpretation of ultrasonograms of the orbit. As dis-cussed in Chapter V, artifacts may be classified into three groups: (1) electronic artifacts (2) reduplication artifacts, and (3) absorption defects.

ELECTRONIC ARTIFACTS. One of the most important electronic artifacts in the orbit is that of "Swiss cheese" due to amplifier overload. The genesis of electronic artifacts is described in the chapter on ocular diagnosis. The effect of amplifier overload is to cause the normally uniformly white retrobulbar fat pattern to appear pockmarked or spongy, thus resembling a Swiss cheese (see Fig. V-12).

REDUPLICATION ARTIFACTS. These artifactual echoes (also known as axial multiple echoes) occur commonly, and usually appear in the central orbit along the axis of the cornea and lens, often in the region of the optic nerve triangle. They represent a "second bounce" of echoes, usually from anteriorly located ocular surfaces. The metal lid

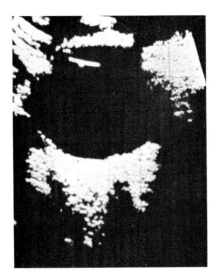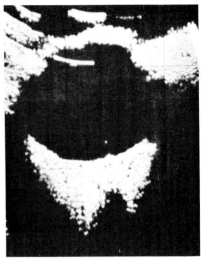

Fig. VI-9. B-scan ultrasonograms taken at 5 MHz (*left*) and 10 MHz (*right*) at comparable sensitivity settings to demonstrate the greater penetration and sensitivity of lower-frequency examination. Echoes from the orbital wall are better portrayed at lower frequencies and internal reflections may be noted.

speculum is another common cause of reduplication echo artifacts. These echoes can be distinguished from real echoes by moving the transducer either away from or toward the eye. This causes movement of the reduplication echo relative to the tissue, allowing it to be readily discerned (Fig. VI-11).

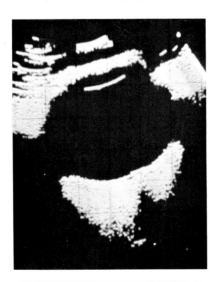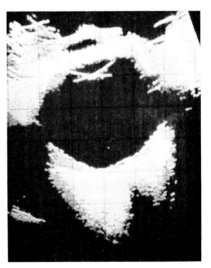

Fig. VI-10. In orbital evaluation, sector scans (*left*) outline the orbital contents quite adequately. Compound scans (*right*) may add to the overall outline of certain structures, especially orbital cysts, but the trade-off in gray scale seldom merits the use of a compound scan technique.

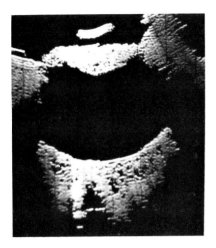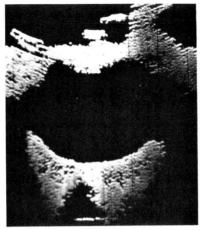

FIG. VI-11. Multiple echoes from the anterior ocular structures in direct alignment with the examining beam can appear in the orbital ultrasonic pattern just as they appear in the vitreous. They are generally lost in the complex of the orbital fat, except when the sonolucent nerve shadow permits them to be seen. If echoes appear within the nerve (*left*), movement of the transducer away from the eye will cause the artifactual echoes to move deeper into the orbit (*right*).

ABSORPTION DEFECTS. Absorption of ultrasound energy by structures located in or in front of the eye may cause abnormal orbital ultrasonic patterns.[7] Since these absorption defects, or "shadows," in the retrobulbar fat pattern may simulate orbital tumors, one must be aware of their existence. Ocular tumors (Fig. VI-12) or dense calcified lenses (see Fig. V-16) are commonly encountered ocular causes of such orbital defects.

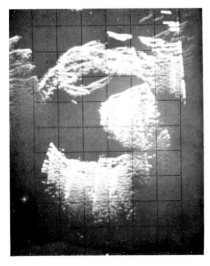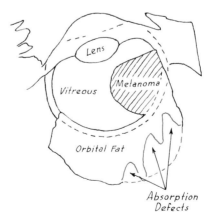

FIG. VI-12. Sound can be absorbed by ocular tumors, blood or inflammatory tissues so that shadowing in the orbit may simulate a tumor mass.

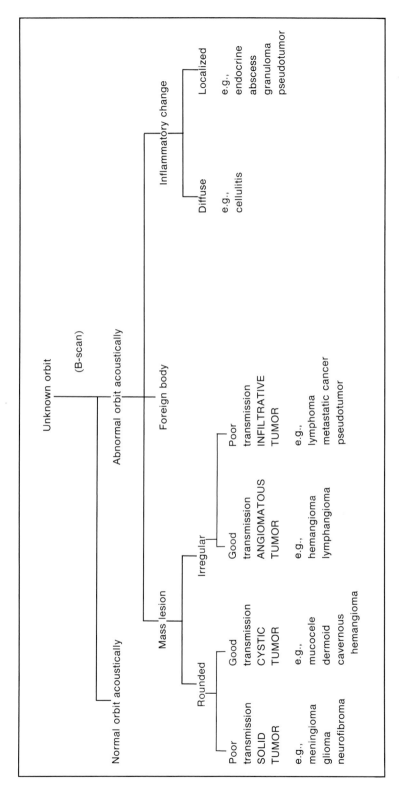

Fig. VI-13. Ultrasonic characterization of patients referred for orbital examination. Schematic flow chart of orbital diagnosis, progressing from distinction of normal from abnormal orbits to differentiation of abnormalities into tumor types or inflammatory tissue, based on criteria of transmission and morphology.

When an abnormal orbital B-scan pattern is encountered, the above artifacts should be ruled out. Recognition is aided by careful monitoring of the A-scan, permitting detection of many electronic artifacts, movement of the transducer toward or away from the eye if a reduplication echo is suspected, and analysis of the ocular B-scan for structures which may cause absorption defects in the orbital pattern.

General Classification of Orbital Abnormality

Ultrasonically, orbital abnormalities can be classified into structural anomalies, mass lesions, inflammatory or congestive changes, or foreign bodies. Each of these categories has several well-defined subdivisions of further classification. A-mode findings in orbital pathology have been described extensively by Ossoinig.[8] B-scan patterns were classified by Purnell[7] and elaborated on by Coleman et al.[9-16] The flow diagram proposed by Coleman[17] (Fig. VI-13) is useful for the examiner in approaching an unknown orbital problem.

Pseudoproptosis of an eye may be accounted for either by a large globe or a shallow bony orbit (Fig. VI-14). A-scan measurement of globe diameters will establish any significant difference between the eyes. A posterior staphyloma may be completely outlined with B-scan. With progressively increasing exophthalmos, even with a unilaterally large globe, complete untrasonography of orbital structures should always be done to evaluate coincident disease.

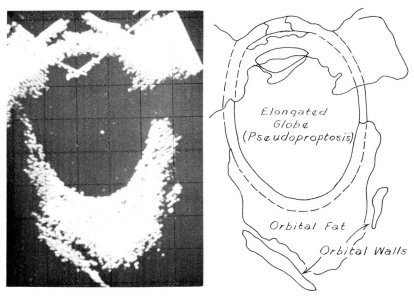

Elongated
Globe
(Pseudoproptosis)

Orbital Fat

Orbital Walls

Fig. VI-14. B-scan ultrasonogram of a markedly enlarged globe demonstrating clearly the ability of ultrasonography to differentiate pseudoproptosis from true proptosis. The orbital fat is normal, though slightly reduced in thickness.

Mass Lesions

A distinct distortion of the retrobulbar fat, optic nerve or rectus muscles by any sort of abnormal contour ultrasonically indicates a mass lesion in the orbit. Purnell[7] first described patterns of the orbit that we have reclassified into four general diagnostic patterns of mass lesions which are identifiable with B-scan ultrasonography:

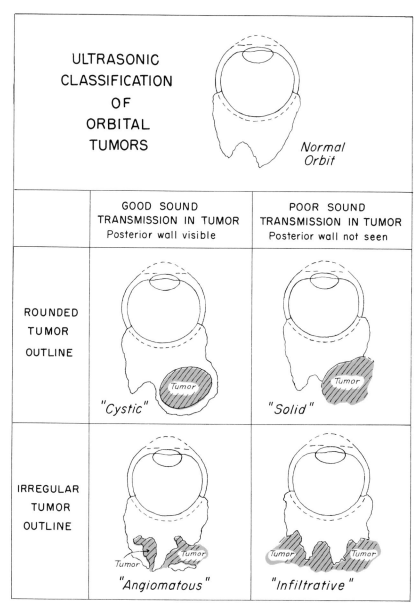

FIG. VI-15. Schematic presentation of the division of orbital tumor patterns based on their outline and transmission properties.

cystic, solid, angiomatous, and infiltrative (Fig. VI-15). Observation of several features of the abnormal area is necessary to categorize the lesion, including its contour, sound transmission, internal echoes, and location (Fig. VI-16). These patterns may be apparent with A-scan examination alone, but they are considerably better defined with B-scan tomography. There is close correlation between the ultrasonographic findings and the morphologic and histologic characteristics of mass lesions.

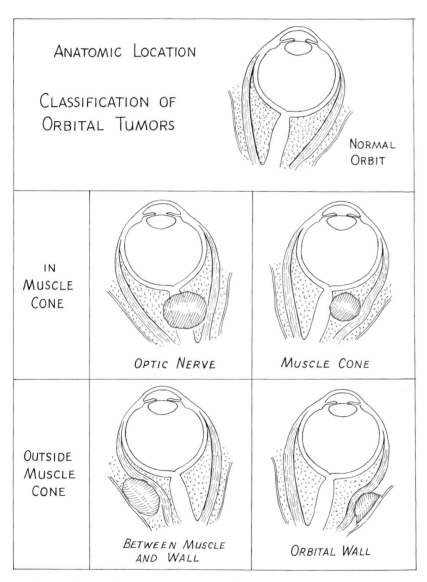

FIG. VI-16. The location of a tumor in the orbit is an important aspect of acoustic evaluation. Tumors within the muscle cone are particularly susceptible to ultrasonic detection.

For example, the contour of an orbital tumor may be smoothly rounded, sharply defined, and compressing adjacent normal structures. If the lesion has good sound transmission, its posterior wall will be clearly evident also. Internally, the lesion may be devoid of echoes, indicating no significant tissue interfaces within the lesion. These findings are characteristics of a fluid-filled cystic lesion such as mucocele or dermoid tumor.

In other cases, a mass lesion may have a contour similar to a cystic lesion. However, its posterior boundary may be indistinct because of poor sound transmission through it. A solid tumor causes significant sound attenuation so that penetration through it is poor. Low-amplitude echoes within the substance of a tumor indicate minor tissue interfaces, characteristic of a homogeneous solid tumor. These findings indicate a well-circumscribed solid tumor, e.g., neurogenic tumor, lacrimal gland tumor and some metastatic tumors. Location of the lesion within the orbit gives further clues to identification. A lesion of this type within the muscle cone and involving the optic nerve is probably one of the neurogenic tumors (glioma, meningioma, or neurofibroma). A similar lesion located in the upper temporal aspect of the orbit is more likely to be a lacrimal gland tumor.

An orbital tumor with an irregular contour suggests a different group of tumors. Angiomatous tumors show finger-like protrusions extending into the orbital fat pattern, usually with a larger mass more posteriorly. The tumor contour may or may not be well defined. The internal structure of angiomatous tumors presents many dense acoustic interfaces from vessel walls and blood-filled spaces comprising the tumor. Ultrasonically, this heterogeneous interior appears as multiple, irregular, high-amplitude echoes throughout the mass, with little sound attenuation. This irregular contour and heterogeneous internal structure is distinctly different from the cystic and solid tumor patterns described previously.

Another irregular orbital tumor, having a more solid character, indicates a solid infiltrative tumor. Although the lesion outline is jagged, it is also sharply defined and distinct. As with other solid tumors, low-amplitude internal echoes are present and sound attenuation is marked, making the posterior tumor margins indistinct. This pattern is associated with infiltrative tumors, particularly lymphomas and sarcomas. Metastatic tumors may show these characteristics also.

Idiopathic granulomas, or pseudotumors, often mimic invasive, solid tumors clinically and ultrasonically. These may be indistinguishable pathologically as well. Orbital hematoma may appear ultrasonically as an infiltrative mass lesion, although it is non-neoplastic.

A history of trauma can be misleading, however, since some tumors are stimulated to bleed with minimal trauma. Follow-up serial ultrasonography will demonstrate gradual resolution of the lesion in the case of solid hematoma.

In our experience, the infiltrative tumor category is the most difficult to identify with certainty, as inflammatory changes, described below, may produce similar appearances, especially when edema involves the optic nerve and the sub-Tenon's space. Scarring from previous orbital surgery may be confused with this category.

It is not always possible to classify orbital tumors into the four categories noted above, since tumors do not always appear the same anatomically. In general, however, the pattern and absorption characteristics outlined have been highly consistent with the tumor types noted. Other ultrasonic techniques can augment the available information. Ballottement of the tumor with a contact probe placed against the eye will demonstrate compression of cystic or angiomatous lesions and resistance to compression with solid tumors. M-scan ultrasound (time-motion study) provides a means of studying vascular pulsations within tumors. Dynamic or kinetic sector scanning will demonstrate motion of orbital structures with changes in gaze position, and often aids in categorization.

Individual tumor types, the variations of ultrasonic patterns associated with them, and the reliability of ultrasonic diagnosis with each tumor type will be discussed more fully as separate topics.

Inflammatory and Congestive Changes

In contrast to orbital mass lesions, inflammatory and congestive processes tend to involve structures that are normally present in the orbit, causing only subtle changes in them. Inflammatory changes may be classified, ultrasonically, as diffuse or as localized to a particular area or tissue in the orbit, depending upon the specific inflammatory process (Fig. VI-17).

A generalized abnormal mottling of the orbital fat pad is indicative of a diffuse orbital inflammation such as cellulitis. Echoes within the fat are more widely spaced than normal and are of high amplitude, giving the fat pad a more heterogeneous appearance without circumscribed borders. A similar acoustic appearance is seen in traumatic orbital hemorrhage. A localized area of such mottling within the fat is seen with abscess or focal granuloma.

Other localized inflammatory findings involve specific orbital structures. Expansion of the sonolucent space between the fat pad and the orbital wall generally indicates enlargement of the extraocular muscles if the finding is present symmetrically all around the

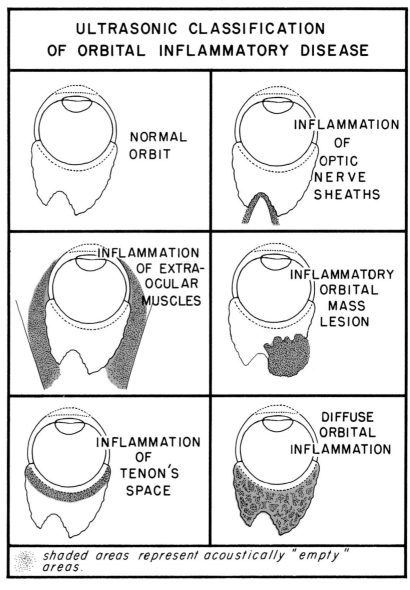

FIG. VI-17. Inflammatory changes along anatomic planes can be ultrasonically identified indicating neuritis, myositis, pseudotumor, scleritis or cellulitis.

orbit. The orbital wall is accentuated in these cases, presumably because tissues are compressed against the bony wall, creating a better reflecting surface than normally present. These findings are particularly characteristic of thyroid-related disease or endocrine exophthalmos, where edema and cellular infiltration of the muscles are present. Other congestive processes may produce similar ultrasound findings (e.g., arteriovenous anomalies, either orbital or intracranial).

Localized inflammation and edema may also involve the optic nerve or the space adjacent to the eye posteriorly. Accentuation of the optic nerve sheath without enlargement indicates an optic neuritis or edema. This is distinctly different from enlargement produced by tumor. These abnormalities resolve with regression of the inflammatory process. Although no pathologic specimens have been examined in the acute stage of retrobulbar neuritis, the ultrasonic findings seem consistent with inflammatory edema of the meningeal sheaths surrounding the nerve. Similar optic nerve findings may be seen with pseudotumor, papilledema or vascular anomalies.

The sub-Tenon's space surrounding the globe may become expanded posteriorly from edema associated with any type of orbital inflammation. Ultrasonically, this appears as a sonolucent area adjacent to the globe wall and connecting to the optic nerve outline. Other inflammatory signs are usually present in the orbit along with this finding. It may accompany some orbital tumors as well, particularly granulomatous tumors or lymphomas. In a normal orbit, this is a potential space and as such is not acoustically evident.

Orbital Tumors

Acoustically "Cystic" Tumors

Acoustically "cystic" orbital tumors are those which have a rounded regular outline and good acoustic transmission. It should be emphasized again at this point that acoustic transmission is a relative phenomenon, and the ability to demonstrate transmission through orbital structures depends on a knowledge of the patterns obtained with one's own equipment and transducers, with careful calibration of receiver gain.

MUCOCELE. Mucoceles are cysts lined by paranasal sinus mucous membranes. They enlarge slowly because of continued secretion and desquamation of lining cells, and cause thinning of the bony walls of the sinus by pressure. They expand in the direction of least resistance, often into the orbit through the medial wall and floor of the frontal sinus, forcing the globe down and out. Common clinical presentations are pain and swelling over the forehead, diplopia and proptosis. Invasion of the orbit by mucoceles of the paranasal sinuses is an important cause of unilateral exophthalmos. In series compiled by radiologists, orbital mucoceles are the most common cause of unilateral exophthalmos, with a figure as high as 15 per cent in the series compiled by Zismor et al.[18] In series compiled by ophthalmologists, orbital mucoceles are a less common but still significant cause of unilateral exophthalmos. In Reese's clinical series of 230 cases, 3 per cent of unilateral exophthalmos was due to orbital invasion by mucoceles.[19]

Ultrasonography gives accurate information as to the location and size of an orbital mucocele. Secondary changes, such as compression of retrobulbar fat and indentation of the posterior pole of the globe, are well shown by ultrasonography.

Mucoceles ultrasonically appear rounded and smooth, or even spherical in contour (Fig. VI-18). They are well demarcated from the surrounding normal orbital tissues. Mucoceles demonstrate a sharply defined, rounded anterior acoustic border which indents the retrobulbar fat. They show definite acoustic hollowness, and A-scans through them show no internal echoes (Fig. VI-19). On B-scan, the interior of a mucocele appears as a solid, black cavity, i.e., a sonolucent space. Little sound energy is absorbed in these cystic structures, and, consequently, ultrasonic radiation can penetrate through the mass, clearly outlining its posterior extent and the orbital walls and orbital apex.

Although X-ray diagnosis is relatively reliable in orbital mucoceles, B-scan ultrasonography adds valuable information as to the soft tissue configuration of the orbit and makes the diagnosis more definite. This facilitates the choice of surgical approach.

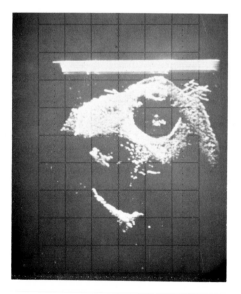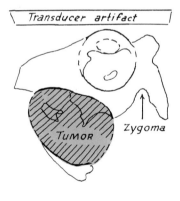

FIG. VI-18.   B-scan ultrasonogram taken at 10 MHz of an orbital mucocele demonstrating the good transmission properties indicated by outlining of the posterior wall of the tumor. The internal echoes seen are the result of organized debris or structural elements within the mucocele.

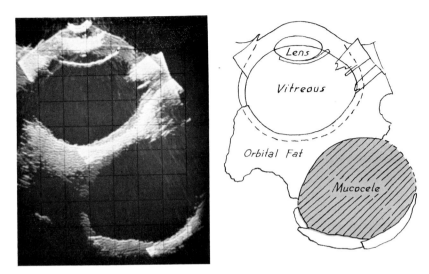

FIG. VI-19. B-scan ultrasonogram of an orbital mucocele with a rounded anterior border and good outlining of the orbital wall. Slight compression of the globe is noted anterior to the tumor.

DERMOID CYSTS. Dermoid cysts are relatively common tumors of aberrant ectodermal tissue. They usually occur in children. When dermoid cysts involve the bony orbital wall, they may be diagnosed on X-ray. However, even in this situation ultrasound is valuable, for it can demonstrate the exact limits of the orbital mass. Often there is no bony involvement, and ultrasound is particularly useful in diagnosing these tumors.

Figure VI-20 demonstrates the B-scan ultrasonogram of a child with unilateral exophthalmos. The pathologic specimen after orbital

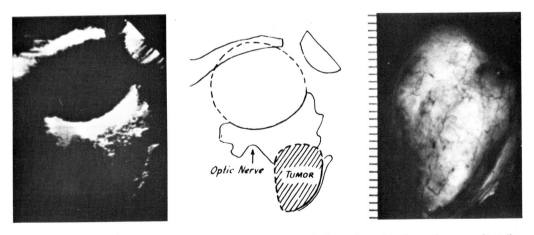

FIG. VI-20. B-scan ultrasonogram (*left*) demonstrating a mass lesion adjacent to the optic nerve along the orbital wall. The mass shows a relatively rounded anterior surface with a discrete border. The pathologic specimen (*right*) illustrates the similarity in histologic and acoustic patterns. This tumor was undetected by X-ray or any other diagnostic study.

biopsy is also presented. X-rays were normal, but ultrasonography showed very accurately the location and rounded nature of this mass. This rounded contour ultrasonically generally indicates encapsulation or pseudoencapsulation of an orbital mass.

CAVERNOUS HEMANGIOMAS. Hemangiomas are the most common of all orbital tumors. Reese described the proportion of hemangiomas to all orbital masses as 12 per cent in a clinical study of 230 consecutive cases, and as 15 per cent in a histopathologic study of 877 cases.[19] The cavernous hemangiomas of adults are by far the most common orbital hemangiomas and have been called the most common primary orbital tumor.

The size and location of cavernous hemangiomas are well demonstrated with B-scan ultrasonography. All cavernous hemangiomas which we have examined were located in the muscle cone. Secondary changes of the globe, such as flattening of the posterior pole, are also demonstrable.

The group of acoustic characteristics of all cavernous hemangiomas includes: (1) a rounded, regular outline, (2) a sharply defined and rounded anterior acoustic border, (3) good demarcation from surrounding structures, (4) low to moderate acoustic absorption (i.e., fair to good sound transmission), (5) appearance alteration with varying transducer frequencies (Fig. VI-21).

Cavernous hemangiomas show a sharply defined anterior acoustic border due to the abrupt transition in acoustic velocities

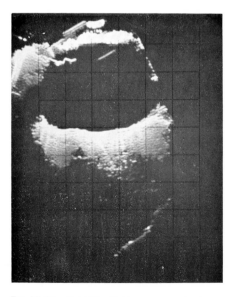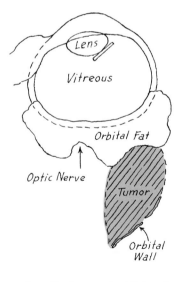

FIG. VI-21. B-scan ultrasonogram of a hemangioma along the temporal orbital wall showing a slightly rounded anterior surface and relatively good sound transmission.

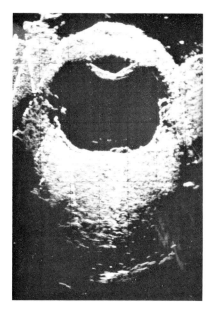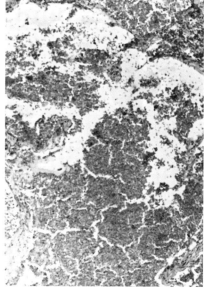

FIG. VI-22. B-scan ultrasonogram (*left*) of an orbital hemangioma. The relatively rounded anterior surface, good sound transmission properities and overall size of the mass are well demonstrated. The histologic section (*right*) demonstrates the marked vascularity of these tumors (original magnification ×40).

between retrobulbar fat and the fluid-filled tumor. These tumors are ultrasonically well demarcated from surrounding normal orbital structures, also due to this marked acoustic discontinuity.

Cavernous hemangiomas are mainly blood filled (Fig. VI-22), are characterized by good sound transmission, but can contain a few low-amplitude internal echoes. Sound transmission is much better than in acoustically solid lesions with high sound absorption (such as optic nerve tumors) but is not quite as high as in the completely acoustically hollow lesions with minimal sound absorption (such as mucoceles). Because of the low level of sound absorption in cavernous hemangiomas, ultrasound energy can penetrate them well, so that the posterior extent of the tumor and the outline of the wall and apex of the orbit are often demonstrated.

Cavernous hemangiomas are best outlined at 10 MHz and 15 MHz. The relatively good outlining of these tumors at 15 MHz helps differentiate them from the group of solid rounded orbital tumors, such as neurogenic tumors.

HEMANGIOPERICYTOMAS. Hemangiopericytomas are much less common than cavernous hemangiomas of the orbit. They contain mostly pericytes rather than endothelial cells. These tumors are blood filled and encapsulated, as are hemangiomas. Their ultrasonic

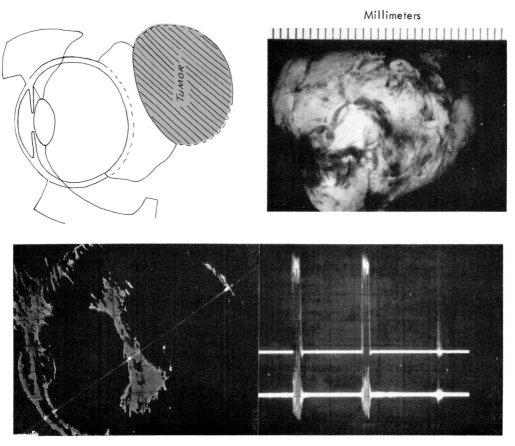

FIG. VI-23. B- and A-scan ultrasonograms of a hemangiopericytoma. The position of the A-scan axis is shown by the bright line on the stored B-scan. The tumor specimen (*right*) demonstrates the encapsulation of the mass.

characteristics are essentially the same as those described for cavernous hemangiomas. Figure VI-23 shows the preoperative B- and A-scan ultrasonograms of a patient with a hemangiopericytoma of the orbit. The tumor is rounded and indents the posterior globe wall. The A-scan shows acoustic hollowness of the mass. The photograph of the surgically excised specimen demonstrates the rounding and marked encapsulation of this tumor.

CYSTIC LYMPHANGIOMAS. Lymphangiomas of the orbit are discussed in more detail in the section on angiomatous tumors. The usual lymphangioma of the orbit is diffuse; however, some are cystic. Hemorrhage into a lymphangioma cavity may cause a hemorrhagic cyst to form. In these cases, the ultrasonic pattern is as has been discussed above, an orbital mass lesion with a rounded outline, and

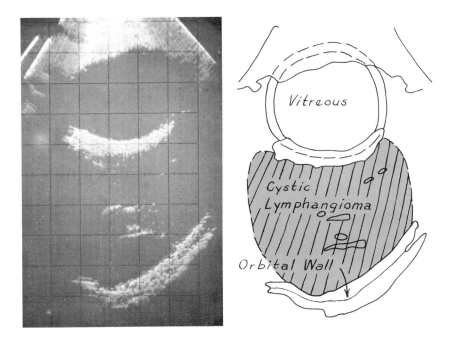

Fig. VI-24. An unusual cystic lymphangioma appearing as a large cystic space in the muscle cone.

good sound transmission through the tumor, permitting outlining of its posterior wall (Fig. VI-24).

Acoustically "Solid" Tumors

Acoustically "solid" orbital tumors have a rounded outline, as do cystic-appearing orbital tumors; however, sound transmission is poor through these masses, and there are multiple internal echoes.

Tumors of the Optic Nerve. Neurogenic tumors are relatively common causes of unilateral exophthalmos. Reese[19] described the proportion of neurogenic tumors to total orbital mass as 11 per cent in a clinical study of 230 cases and as 10.6 per cent in a histopathologic study of 877 cases. Silva[20] found 32 neurogenic tumors in a series of 300 consecutive cases of orbital masses, a proportion of 10.9 per cent. This group of tumors may require a neurosurgical approach for optimum removal and, thus, differentiation from other orbital tumors is clinically important. This differentiation is aided by B-scan ultrasonography.

The location and size of optic nerve tumors are depicted accurately with B-scan ultrasonography. Secondary changes, such as flattening of the posterior pole of the globe and papilledema, are also well shown (Figs. VI-25 and VI-26).

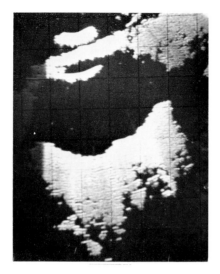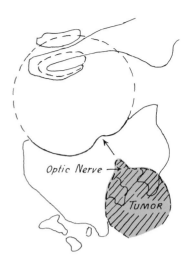

Optic Nerve

TUMOR

FIG. VI-25. B-scan ultrasonogram of a solid neurogenic tumor (meningioma) demonstrating compression of the globe and a prominent optic nerve head. The mass lesion is typified by an abnormal nerve pattern in addition to a rounded outline surrounding the nerve. Kinetic scans may aid in differentiating these tumors from those immediately adjacent to the nerve, since movement of the nerve may be inhibited.

Acoustic characteristics of this group of tumors are as follows: (1) rounded configuration, (2) good demarcation from surrounding orbital structures, (3) acoustic solidity and high acoustic absorption, and (4) lack of acoustic homogeneity, with multiple internal reflections.

All optic nerve tumors have sharply defined anterior borders and are relatively well demarcated from the surrounding orbital tissues, except in orbits which have undergone prior surgical exploration.

Optic nerve tumors show acoustic solidity. Sound energy absorption does not permit good outlining of the orbital walls. The posterior extent of the tumor often cannot be acoustically delimited.

In the interior of these solid masses, scattered low-amplitude echoes (or internal reflections) occur due to occasional acoustic discontinuities in the tumor mass. These are best demonstrated on the A-scan presentation. The presence of interfaces between tumor cell planes, collagenous connective tissue septae, and large blood vessels in the tumor provides a possible histologic basis for these acoustic discontinuities.

Tumors of the optic nerve often produce a smooth indentation of the anterior retrobulbar pattern of the nerve. Enlargement of the normal optic nerve shadow, however, is the most important feature in the diagnosis. The normally acutely angled optic nerve shadow is converted into an obtuse-angled or smoothly convex shadow (Fig. VI-27).

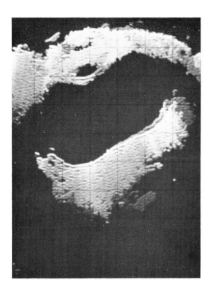
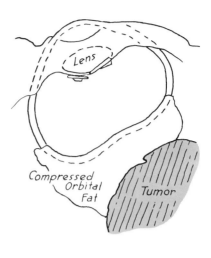

FIG. VI-26. B-scan ultrasonogram of a rounded, well-encapsulated orbital tumor compressing the globe. Poor transmission properties are noted, and no acoustic details are available posterior to the leading edge of the tumor. This tumor was a meningioma. The optic nerve could not be isolated on serial scanning.

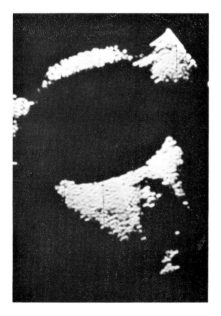
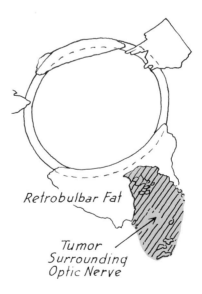

FIG. VI-27. B-scan ultrasonogram of a glioma of the optic nerve. Both glioma and meningioma appear as a solid tumor in the region of the optic nerve, producing a marked widening of the normal nerve shadow. This tumor appears sonolucent, indicating marked homogeneity. The enlargement of the nerve sheath and displacement of the adjacent orbital fat indicate a neurogenic tumor.

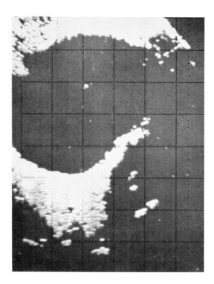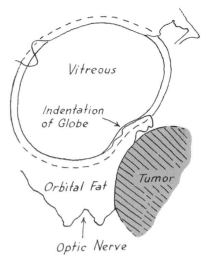

FIG. VI-28. B-scan ultrasonogram of a leiomyoma adjacent to the optic nerve with a similar acoustic pattern to a neurogenic tumor. This tumor demonstrates compression of the globe and an encapsulated or rounded outline with poor acoustic transmission. The mass has low-amplitude echoes within its structure, indicating moderate solidity.

These solid tumors show a similar appearance at the examining frequencies of 5, 10, 15 and 20 MHz. However, poor penetration of the orbit occurs at higher examining frequencies. In general, 10 MHz provides the best compromise of penetration and resolution in outlining of these tumors.

Peripheral nerve tumors (neurilemmomas and neurofibromas) differ significantly from the tumors involving the optic nerve in their ultrasonic patterns. These tumors are located randomly in the orbit, are often poorly encapsulated or not encapsulated, and thus may show an infiltrative type of ultrasonic pattern, as will be discussed in a later section.

LEIOMYOMAS. We have examined one patient with unilateral exophthalmos who proved to have the rare condition of orbital leiomyoma.[19] This tumor showed an ultrasonic pattern indicative of a solid tumor; however, the tumor was not located in the optic nerve region, yet had a rounded anterior border and demonstrated very poor sound transmission (Fig. VI-28). Upon gross pathologic examination, it was found to be rounded and well encapsulated.

Acoustically "Angiomatous" Tumors

Acoustically "angiomatous" orbital tumors have irregular outlines, as compared to the previously discussed tumors with rounded outlines. In these orbital tumors, as in the cystic group of tumors, there is good sound transmission through the mass lesion.

DIFFUSE LYMPHANGIOMA. Lymphangiomas in the region of the eye are uncommon.[21] Reese[19] described the proportion of lymphangiomas to total orbital masses as 1.8 per cent in a histopathologic study of 877 cases, and Silva[20] found three lymphangiomas in a series of 300 consecutive orbital masses, a proportion of 1 per cent. The clinical differentiation of lymphangiomas from other orbital tumors, which is difficult when lid conjunctival involvement is absent,[21] may be aided by ultrasonography.

The location, size and outline of lymphangiomas may be well demonstrated with B-scan ultrasound (Fig. VI-29). All diffuse lymphangiomas exhibit a highly irregular outline because the tumor is not encapsulated and extends diffusely through the orbit. Numerous finger-like or lobate projections of the tumor into the retrobulbar fat pattern are seen ultrasonically. Occasionally these projections are sectioned transversely by the examining ultrasound beam, giving the appearance of a tiny cyst in the retrobulbar fat pattern (Fig. VI-30). The acoustic borders of these diffuse lymphangiomas are moderately well defined, and they are acoustically well demarcated from surrounding orbital structures because of the abrupt acoustic discontinuity between fat and muscle tissue and the fluid-filled lymphangioma. Lymphangiomas demonstrate definite acoustic hollowness. Sound transmission through these fluid masses is good, and little sound attenuation occurs. As a result, the posterior extent of

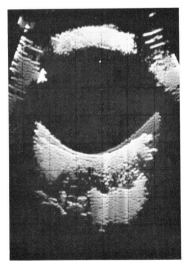
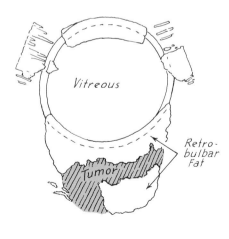

FIG. VI-29. B-scan ultrasonographic section of a lymphangioma demonstrating the irregular outline and good acoustic transmission properties of these tumors.

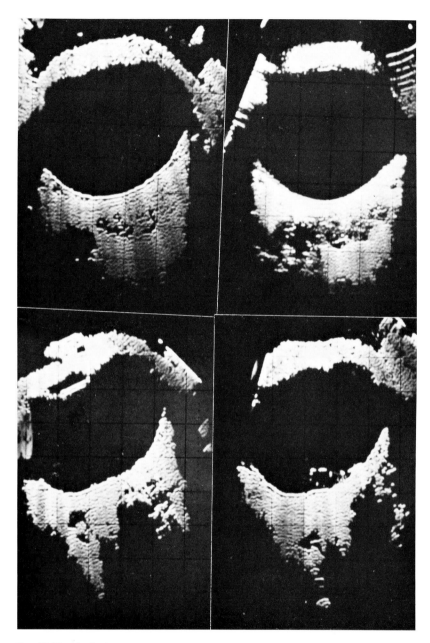

FIG. VI-30. A single sector B-scan ultrasonogram may not adequately portray the multiple finger-like projections of a lymphangioma, and may resemble an isolated cyst in the retrobulbar fat. Serial cuts will demonstrate the full extent of the tumor.

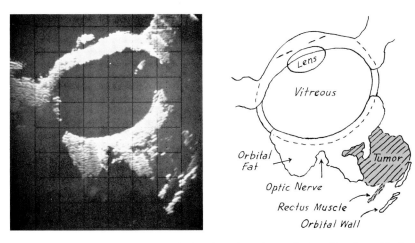

FIG. VI-31. B-scan ultrasonogram of a lymphangioma located primarily adjacent to the temporal orbital wall.

the tumor is well outlined acoustically (Fig. VI-31). M-scans through these tumors may show pulsatile activity.

NONENCAPSULATED HEMANGIOMAS. Figure VI-32 demonstrates the preoperative ultrasonogram of a child with unilateral exophthalmos, who was found at surgery to have a hemangioendothelioma of the orbit. The ultrasonogram of the tumor demonstrated an irregular outline with good sound transmission and outlining of the orbital wall temporally. The tumor was found at surgery to be diffuse, and on pathologic examination to be nonencapsulated.

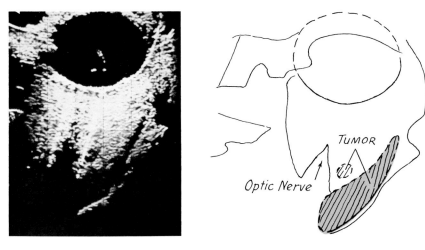

FIG. VI-32. B-scan ultrasonogram of a hemangioendothelioma showing extension of the tumor along the temporal orbital wall from the orbital apex. A single section will often demonstrate isolated cystic vacuoles and serial scanning should be utilized to delineate the extent of the mass.

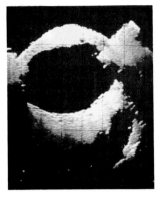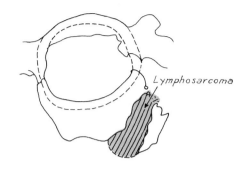

FIG. VI-33. B-scan ultrasonogram of a lymphosarcoma with an irregular outline and poor acoustic transmission.

Acoustically "Infiltrative" Tumors

Acoustically "infiltrative" tumors of the orbit demonstrate a highly irregular outline, in contrast to the cystic and solid groups of tumors. In contrast to the cystic and angiomatous groups of tumors, there is very poor sound transmission through these masses. A number of tumors demonstrate this ultrasonic pattern, and, as will be mentioned, the pattern is also seen in certain orbital pseudotumors.

LYMPHOMAS. Malignant lymphomas are a relatively common cause of unilateral exophthalmos. Reese[19] described the proportion of malignant lymphomas to total orbital masses as 10 per cent in a clinical study of 230 cases and as 14 per cent in a histopathologic study of 877 cases. Silva[20] found 21 lymphomas in a series of 300 consecutive orbital masses, a proportion of 7 per cent. This group of tumors requires radiation therapy rather than surgical excision. Tissue biopsy is essential for definitive diagnosis, but preoperative ultrasonic differentiation of lymphomas from other orbital tumors is useful clinically. A minimally traumatic surgical approach can be planned since excision is not indicated.

Lymphomas of the orbit on pathologic examination are non-encapsulated and are poorly demarcated from the surrounding orbital structures. These properties permit their ultrasonic distinction from rounded, discrete, encapsulated orbital tumors such as cavernous hemangiomas and orbital cystic lesions.

Lymphomas are randomly located in the orbit, and most are fairly large when examined. Secondary changes of the globe, such as flattening of the posterior pole, are demonstrable by ultrasonography.

The group of orbital acoustic features characteristic of all

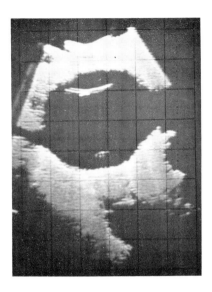
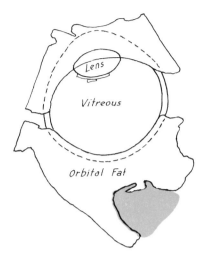

FIG. VI-34. B-scan ultrasonogram of a lymphosarcoma extending into the orbit, again with poor acoustic transmission and an irregular outline.

lymphomas (whether lymphocytic lymphomas or reticulum cell lymphomas) include: (1) irregular contour, (2) scalloped or lobulated outline, (3) demarcation from surrounding structures, (4) acoustic solidity, with high acoustic absorption, and (5) acoustic homogeneity (Figs. VI-33, VI-34 and VI-35).

All orbital lymphomas demonstrate definite acoustic solidity.

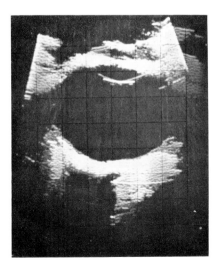
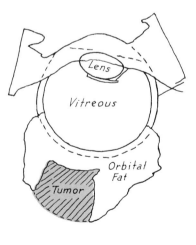

FIG. VI-35. B-scan ultrasonogram showing an irregularly outlined tumor adjacent to the optic nerve. The tumor surrounds the nerve and appears to have extensions from the nerve into Tenon's space. This tumor shows poor acoustic transmission. Histologic examination revealed a lymphosarcoma.

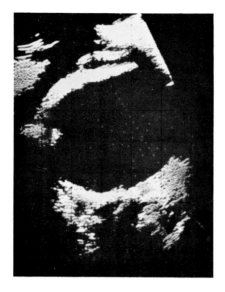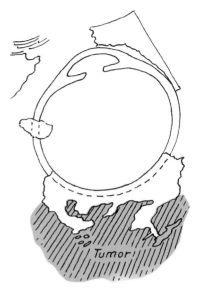

FIG. VI-36. B-scan ultrasonogram of a metastatic carcinoma with irregular outline and relatively poor sound transmission. The irregular echoes seen posteriorly represent irregular internal echoes rather than a delineation of the mass's posterior extent.

Sound energy is readily absorbed in these masses and does not penetrate through them to outline the posterior extent of the tumor, the orbital walls or the apex of the orbit.

In the interior of these solid masses, acoustic echoes or internal reflections do not occur. The monotonous, highly cellular tumor pattern does not provide acoustic discontinuities. Poor acoustic penetration of the orbit occurs with high ultrasound examining frequencies, and lymphomas are best outlined at 5 and 10 MHz.

METASTATIC CARCINOMAS. Figure VI-36 is the ultrasonogram of a patient with disseminated breast carcinoma and known orbital metastasis. The ultrasonogram demonstrates the typical pattern in metastatic carcinoma, that of irregular acoustically empty (black) spaces infiltrating the retrobulbar fat pattern. This patient exhibited unilateral enophthalmos rather than exophthalmos. Adenocarcinoma commonly appears as enophthalmos.

FIBROUS HISTIOCYTOMA. Fibrous histiocytomas are non-encapsulated, locally invasive tumors which tend to recur after surgery. These tumors demonstrate a similar ultrasonic pattern to that seen in lymphomas and metastatic carcinomas (Fig. VI-37).

RHABDOMYOSARCOMA. Rhabdomyosarcoma is the most common malignant neoplasm of mesenchymal origin in the orbit.[19] It occurs

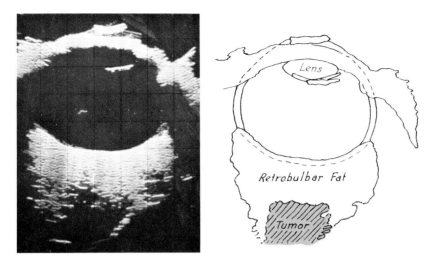

FIG. VI-37. B-scan ultrasonogram of an irregular tumor extending into the orbital fat demonstrating a relatively poor transmission pattern and extensions of the tumor into adjacent areas along the orbital wall. This tumor was classified as a histiocytoma (fibrous histiocytoma).

predominantly in Caucasians in the first decade of life. These tumors ultrasonically appear similar to the previously described types of infiltrative tumors. They are irregular in outline, and acoustically solid (Fig. VI-38). They may become very large. Ultrasonography can demonstrate serial changes in rhabdomyosarcoma over time (Fig. VI-39).

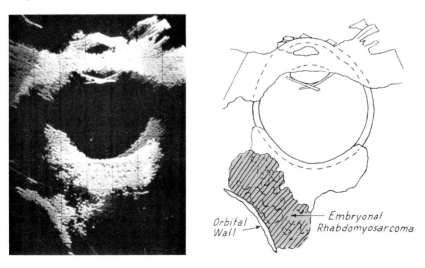

FIG. VI-38. B-scan ultrasonogram showing marked accentuation of the orbital wall with a mass compressing the temporal wall of the globe. This embryonal rhabdomyosarcoma was not easily differentiated from similar acoustic patterns of muscle infiltration. A hematoma secondary to trauma may also present a similar acoustic appearance.

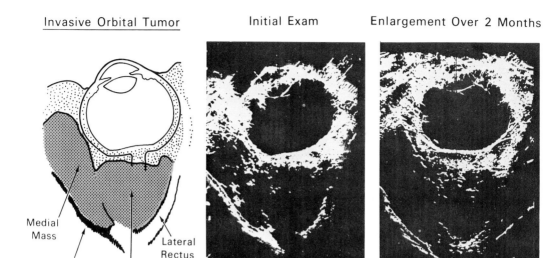

Invasive Orbital Tumor   Initial Exam   Enlargement Over 2 Months

Medial Mass

Bony Wall   Intraconal Mass

Lateral Rectus

FIG. VI-39. B-scan ultrasonogram of a rhabdomyosarcoma showing enlargement of the mass over a two-month time period. (Courtesy of Dr. R. Dallow.)

PSEUDOTUMORS. The mass lesion type of orbital pseudotumor presents an ultrasonographic appearance which is similar to the infiltrative tumor pattern which has been discussed. This is a difficult area in ultrasonic differential diagnosis. The patterns in orbital pseudotumors will be discussed with orbital inflammation.

Lacrimal Gland Tumors

Tumors of the lacrimal gland can be benign or highly neoplastic. Benign pseudotumors are confined to the gland, although inflammation may invade adjoining muscle. Adenocarcinoma or squamous carcinoma involving the lacrimal gland may invade other tissues. Since only the anterior tip of these tumors can be palpated, ultrasonography is useful in determining the size, extent and configuration of tumors in this area.

Lacrimal gland tumors generally appear as solid tumors with well-demonstrated contours, poor sound transmission and few internal echoes. The size and shape are highly variable and, because of bony overhang from the superior orbital rim, may not be easily outlined to their full extent with B-scan. The most useful aspect of the ultrasonic evaluation is in determining the posterior extention of the tumor and the lateral enlargement of invading orbital tissue (Fig. VI-40). This finding is an ominous indication of a probable malignant lesion.

It is best to use contact A-scan techniques to complete the evaluation of the lacrimal gland area.

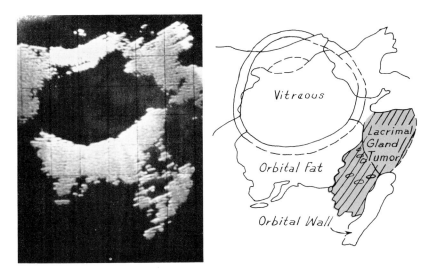

FIG. VI-40. B-scan ultrasonogram of a lacrimal gland tumor showing indentation of the normal orbital fat pattern. Localized tumors of this type are usually best evaluated with a contact A-scan technique since the ultrasonic beam can be more precisely directed. Extensions of a lacrimal gland tumor are better seen on the B-scan display since accentuation of the orbital wall and indentation of the orbital fat can be graphically portrayed.

Orbital Inflammation

Ultrasonography can reliably show inflammation of the extraocular muscles, of the optic nerve, of Tenon's space, localized inflammatory lesions (pseudotumors), and other forms of localized and diffuse orbital inflammation (see Fig. VI-17). These five different topographic types of inflammation may exist singly or together.

Presurgical differentiation of these inflammatory processes from mass lesions of the orbit is difficult on clinical or radiographic criteria alone, and ultrasonic identification of an inflammatory process may obviate the need for surgical biopsy or, alternately, direct its route.

Inflammation of the Extraocular Muscles (Myositis)

In the normal orbit, using our equipment, only a small portion of either orbital wall is usually seen. The extraocular muscles are represented acoustically as black spaces between the retrobulbar fat and the occasional low-amplitude echoes from the orbital wall. The extraocular muscles in the normal orbit appear acoustically clear, because of the highly ordered structure of muscle, and because muscle fibers and connective tissue septae lie parallel to the examining ultrasound beam so that no echoes are returned to the transducer.

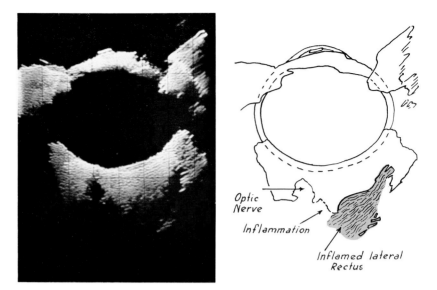

FIG. VI-41. B-scan ultrasonogram of a patient with myositis of unknown etiology. The lateral rectus muscle and the adjacent orbital wall are abnormally accentuated for the full course of the muscle although only the posterior portion of the muscle is significantly enlarged.

NONSPECIFIC MYOSITIS. Although Graves' disease is the most common cause of unilateral exophthalmos, a myositis of nonspecific etiology may cause the ultrasonic picture to show accentuation of the orbital wall and enlargement of only a portion of any one of the rectus muscles.

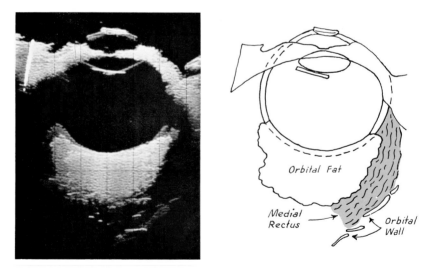

FIG. VI-42. The lateral rectus muscle in this patient with chronic granulomatous episcleritis is markedly enlarged along its entire path in an acoustic pattern indistinguishable from the myositis of Graves' disease.

In general, such a localized inflammation would appear acoustically as a bulbous or globular enlargement of the muscle in its posterior portion, with less involvement of the more anterior portion of the muscle (Fig. VI-41). Indentation of the apical orbital fat pattern by an enlarged portion of an extraocular muscle may simulate a rounded tumor. This common misinterpretation may be avoided by serially delineating the exact extent of muscle enlargement. If, however, a single muscle is enlarged along its entire course, in cases of myositis such as chronic granulomatous episcleritis (Fig. VI-42), acoustic differentiation from Graves' disease cannot be made.

GRAVES' DISEASE. The severe ocular changes which occur with toxic diffuse goiter (Graves' disease) have been described as "progressive exophthalmos," "malignant exophthalmos," "thyrotropic exophthalmos" and "endocrine exophthalmos." Recently, the American Thyroid Association[22] has suggested the term "eye changes of Graves' disease," which we presently use. Graves' disease is the most frequent cause of unilateral exophthalmos, and by far the most common cause of bilateral exophthalmos.[19]

The eye changes in hyperthyroidism result from an increase in volume in orbital tissues. The ground substance of orbital connective tissue increases in amount, mast cells and lymphocytes become prominent, and extraocular muscles increase greatly in volume (up to eight times that of normal). Electron microscopy of muscles so involved has shown marked infiltration of inflammatory cells and interstitial edema, with little muscle fiber involvement.[23] One of the most important uses of diagnostic orbital ultrasonography is the demonstration of changes in both orbital fat and extraocular muscles which occur in the active eye changes of Graves' disease.

Clinically, it is known that the inferior rectus muscle is involved most commonly in Graves' disease. Ultrasonically, however, it is easier to demonstrate the medial and lateral rectus muscles, since the medial and lateral orbital walls are less obstructed by bony overhang than the superior and inferior orbital walls. Ultrasonography may show muscle swelling without clinical evidence of impairment of muscle function and, indeed, with no signs or symptoms.

In Graves' disease, a large portion of the orbital wall is usually evident ultrasonically (Fig. VI-43), and, occasionally, both orbital walls are demonstrated (Fig. VI-44). The extraocular muscles still appear acoustically clear, but the space between retrobulbar fat and the orbital wall is increased, indicating enlargement of the muscles in this condition. This enlargement ranges from minimal to marked, and when the scan plane is adjusted to pass through the greatest diameter of the muscle the enlargement can be to some degree quantified.

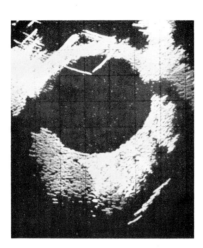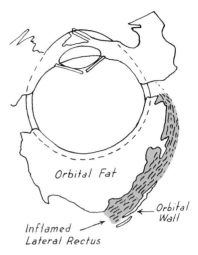

Orbital Fat

Orbital Wall

Inflamed Lateral Rectus

FIG. VI-43. B-scan ultrasonogram of a patient with Graves' disease showing accentuation of the temporal orbital wall and minimal thickening of the lateral rectus muscle along its full course. These changes must be noted to suggest Graves' disease. The orbital wall can be seen on normal scans when the transducer is directed in the proper orientation to the wall and the sensitivity is high enough at 10 MHz and can also be seen at 5 MHz. However, the boundary between muscle and orbit is accentuated when the muscle becomes edematous as in the eye changes of Graves' disease.

The posterior outline of the retrobulbar fat also often appears "scalloped" or indented (Fig. VI-45) because of compression of the retrobulbar fat by markedly enlarged extraocular muscles. There is no obvious increase in volume of the retrobulbar fat, nor any apparent difference in the echo pattern produced in its interior (i.e., its acoustic texture) as compared to the normal orbit.

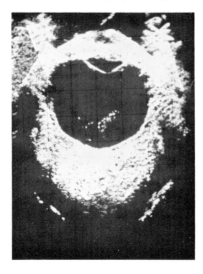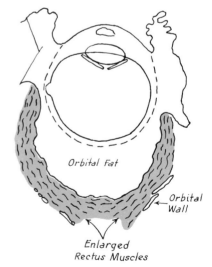

Orbital Fat

Orbital Wall

Enlarged Rectus Muscles

FIG. VI-44. Both medial and lateral rectus muscles are seen in this B-scan ultrasonogram.

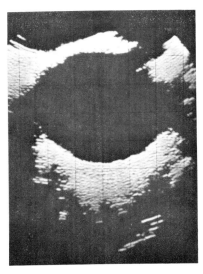
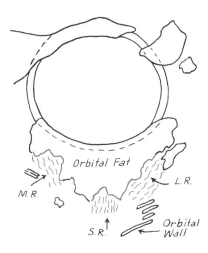

FIG. VI-45. Three rectus muscles are evident in this B-scan of a patient with Graves' disease. The medial and lateral rectus muscles are enlarged, showing an irregular boundary with the retrobulbar fat. The scalloped indentation of the fat outline adjacent to the optic nerve indicates the presence of an inflamed superior rectus muscle.

Changes in extraocular muscle enlargement over time or during steroid treatment can be monitored with ultrasonography (Fig. VI-46).

In advanced orbital involvement, edematous changes about the optic nerve may be shown ultrasonically (Fig. VI-47). These perineural changes are demonstrated ultrasonically as definite (though

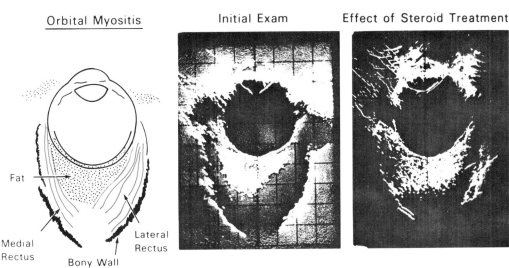

FIG. VI-46. B-scan ultrasonogram (*center*) of thickened rectus muscles indicative of myositis. *Right:* The same patient following steroid therapy evidences resolution of the swelling noted previously. (Courtesy of Dr. R. Dallow.)

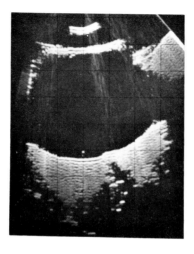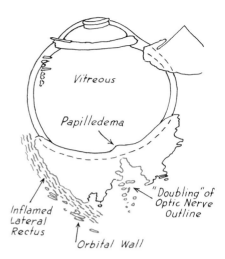

Vitreous

Papilledema

"Doubling" of
Optic Nerve
Outline

Inflamed
Lateral
Rectus

Orbital Wall

FIG. VI-47. B-scan ultrasonogram of a patient with Graves' disease showing a slight papilledema, doubling of the optic nerve shadow and thickening of the lateral rectus muscle. This patient was considered to have grade-6 Graves' disease.

often subtle) duplication echoes of the optic nerve outline. Optic neuritis of origin other than Graves' disease will be discussed in a later section.

Most patients with Graves' disease and exophthalmos present no problem diagnostically. However, the appearance of unilateral exophthalmos may raise the question of conditions such as orbital tumors, orbital granulomas, and carotid-cavernous fistula. Reese[19] has stated:

> Because most tests cannot confirm the diagnosis adequately, and because sometimes the unilateral cases mimic expanding neoplastic lesions so accurately, it may be advisable to palpate the orbit through an external canthotomy. If no tumor is present and the extraocular muscles are enlarged, then the diagnosis is established.

However, surgical exploration of the orbit involves the risk of hemorrhage or optic nerve damage. The ability of B-scan ultrasonography to differentiate Graves' disease from most of these other disorders will dismiss, in most instances, the need for performing operative procedures.

In examining a large number of patients with various thyroid abnormalities with Dr. Sidney Werner[24] of Columbia University, we have found that a certain number of patients with nontoxic nodular goiter and myxedema may show the enlargement of extraocular muscles as seen in Graves' disease. The reason for myositis to be present in thyroid conditions other than Graves' disease is not understood and is currently under investigation.

As a final note, it should be mentioned that patients with clinically obvious Graves' disease may also have orbital tumors. Dallow[25] has had experience with a small number of such patients. Ultrasonography should not be neglected in these patients, for it may show an orbital tumor in a patient who has been followed for many years with the diagnosis of exophthalmos due to Graves' disease.

Inflammation of the Optic Nerve

As Coleman and Carroll[26] first demonstrated, inflammatory change around the optic nerve can be shown utilizing B-scan ultrasonography. This condition can manifest itself as a single disease state, such as optic neuritis, or as a secondary complication of pathology such as Graves' disease or pseudotumor.

The outline of the normal optic nerve shadow is single walled, forming a white line which blends smoothly with the retrobulbar fat pattern. In cases of optic inflammatory change, there is doubling of the optic nerve shadow or acoustic accentuation of the optic nerve outline.

Inflammatory states of the optic nerve may produce a variety of anomalous echoes. We have noted three typical acoustic patterns. The first is accentuation of the optic nerve sheath, which may appear as uniformly spaced linear echoes or as a more visually apparent

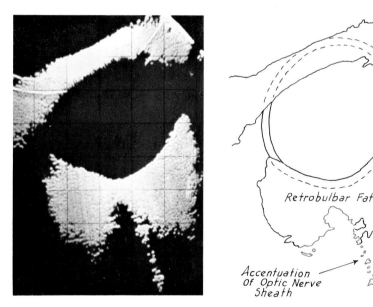

Retrobulbar Fat

Accentuation
Of Optic Nerve
Sheath

FIG. VI-48. B-scan ultrasonogram of a patient with optic neuritis demonstrating accentuation of the optic nerve sheath beyond the retrobulbar fat, nearly to the orbital apex. This unusual accentuation pattern is one of three patterns commonly seen with inflammation or congestion of the optic nerve.

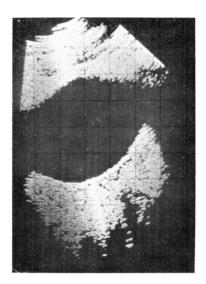
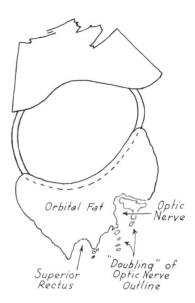

Orbital Fat

Optic Nerve

Superior Rectus

"Doubling" of Optic Nerve Outline

FIG. VI-49. B-scan ultrasonogram of a patient with optic neuritis showing a definite tissue plane separation or doubling of the optic nerve echo, separating it, presumably, from the meningeal sheath which blends acoustically with the orbital fat. This pattern is the most commonly seen with inflammation of the optic nerve.

configuration in which one or both sides of the nerve appears doubled (Fig. VI-48). The second finding, closely related to doubling, is the demonstration of a "half-ring" around the distal (globe) end of the optic nerve, but without a marked posterior extension (Fig. VI-49). Finally, random echoes may be noted lying perpendicular to

O.D.

O.S.

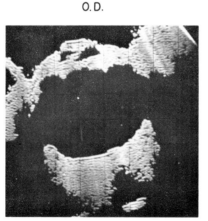
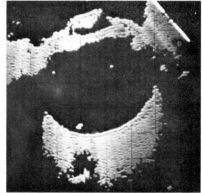

FIG. VI-50. B-scan ultrasonograms of both orbits of a patient with bilateral optic neuritis demonstrating the third type of optic nerve change seen in optic nerve inflammation. (The right nerve also shows the doubling pattern as seen in Fig. VI-49.) This third pattern shows a high-amplitude line or plane originating within the nerve. It must be identified as not artifactual from a reduplication echo of the cornea by moving the transducer in relation to the eye. This pattern may result from oblique sectioning of the inflamed nerve.

the path of the nerve, within the normally sonolucent nerve shadow (Fig. VI-50). Although this pattern may be initially interpreted as an artifact (see Fig. VI-12) on testing, the echoes are real and may be reproduced in varying scan angles. Figure VI-50 shows the ultrasonograms of a patient with bilateral optic neuritis. Evaluation of the left eye revealed an eccentric yet reproducible abnormality within the nerve, and upon comparative examination of the fellow eye a similar subtle change was noted. This finding of optic nerve change is of great interest, since ultrasonography has proven to be the only available method of clinically demonstrating the orbital optic nerve changes in retrobulbar neuritis.

In a study on the reproducibility of this finding, Coleman and Carroll[27] found that 90 per cent of patients with clinically confirmed retrobulbar neuritis demonstrated ultrasonic evidence of optic nerve abnormalities.

The ultrasonic characteristics demonstrating inflammatory or edema-like changes around the optic nerve are not specific for optic neuritis. They may be noted in Graves' disease with optic nerve involvement, in pseudotumor with involvement of the optic nerve, in venous congestion of the orbit and optic nerve, and with carotid cavernous fistulas. A somewhat similar pattern was also observed in a patient found to have an aneurysm of the ophthalmic artery.

In an attempt to portray these inflammatory accentuations of the optic nerve ultrasonically, positions of gaze, sensitivity settings and transducer angulation should be varied to establish the acoustic patterns. However, even in a normal nerve, extreme positions of gaze may bring portions of the nerve sheath more perpendicular to the examining ultrasound beam and produce a doubling of the sheath which may be erroneously interpreted as a pathologic condition.

The precise source of redundant echoes outlining the optic nerve in these cases is not known. Since the optic nerve abnormalities seen acoustically have all resolved with resolution of the inflammatory disease, no pathologic optic nerves have been available for study. The acoustic pattern seen seems most consistent with inflammatory edema of the meningeal space and spreading of the meningeal sheaths.

Inflammation of the Retrobulbar Fat and Tenon's Space

Primary inflammatory changes of orbital tissues have their own unique ultrasonic appearance.

Episcleritis or panophthalmitis can produce an inflammatory edema of the potential space of Tenon (Fig. VI-51). A diffuse mottling

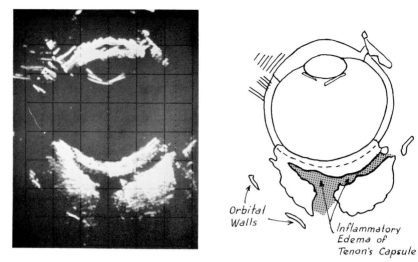

FIG. VI-51. Marked accentuation of the potential space of Tenon is shown in this scan of an orbit of a patient with episcleritis. Accentuation of this area is commonly seen in globes showing signs of phthisis bulbi.

of the orbital fat pattern acoustically is pathognomonic of orbital cellulitis (Fig. VI-52).

Some cases of orbital cellulitis may have discrete cavities that can be acoustically outlined. Almost invariably, associated inflammatory changes are also seen.

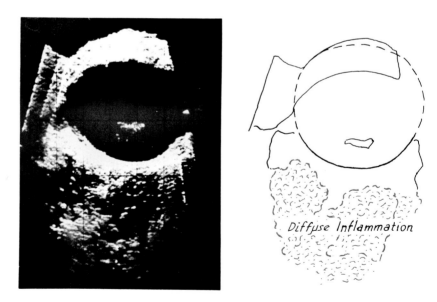

FIG. VI-52. Orbital cellulitis may evidence a diffuse orbital moth-eaten appearance as shown here, or there may be focal cavities, presumably abscess pockets.

The term "orbital pseudotumor" is used to describe "inflammatory lesions of the orbital tissues of unknown cause, simulating in their clinical picture a neoplasm of the orbit."[28] Pseudotumors are some of the most frequent causes of unilateral exophthalmos (16 per cent in Reese's series),[19] and are a significant cause of bilateral exophthalmos. Pseudotumors occur predominantly in older individuals and are infrequent in childhood and youth.

Orbital pseudotumors have been subdivided into "specific" types (i.e., those with a known, specific cause such as sarcoidosis, collagen disease, xanthogranuloma, foreign body) and "nonspecific" types (i.e., those with no demonstrable etiologic agent). The nonspecific pseudotumors may be divided further into pathologic types such as lymphoid hyperplasia, myositis, vasculitis, lipogranulomas, and dacryoadenitis.[29] Reese[19] uses the term "orbital pseudotumor" only for the nonspecific, idiopathic types of orbital inflammation and as a diagnosis of exclusion after known causes (especially the eye changes of Graves' disease) are ruled out. We use the term "orbital pseudotumor" to refer to the idiopathic orbital inflammatory lesions only, after Reese's classification.

Reese has described the following clinical features which should suggest pseudotumor in cases of exophthalmos: (1) later age of onset than primary neoplasms, (2) more acute onset than primary neoplasm, (3) sometimes bilateral, (4) pain and edema of lids or conjunctiva in 50 per cent of cases, and (5) regression of exophthalmos with steroid therapy. These features, however, are not diagnostic. Ultrasonography is of great benefit to the clinician in diagnosing these orbital conditions.

Orbital B-scan ultrasonography in cases of orbital pseudotumor may show two characteristic types of orbital abnormality: inflammatory mass lesions of the orbit and inflammatory edema of normally present orbital structures.

The size and location of pseudotumors are determined, as in all orbital conditions, by serial acoustic sectioning of the orbit. Pseudotumors of the orbit usually demonstrate many of the characteristics of lymphomas and metastatic carcinomas, including an irregular outline and acoustic solidity with high acoustic absorption. Pseudotumors may appear as a dark area encroaching on the normal retrobulbar fat pattern from its periphery. The dark area usually has an irregular anterior border (Fig. VI-53), but on occasion may have a rounded one (Fig. VI-54).

Pseudotumors may also appear as acoustically empty (black) areas, diffusely infiltrating the retrobulbar fat (Fig. VI-55).

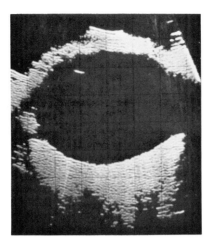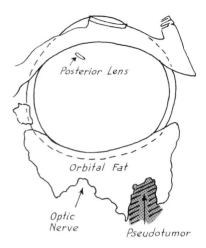

FIG. VI-53. The typical pseudotumor pattern seen acoustically is an irregular notching of the orbital fat by a sonolucent mass. Inflammatory granulomas absorb sound to such a degree that internal echoes are not usually seen.

Pseudotumors of the "en plaque" type, formed on the orbital wall, may be visualized ultrasonically. Figure VI-56 shows the ultrasonogram of a patient with an "en plaque" pseudotumor along the orbital roof. Results of orbital X-rays and tomograms were normal, and only ultrasonography demonstrated the presence of this extensive flattened mass.

Another morphologic variant of the orbital pseudotumor is a tumor which surrounds the area of the optic nerve, as shown in Figure VI-57. This is readily differentiable from an optic nerve tumor: the edges of the area are irregular and signs of inflammatory edema of the optic nerve and Tenon's space are usually demonstrable.

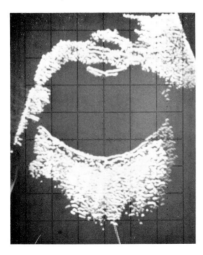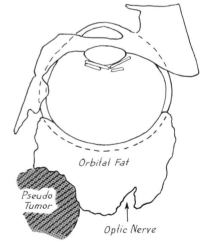

FIG. VI-54. A pseudotumor is shown in this B-scan ultrasonogram, producing a more rounded indentation of the orbital fat.

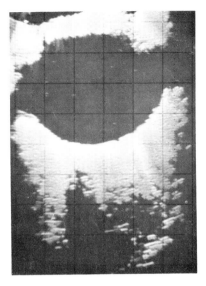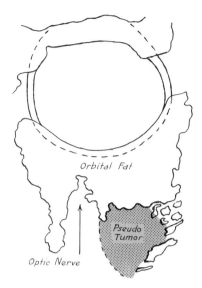

FIG. VI-55. Orbital granuloma exhibiting a diffuse, mottled leading edge as it encroaches into the orbital fat. Almost invariably, granulomas seen to extend into the orbit from the orbital wall will not exhibit good sound transmission.

Most pseudotumors demonstrate definite acoustic solidity. Sound energy is highly attenuated by these masses, and usually does not penetrate through them to clearly outline the posterior extent of the tumor or the orbital wall (Figs. VI-53 and VI-54). An exception to this is the lymphoid pseudotumor shown in Figure VI-58.

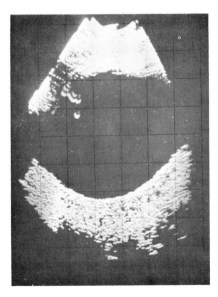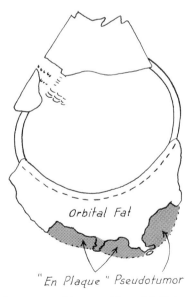

FIG. VI-56. An "en plaque" pseudotumor extending over a wide area of the orbital fat. This appearance also may be seen with sphenoidal ridge meningiomas.

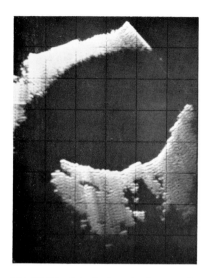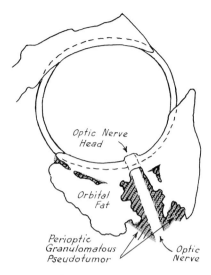

FIG. VI-57. A typical perioptic granulomatous pseudotumor is demonstrated in this B-scan, which shows doubling of the optic nerve sheath as well as accentuation of Tenon's space. This photograph demonstrates the classic signs of inflammation of both the nerve and sclera.

Solid orbital mass lesions of irregular outline (such as lympho-sarcoma and metastatic carcinoma) are similar in appearance acoustically to pseudotumor and form the category most likely to be misinterpreted as pseudotumor. Conversely, pseudotumor may be mistaken for a neoplastic tumor of this type. Figure VI-58 shows a lymphoid pseudotumor indistinguishable acoustically from a true lymphoma.

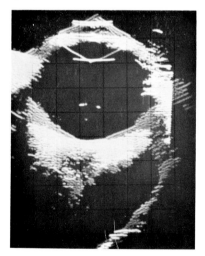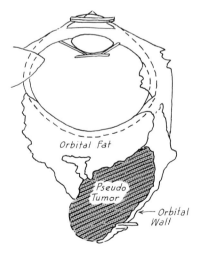

FIG. VI-58. A lymphoid pseudotumor appearing as a large mass along the orbital wall is shown in this B-scan ultrasonogram. This pseudotumor shows unusually good sound transmission and resembles a lymphoma or a lymphosarcoma. The presence of an inflammatory satellite near the nerve suggests pseudotumor.

Changes due to inflammatory edema may often be noted acoustically in adjacent orbital structures, thus indicating the inflammatory character of the mass lesion. These changes may be noted in the optic nerve, the extraocular muscles or Tenon's space.

Inflammatory enlargement of the extraocular muscles is demonstrable ultrasonically and may be seen in the presence or absence of a mass lesion. Enlargement of a muscle may also be mistaken for a mass lesion (Fig. VI-59).

Inflammation of Tenon's capsule with enlargement of the potential Tenon's space by edema fluid may be seen ultrasonically in the presence of a mass lesion (Fig. VI-57) or in the absence of a mass lesion (Fig. VI-51).

Pseudotumors are the most difficult "tumors" of the orbit to diagnose acoustically and account for the majority of differential problems in orbital ultrasonic evaluation. In a recent series of 100 orbital cases evaluated for reliability of orbital ultrasonic diagnosis,[17] seven cases classed ultrasonically as tumor were classed as false-positive diagnoses, since only diffuse inflammatory tissue was found at biopsy. In addition, of the 52 tumor cases classed as correct diagnoses, 12 cases showed mass lesions easily identified at surgery, but these histologically were classed as "nonspecific granulomas" or "lymphoid pseudotumors."

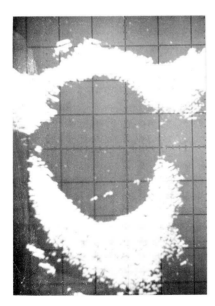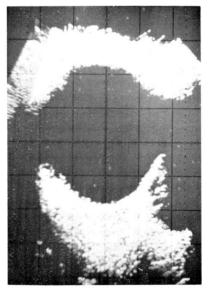

FIG. VI-59. These B-scans of the same patient demonstrate the effect of obliquely sectioning an enlarged rectus muscle (*right*) from Graves' disease. This figure again emphasizes the necessity of serial sections of any abnormal lesion seen in the orbit so that its full extent can be appreciated. The ultrasonogram on the left shows the "mass," which is actually muscle, extending to the orbital apex.

It is not surprising that this large group of orbital inflammatory lesions, which covers such a wide spectrum of pathologic manifestations, should have a range of varying appearances in ultrasonic B-scans. These inflammatory orbital mass lesions may ultrasonically mimic certain neoplastic tumors such as lymphoma and metastatic carcinoma. They usually appear as solid masses, with poor acoustic transmission, and cause irregular indentation of the retrobulbar fat pattern. Thus, they may be erroneously classified as "irregular, solid" tumors. Since lymphoid hyperplasia is often difficult to differentiate from lymphoma under the microscope, lymphoid pseudotumors may be identical to lymphomas on B-scan ultrasonographic examination. Similarly, diffuse inflammation of the retrobulbar fat closely resembles the patterns produced by a metastatic carcinoma.

B-scan ultrasonography cannot differentiate between inflammatory mass lesions and "solid, irregular" neoplastic lesions unless acoustic signs of inflammatory edema are found. Signs of myositis, sclerotenonitis, and optic nerve inflammation must be carefully sought whenever the "irregular, solid" tumor pattern is seen, since we believe that these signs are usually indicative of a primary inflammatory process.

Arteriovenous Orbital Anomalies

Patients with arteriovenous abnormalities exhibit several clinical signs. They may or may not have exophthalmos, and, if present, it may be intermittent or patient induced. Occasionally, the patient will note intermittent or more chronically apparent ectasia and/or discoloration in the ocular adnexa. Bruits may be noted by either the examiner or the patient.

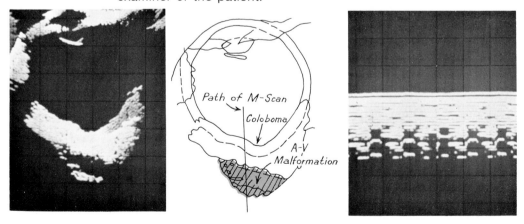

FIG. VI-60. Cystic space apparent in the orbital apex of the B-scan (*left*) is seen to have a pulsatile component which can be seen in the M-scan taken along the path noted in the schematic diagram (*center*). M-scan of the orbit (*right*) graphically shows the arterial pulsations within this arteriovenous malformation.

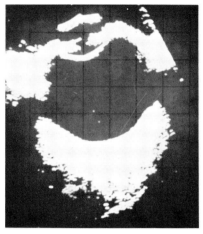 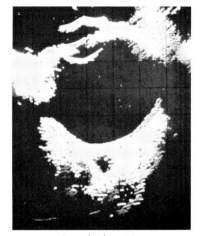

Resting State   With Valsalva Maneuver

FIG. VI-61. *Left:* A patient with venous varices exhibited small cystic spaces in the orbital fat in his normal resting state. *Right:* Upon performing a combined Mueller-Valsalva maneuver, blood pooled in the orbit, enlarging the cystic spaces.

In many patients with these conditions, no ultrasonographic abnormalities can be discerned in the orbit. However, gross abnormalities, such as those with poolings of blood, are readily demonstrable on B-scan, but must be differentiated from simple cystic masses. The A-scan should be carefully monitored for vascular pulsations, which may then be further characterized with M-scan studies (Fig. VI-60). The combined Mueller-Valsalva maneuver may be implemented in certain cases to markedly alter the venous flow, which thereby increases the size of the cystic spaces portrayed on the B-scan (Fig. VI-61).

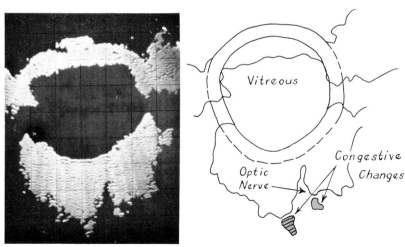

FIG. VI-62. Venous congestive changes often reveal only subtle deviations from the normal orbital fat outline, as shown here by the discrete echoes adjacent to the optic nerve.

Most patients with arteriovenous anomalies will demonstrate only subtle ultrasonic changes (Fig. VI-62). These are most often minimal irregularities in the posterior fat outline and may appear in any quadrant. If they occur adjacent to the optic nerve they may simulate an inflammatory or atrophic state of the optic nerve.

Vascular pulsations are not necessarily apparent on A- or M-scan and thus this valuable differential aid is frequently not available. If this type of abnormality is clinically suspected and routine horizontal examinations are inconclusive, vertical scanning may detect an orbital varix obscured by the orbital rim.

Orbital Trauma

Orbital trauma causes a variation in echo patterns requiring careful ultrasonic analysis. This section on orbital trauma will discuss ultrasonic localization and characterization of orbital foreign bodies, optic nerve damage and orbital hemorrhage. The latter two types of traumatic change can occur with foreign bodies, lacerations or concussion.

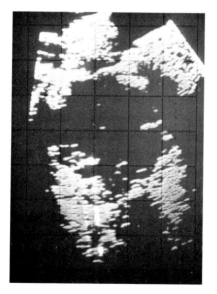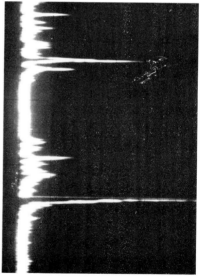

Fig. VI-63. The orbital foreign body present in this severely traumatized patient is not differentiable in the B-scan on the left. By lowering the gain, the high-amplitude spike from the metallic foreign body stands out from the retrobulbar echo complex in the A-scan on the right. The line of bright dots in the retrobulbar region of the B-scan indicates the path of the A-scan. The photographic record was obtained by double exposing the B-scan: first with the gain low and the transducer held on the foreign body echo, and then with the shutter open a second time for the normal B-scan sweep.

Ultrasonic detection of orbital foreign bodies, whether radio-paque or radiolucent, depends on their size, location, orientation and the presence of associated inflammatory change. Orbital foreign bodies are by no means always demonstrable by ultrasound. If a foreign body of any size lies along the posterior sclera or in the retrobulbar fat, echoes from the foreign body may be lost in the retrobulbar echo complex. Very small orbital foreign bodies are not usually seen with present ultrasonographic techniques.

Some metallic foreign bodies may be located by selectively decreasing the gain (Fig. VI-63) and by study of high-amplitude spikes or ringing patterns. Smaller metallic orbital foreign bodies may be detected with use of more subtle ultrasonic techniques if prior radiographic localization has been performed (Fig. VI-64).

Vegetable material, on the other hand, usually returns lower-amplitude echoes that are not identifiable amidst the echoes from the fat. If, however, the vegetable foreign body is surrounded by hemorrhage, edema, or purulence, the cystic area may enhance the outline of the foreign body (Fig. VI-65).

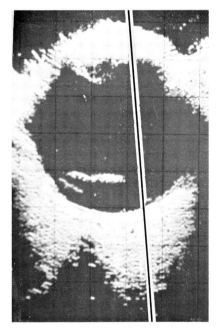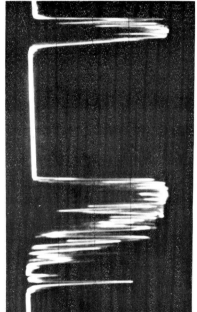

FIG. VI-64. These ultrasonograms are of a patient with a small orbital foreign body that was radiographically localized prior to the scan. The B-scan (*left*) appears acoustically normal. An A-scan (*right*), however, along the path indicated by the line on the B-scan, reveals a high-amplitude spike in the orbital apex that represents the foreign body.

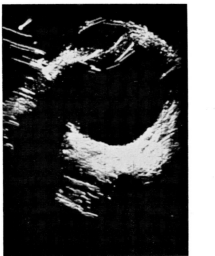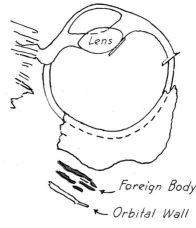

Lens

Foreign Body

Orbital Wall

FIG. VI-65. A B-scan ultrasonogram showing the doubled outline of a wood foreign body surrounded by a sonolucent area of inflammation. In the absence of secondary edema, a wood foreign body may be difficult to localize, since the acoustic impedance of wood does not differ greatly from that of the orbital fat.

Orbital Hemorrhage

The ultrasonic patterns seen in hemorrhage of the orbit, whether traumatic or postsurgical, fall into two general groups. We have found the most common pattern to be that of a mass lesion of the orbit, appearing much as a solid tumor. In this pattern, there is an acoustically empty (black) area replacing an area of orbital fat (Fig. VI-66). Its contour may be regular or irregular, it is relatively well demarcated from surrounding structures, and there is moderate sound transmission through the area. In children with unilateral proptosis and a history of trauma, ultrasonography cannot definitely differentiate between rhabdomyosarcoma and a massive orbital hemorrhage, as these often have a similar ultrasonic appearance. In this situation, follow-up over a short period of time and repeated ultrasonography will usually provide the correct diagnosis, since the hemorrhage should clear, and a rhabdomyosarcoma would enlarge rapidly. Another ultrasonic pattern seen in orbital hemorrhage is the "diffuse inflammatory disease pattern," as is seen in certain cases of orbital cellulitis and orbital pseudotumor. In our experience, this pattern is much less commonly seen than the mass lesion pattern described previously. If the hemorrhage is anterior in the orbit, it may infiltrate Tenon's space, simulating inflammation. Small orbital hemorrhage will show minimal irregularity of the posterior fat pattern.

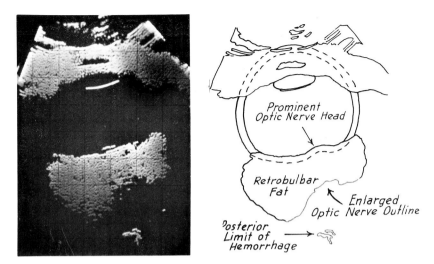

Fig. VI-66. B-scan ultrasonogram of a patient who had demonstrated loss of vision subsequent to a penetrating foreign body of the orbit. No light perception was noted for 48 hours. The B-scan shows a marked enlargement of the optic nerve shadow with good acoustic transmission, indicating a hemorrhage in the region superior to the optic nerve. The hemorrhage was drained with a 17-gauge needle and the patient recovered light perception vision. The foreign body is not seen in this scan plane.

Optic Nerve Trauma

We have made an attempt to determine whether ultrasonography can demonstrate any orbital changes in traumatic cases with avulsion of the optic nerve. In the cases examined, the V-shaped optic nerve shadow in the retrobulbar fat moved well with change of gaze, and there were no acoustic changes seen unless an orbital hemorrhage was present in addition to the optic nerve damage. The optic nerve, when avulsed, apparently is still held in position by the meninges and surrounding retrobulbar fat, and moves on the kinetic scan in a fashion identical to that seen in the normal orbital ultrasonographic examination.

Usefulness, Reliability and Limitations
of Orbital Ultrasonography

Orbital ultrasonography exceeds all other diagnostic techniques in demonstrating soft tissue abnormalities of the orbit. Comments in this section refer to high-resolution B-scan tomographic methods of ultrasound examination with water immersion.

The diagnostic accuracy of B-scan ultrasonic tomography has been documented by Coleman[17] in a series of 100 consecutive orbital cases.

In this series, the ultrasonograms in 59 cases were considered to exhibit evidence of tumor. In 11 cases, findings were considered normal, and in 1 case a foreign body was localized in the orbit. In the remaining 29 cases, ultrasonograms were classified as showing inflammatory changes, or as simply being abnormal but nonspecific for possible tumor.

In the presumed group of 59 tumors in this series, the presence of a neoplastic orbital tumor was confirmed surgically in 40 cases, and 12 cases were found to have tumors of an inflammatory nature. In the other 7 cases, either no tumor was found on attempted biopsy or the patient had clinical remission of signs on corticosteroid therapy. Two cases classified ultrasonically as nonspecifically abnormal, but possibly tumor, were later found to be orbital tumors. No case classified as normal or inflammatory by ultrasonic criteria was later found to be tumorous.

This series thus presents 88 per cent reliability in diagnosing orbital tumors. The false-positive rate for tumor diagnosis was 12 per cent. It is noteworthy that seven tumors in the series were detected only by ultrasonography, although a battery of other diagnostic tests had been employed in each case. There were no false-negatives in tumor detection, but in two cases ultrasonography was classified only as suspicious. The false-positive diagnoses were presumed to be caused by inflammatory tissue such as focal granuloma, pseudotumor, or myositis which did not appear as discrete tumor masses at the time of surgical exploration. Usually additional ultrasonic inflammatory signs accompany such lesions and suggest the inflammatory nature of the disease.

In more extensive experience with several thousand examinations since this report, the limitations of the technique have become more explicit.

Orbital mass lesions greater than 3 mm in diameter can be shown if they are isolated and discrete. Larger masses usually present no problem for identification. Tumors located at the orbital apex are difficult to recognize, because of the confluence of optic nerve and muscles which are inseparable ultrasonically. Tumors originating or extending along the bony wall of the orbit in an "en plaque" configuration, as with meningioma, osteoma or pseudotumor, do not present a reflecting surface perpendicular to the ultrasonic beam, and consequently do not produce distinct echoes. An enlarged space between retrobulbar fat and bony orbital wall in a localized area may suggest tumor, but absolute demonstration may not be possible. This problem is particularly evident in tumors along the orbital roof, which is poorly accessible ultrasonically.

Ultrasonic signs of generalized inflammation and congestion are nonspecific and may appear with several types of disease processes, including cellulitis, pseudotumor, and passive venous congestion from arteriovenous abnormalities. Inflammatory signs localized to one tissue element, such as optic neuritis, focal granuloma, or orbital myositis, are, however, more specific. Orbital changes of infiltrative tumor and pseudotumor overlap considerably, making this the most difficult tumor category to diagnose definitively.

Floor fractures and surgical defects of the orbital wall, as well as hyperostosis of bone, are not detectable reliably with ultrasonic techniques and radiographic supplementation is required to augment the soft tissue information best obtained with ultrasound.

The reliability and limitations of B-scan ultrasonography of the orbit can be succinctly summarized as a means of providing unique information concerning soft tissue abnormalities, identifying tumors and inflammatory processes. Only rarely will any significant orbital abnormality be undetectable with ultrasonography. Inflammatory changes may produce morphologic tissue changes not acoustically identified from neoplasm, giving a false-positive tumor diagnosis, but still providing 85 per cent accuracy in tumor diagnosis. Ultrasonography graphically indicates the location, size, extent and basic tissue type of detected lesions. It has proven an invaluable aid to orbital diagnosis and surgery.

References Cited

1. Coleman, D. J., Konig, W. F., and Katz, L.: A hand operated ultrasound scan system for ophthalmic evaluation. Am. J. Ophthalmol., 68:256–263, 1969.
2. Ossoinig, K.: Clinical echo-ophthalmography. In: Current Concepts in Ophthalmology. Edited by F. C. Blodi. St. Louis, C. V. Mosby Co., 1972, pp. 101–130.
3. Dallow, R.: Ultrasonography of the eye and orbit. Appl. Radiol., May–June, 1975.
4. Buschmann, W., Voss, M., and Kemmerling, S.: Acoustic properties of normal human orbit tissues. Ophthalmol. Res., 1:354–364, 1970.
5. Trokel, S. L.: Radiology and ultrasonography in the diagnosis of orbital lesions. Trans. Pa. Acad. Ophthalmol. Otolaryngol., 27:10–14, 1974.
6. Guibor, P., and Keeney, A.: Thermography and ophthalmology. Trans. Am. Acad. Ophthalmol. Otolaryngol., 74:1032–1043, 1970.
7. Purnell, E.: Ultrasonic interpretation of orbital disease. In: Ophthalmic Ultrasound. Edited by K. Gitter, et al. St. Louis, C. V. Mosby Co., 1969, pp. 249–255.
8. Ossoinig, K., and Till, P.: A ten year study of clinical echography in orbital disease. In: Ultrasonography in Ophthalmology. Edited by J. Francois and F. Goes. Basel, S. Karger, 1975, pp. 200–216.
9. Coleman, D. J., Jack, R. L., and Franzen, L. A.: High resolution B-scan ultrasonography of the orbit. Part 1: The normal orbit. Arch. Ophthalmol., 88:358–367, 1972.
10. Coleman, D. J., Jack, R. L., and Franzen, L. A.: High resolution B-scan ultrasonography of the orbit. Part II: Hemangiomas of the orbit. Arch. Ophthalmol., 88:368–374, 1972.

11. Coleman, D. J., Jack, R. L., and Franzen, L. A.: High resolution B-scan ultra-sonography of the orbit. Part III: Lymphomas of the orbit. Arch. Ophthalmol., 88:375–379, 1972.
12. Coleman, D. J., Jack, R. L., and Franzen, L. A.: High resolution B-scan ultra-sonography of the orbit. Part IV: Neurogenic tumors of the orbit. Arch. Ophthalmol., 88:380–384, 1972.
13. Coleman, D. J., Jack, R. L., Franzen, L. A., and Werner, S.: High resolution B-scan ultrasonography of the orbit. Part V: Eye changes of Graves' disease. Arch. Ophthalmol., 88:465–471, 1972.
14. Coleman, D. J., Jack, R. L., Jones, I. S., and Franzen, L. A.: High resolution B-scan ultrasonography of the orbit. Part VI: Pseudotumors of the orbit. Arch. Ophthalmol., 88:472–480, 1972.
15. Coleman, D. J., Jack, R. L., and Franzen, L. A.: B-scan ultrasonography of orbital lymphangiomas. Br. J. Ophthalmol., 57:193–198, 1973.
16. Coleman, D. J., Jack, R. L., and Franzen, L. A.: B-scan ultrasonography of orbital mucocoeles. Eye Ear Nose Throat Mon., 51:207–211, 1972.
17. Coleman, D. J.: Reliability of ocular and orbital diagnosis with B-scan ultrasound. 2. Orbital diagnosis. Am. J. Ophthalmol., 74:704–718, 1972.
18. Zismor, J., Fasano, C., Smith, B., and Rabbett, W.: Roentgenographic diagnosis of unilateral exophthalmos. J.A.M.A., 197:343–346, 1966.
19. Reese, A.: Tumors of the Eye, 2nd ed. New York, Harper and Row, 1963, pp. 532–537.
20. Silva, D.: Orbital tumors. Am. J. Ophthalmol., 65:318–339, 1968.
21. Jones, I. S., and Cleasby, G. W.: Hemangioma of the choroid: a clinicopathologic analysis. Am. J. Ophthalmol., 48:612–628, 1959.
22. Werner, S.: Classification of the eye changes of Graves' disease. J. Clin. Endocrinol. Metab., 29:982, 1969.
23. Kroll, A., and Kubara, T.: Dysthyroid ocular myopathy. Arch. Ophthalmol., 76:244, 1966.
24. Werner, S. C., Coleman, D. J., and Franzen, L. A.: Ultrasonographic evidence of a consistent orbital involvement in Graves' disease. N. Engl. J. Med., 290:1447–1450, 1974.
25. Dallow, R.: Evaluation of unilateral exophthalmos with ultrasonography: Analysis of 258 consecutive cases. Laryngoscope, 85:1905–1919, 1975.
26. Coleman, D. J., and Carroll, F. D.: A new technique for evaluation of optic neuropathy. Am. J. Ophthalmol., 74:915–920, 1972.
27. Coleman, D. J., and Carroll, F. D.: A new technique for evaluation of optic neuropathy. Trans. Am. Ophthalmol. Soc., 70:154–163, 1972.
28. Blodi, F., and Gass, J.: Inflammatory pseudotumors of the orbit. Trans. Am. Acad. Ophthalmol. Otolaryngol., 71:303–323, 1967.
29. Hogan, M., and Zimmerman, L.: Ophthalmic Pathology. Philadelphia, W. B. Saunders, 1962, p. 763.

Additional References

Orbital Tumors

Baum, G., and Greenwood, I.: Orbital lesion localization by three dimensional ultra-sonography. N.Y. State J. Med., 61:4149–4157, 1961.
Bellone, G., and Gallenga, P. E.: Echography of mixed tumors of the lacrimal gland. Ophthalmologica, 166:156–160, 1973.
Bock, J.: Orbital tumor clinic. In: Ultrasonographia Medica (SIDUO III). Edited by J. Bock and K. Ossoinig. Vienna, Verlag der Weiner Med. Akad., 1971, pp. 367–370.

Dakters, J. G.: Ultrasonography for diagnosis of orbital tumors. J.A.M.A., 203:803–805, 1968.

Francois, J.: Tumor caused exophthalmos. Ann. Ocul., 1:57–62, 1969.

Francois, J., and Goes, F.: Dermoid cyst of the orbit. Bull. Soc. Belge. Ophtalmol., 161:738–748, 1972.

Griffith, D. G., Passmore, J. W., and Penner, R.: Ultrasonographic discovery of cyst formation in metastatic neuroblastoma. Am. J. Ophthalmol., 63:313–316, 1967.

Kruger, E. G., Polifrone, J. C., and Baum, G.: Retrobulbar orbital myxoma and its detection by ultrasound. J. Neurosurg., 26:87–91, 1967.

Mandelcorn, M., and Shea, M.: Primary orbital perioptic meningioma. Can. J. Ophthalmol., 4:293–297, 1971.

Massin, M., and Poujol, J.: Report of a case of orbital tumor examined by B-mode echography. Bull. Soc. Ophtalmol. Fr., 68:30, 1968.

Ossoinig, K., and Seher, K.: Results of diagnostic ultrasound for orbital tumors. Klin. Monatsbl. Augenheilkd., 151:519–524, 1967.

Ossoinig, K.: Basics, methods, and results of ultrasonography used in diagnosis of intraorbital tumors. *In:* Ophthalmic Ultrasound. Edited by K. Gitter, et al. St. Louis, C. V. Mosby Co., 1969, pp. 282–293.

Ossoinig, K., and Valencak, E.: Ultrasonography and other diagnostic methods: importance in orbital tumors. *In:* Ophthalmic Ultrasound. Edited by K. Gitter, et al. St. Louis, C. V. Mosby Co., 1969, pp. 301–305.

Ossoinig, K. C.: Enophthalmos—a symptom of orbital tumor. Ber. Dtsch. Ophthalmol. Ges., 70:82–85, 1969.

Ossoinig, K., Keenan, T. P., and Bigar, F.: Cavernous hemangioma of the orbit. A differential diagnosis in clinical echography. *In:* Ultrasonography in Ophthalmology. Edited by J. Francois and F. Goes. Basel, S. Karger, 1975, pp. 236–245.

Psilas, K., Soriano, H. M., Itin, W., and Brawand, L. C.: The usefulness of the echography in the differential diagnosis of tumor and pseudo-glioma. Arch. Ophtalmol., 29:753–763, 1969.

Psilas, K., Houber, J. P., and Soriano, H.: Diagnosis by echography of histologically verified unilateral exophthalmia. Bull. Mem. Soc. Fr. Ophtalmol., 83:434, 1970.

Sayegh, R., Hallerbach, H., and Trier, H.: Echography (A- and B-modes) in comparison to roentgen diagnosis in space occupying orbital processes. *In:* Ultrasonographia Medica (SIDUO III). Edited by J. Bock and K. Ossoinig. Vienna, Verlag der Weiner Med. Akad., 1971, pp. 407–422.

Sayegh, F., and Trier, H. G.: The importance of diagnosis ultrasound (A- and B-mode) of the orbit in cases with suspicious tumors in the paranasal sinus region. Ophthalmol. Res., 2:183–188, 1971.

Tane, S., Noguchi, J., Ishibashi, T., Shiba, Y., and Kobayashi, Y.: A case of reticulum cell sarcoma of the orbit. Folia Ophthalmol., 7:678–680, 1969.

Till, P., and Ossoinig, K.: Echography evaluation of the penetration of supramaxilla tumors into the orbit. Monatsschr. Ohrenheilkd Laryngorhinol., 106:442–448, 1972.

Orbital Arteriovenous Abnormalities

Buschmann, W.: Ultrasonic examination of arteries and veins. *In:* Ultrasonics in Ophthalmology. Edited by R. Goldberg and L. Sarin. Philadelphia, W. B. Saunders, 1967, pp. 183–186.

Buschmann, W.: Ultrasonic diagnosis of superficial arteries. Wiss. Z. Humboldt Univ. Berlin [Math. Naturwiss.], 14:223–224, 1965.

Buschmann, W.: Diagnosis of carotid thrombosis. Graefe. Arch. Ophthalmol., 166:519–529, 1964.

Ossoinig, K.: The ultrasonic diagnosis of orbital vascular processes. Klin. Monatsbl. Augenheilkd., 158:526–533, 1971.

Valencak, E., and Ossoinig, K.: Arterio-venous fistulas of the orbit in A- and B-mode echograms. Neurochirurgie, 4:549–552, 1968.

Orbital Trauma

Bellone, G., and Gallenga, P. E.: Diagnostic echography of ophthalmic foreign bodies. Part III. Foreign bodies located in the orbit. Arch. Rass. Ital. Ottal., 2:122–133, 1970.

Ossoinig, K., Bigar, F., Kaefring, S., and McNutt, L.: Echographic detection and localization of BB shots in the eye and orbit. *In:* Ultrasonography in Ophthalmology. Edited by J. Francois and F. Goes. Basel, S. Karger, 1975, pp. 109–118.

Runyan, T. E., and Penner, R.: Comparison of localization of orbital foreign bodies by radiologic and ultrasonic methods. Arch. Ophthalmol., 4:512–517, 1969.

Till, P.: Echography in orbital trauma. *In:* Ultrasonographia Medica (SIDUO III). Edited by J. Bock and K. Ossoinig. Vienna, Verlag der Weiner Med. Akad., 1971, pp. 437–442.

Till, P.: Ultrasonic diagnosis of retrobulbar hematomas. Klin. Monatsbl. Augenheilkd., 158:723–727, 1971.

General Orbital Diagnosis

Abramson, D. H., Coleman, D. J., and Franzen, L.: Ultrasonic diagnosis of optic nerve lesions. *In:* Ultrasonography in Ophthalmology. Edited by J. Francois and F. Goes. Basel, S. Karger, 1975, pp. 231–235.

Baum, G.: A reappraisal of orbital ultrasonography: Series II. Trans. Am. Acad. Ophthalmol. Otolaryngol., 69:943–958, 1965.

Baum, G., and Greenwood, I.: Present status of orbital ultrasonography. Am. J. Ophthalmol., 56:98–105, 1963.

Buschmann, W.: Problems of ultrasound diagnosis in the orbit. *In:* Diagnostica Ultrasonica in Ophthalmologia (SIDUO II). Edited by J. Vanysek. Brno, University of Brno, 1968, pp. 109–116.

Coleman, D. J.: Orbital ultrasonic tomography (B-scan). Trans. Am. Acad. Ophthalmol. Otolaryngol., 78:577–580, 1974.

Fridman, F. E.: The use of acoustic tomography in the diagnosis of certain orbital diseases. Vestn. Oftalmol., 81:30, 1968.

Gitter, K. A., Meyer, D., Goldberg, R., and Sarin, L. K.: Role of ultrasound in diagnosis of unilateral proptosis. *In:* Diagnostica Ultrasonica in Ophthalmologia (SIDUO II). Edited by J. Vanysek. Brno, University of Brno, 1968, pp. 327–331.

Gitter, K. A., Meyer, D., Goldberg, R., and Sarin, L. K.: Ultrasonography in unilateral proptosis. Arch. Ophthalmol., 79:370–375, 1968.

Gitter, K. A.: Time-amplitude (A-mode) ultrasonography in the diagnosis of unilateral proptosis. *In:* Ultrasonics in Ophthalmology. Edited by R. Goldberg and L. Sarin. Philadelphia, W. B. Saunders Co., 1967, pp. 201–203.

Hamard, H., and Bregeat, P.: Orbital echo-tomography. Arch Ophtalmol., 31:137–144, 1971.

Hildebrandt, I.: The positional relationship between the middle point of the bulb and the temporal edge of the orbit in exophthalmos. Wiss. Z. Humboldt Univ., Berlin [Math. Naturwiss.], 14:213–216, 1965.

Meier, J., Staudt, J., Wilcke, G., and Buschmann, W.: Topographical and anatomical foundations of ultrasonic diagnosis in the region of the orbit. Anat. Anz., 126:21–32, 1970.

Oksala, A.: Diagnosis by ultrasound in acute dacryocystitis. Acta Ophthalmol., 37:176–179, 1959.

Oksala, A.: Echogram in some palpebral conditions. Acta Ophthalmol., 38:100–108, 1960.

Oksala, A., and Hakkinen, L.: Comparative experiments on the attenuation of ultrasound in muscular and fat tissue. Acta Ophthalmol., 47:735, 1969.

Oksala, A., and Niiranen, A.: Experimental observations of the reflection and interference phenomenon of the ultrasound caused by orbital fat and muscular tissues. Acta Ophthalmol., 48:481–486, 1970.

Oksala, A., Hadidi, M. A., and Jaaslahiti, S.: Experimental observations on the echograms of the optic nerve and the effects of some tissues upon them. Acta Ophthalmol., 50:360–366, 1972.

Oskala, A.: The effect of retrobulbar tissues on the ultrasonic field. Acta Ophthalmol., 50:247–254, 1972.

Ossoinig, K.: The echographic picture presented by a healthy orbit. *In:* Diagnostica Ultrasonica in Ophthalmologia (SIDUO II). Edited by J. Vanysek. Brno, University of Brno, 1968, pp. 101–107.

Ossoinig, K. C.: Routine ultrasonography of the orbit. Int. Ophthalmol. Clin., 9:667–683, 1969.

Ossoinig, K.: Echography for the diagnosis of exophthalmos in children. Ber. Dtsch. Ophthalmol. Ges., 69:98–104, 1969.

Ossoinig, K.: Orbital ultrasonography—method of choice for the diagnosis of unilateral exophthalmos. Schweiz. Med. Wochenschr., 99:1033, 1969.

Ossoinig, K.: Clinical echo-ophthalmology in diseases of the orbit. *In:* Ultrasonographia Medica (SIDUO III). Edited by J. Bock and K. Ossoinig. Vienna, Verlag der Weiner Med. Akad., 1971, pp. 423–436.

Poujol, J.: A-scan ultrasound accuracy of diagnosis in orbital disease. Mod. Prob. Ophthalmol., 14:250–253, 1975.

Purnell, E. W.: B-mode orbital ultrasonography. Int. Ophthalmol. Clin., 9:643–665, 1969.

Purnell, E. W., Cappaert, W. E., and Sokollu, J. K.: B-scan ultrasonography during orbital surgery. J. Clin. Ultrasound, 1:32–36, 1973.

Smith, M. E.: The differential diagnosis of unilateral exophthalmos. Int. Ophthalmol. Clin., 7:911, 1967.

Staudt, J., Kunz, G., Wilcke, G., and Buschmann, W.: Topographic, anatomical and statistical examination in orbital diagnosis. Anat. Anz., 131:88–96, 1972.

Uchida, H.: Analysis of retrobulbar echo in ultrasonography. Folia Ophthalmol. Jap., 20:947–951, 1969.

Vanysek, J., and Preisova, J.: The possibilities of examining the orbital region by means of ultrasound. Wiss. Z. Humboldt Univ. Berlin [Math. Naturwiss.], 14:179–184, 1965.

Appendix

Techniques of Ultrasonic Examination

ULTRASONIC evaluation of the eye can be performed with either contact or immersion techniques. The contact method is the simplest and most direct way of viewing the eye. In the contact method, the A- or B-scan transducer is applied to the closed lid, with methylcellulose to provide an acoustic couplant, and the globe is systematically searched. Use of proparacaine to anesthetize the surface of the globe can allow direct application of the transducer to the eye for improved resolution. For more complete evaluation, an immersion method is preferred, and when the anterior segment is to be examined an immersion system is required. Regardless of the equipment used, a water bath technique may form part of the examination.

We have found that a description of the technique to the patient allays any fears he might have and encourages cooperation. The explanation is of the following type:

> This test is called an ultrasonogram. We use sound waves that are much the same as my voice, but which are of higher frequency, to provide echoes from the tissues within your eye, much like sonar is used to map out an ocean floor. Examination is painless. You do not feel the sound, and it does not cause any tissue damage. We do use a water bath around your eye to conduct the sound. The water is a sterile salt solution and the feeling will be much the same as if you were to open your eye under water while swimming. We will put a drop of anesthetic into your eye, so it will not be uncomfortable, and we will hold your eyelids open so you do not have to exert any effort.

With the patient supine on the examination table, we place a plastic Steri-drape around the eye to provide the container for the water bath (Fig. 1). The Steri-drape is an ocular drape that has a central opening so that no plastic comes between the transducer and the eye. The drape may be applied directly to the skin, but we have found that perspiration, oily skin or heavy makeup prevents a water-tight seal. Therefore, we routinely elect to paint a ring of

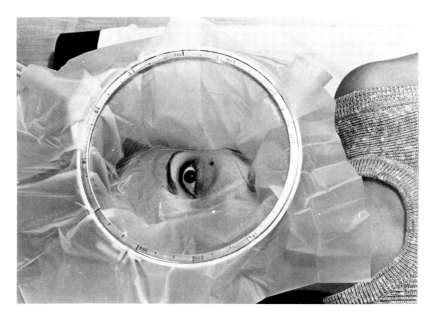

FIG. 1. The plastic Steri-drape water bath system developed by Coleman for routine immersion scanning. An ocular Steri-drape is placed about the eye and approximately 400 cc of normal saline solution provide an easily accessible acoustic view of the eye and orbit.

collodion around the patient's eye, using a cotton-tip swab. Leakage of saline occasionally occurs inside the nasolabial fold or between the eyebrows, and care should be taken to allow at least a quarter inch of plastic material to cover these areas. The collodian should never be passed directly over the patient's open eye, and, for extra caution, the patient is instructed to keep his eyes closed.

Once the drape is in position, a metal hoop is centered over the patient's eye. The edges of the drape are brought up through the hoop, but the hoop is not clamped. A drop of Ophthaine is placed in the patient's eye and a sterile Barraquer speculum is then gently inserted to hold the eyelids open. On occasion, the patient will move his head during this process and, if the drape had been clamped, it might be torn loose.

Following the insertion of the speculum, the clamp is used to secure the edges of the plastic, and sterile warmed saline is poured into the edge of the drape, but not directly onto the eye. We preheat the saline to body temperature in a water bath to minimize discomfort to the patient. For the experienced examiner, this initial patient preparation usually takes two minutes.

The transducer is then swung into position above the eye (Figs. 2 and 3) and the transducer is dipped to just below water level. Horizontal scans are then made across the eye and the display is

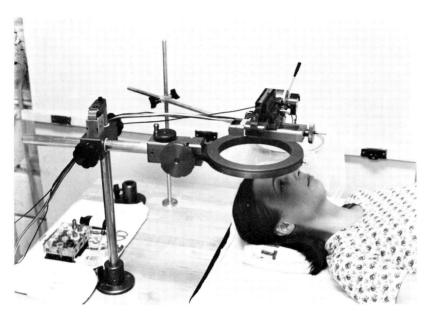

FIG. 2. The manually operated scan carriage used to provide the illustrations in this book. Serial, compound and linear B-scans can be made through any meridian of the globe or orbit using the water bath shown in Figure 1.

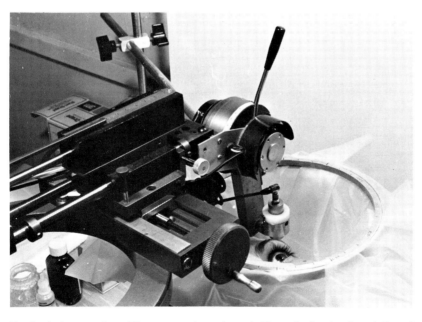

FIG. 3. A close-up view of the scan carriage shown in Figure 2, showing the relation of the transducer to the eye. The transducer can be lifted out of its holder to permit hand-held A-scanning and to detect artifacts.

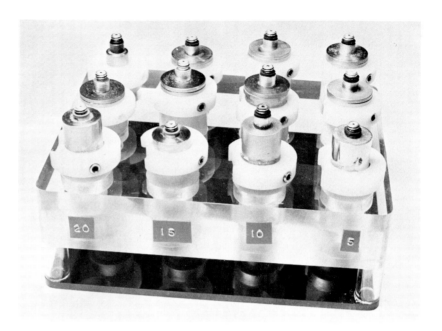

FIG. 4. A selection of transducers of different frequencies (5, 10, 15, 20 MHz), both focused and unfocused, can be easily interchanged to allow maximum flexibility in displaying tissues.

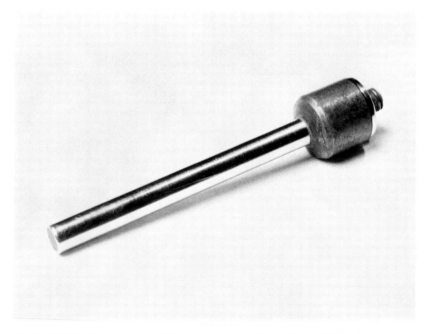

FIG. 5. 10-MHz transducer used for A-scan evaluation which is $\frac{3}{16}''$ in diameter and can be sterilized for use in the operating room.

Horizontal scans are then made across the eye and the display is observed. Vertical scans are employed in selected cases to better portray the situation. The two-dimensional pictures on the oscilloscope provide a real time monitor for the procedure. The examiner continually observes the A- and B-scan traces to abstract maximum acoustic information.

By changing transducer frequencies certain features more amenable to greater resolution (higher frequency and/or focused transducers) or greater sensitivity (lower sensitivities and/or unfocused transducers) may be portrayed (Fig. 4). In rare instances, a hand-held A-scan unit may be held directly against the globe to ballotte or visualize obstructed orbital areas (Fig. 5).

The examination is primarily a visual one, but photographs are essential for documentation. Best resolution is obtained with 35-mm photographs, but we have primarily used Polaroid pictures since they provide an immediate record of adequate clarity.

Photographs can be made either of the storage oscilloscope or of a single or compound sweep in nonstored mode, with the camera shutter open during the entire sweep. We prefer the latter method. Experience is required to make a smooth manual sector scan without dwelling in any position in the scan, but the technique is quickly learned, and has provided the scans used in most of the illustrations in this book.

The total examination time varies according to the difficulty of the case. A simple precataract extraction screening procedure can take as little as four to five minutes, while a thorough tumor differentiation study employing multiple frequencies can last up to 35 minutes. The total examination time should not exceed this period, as the anesthetic becomes ineffective and the patient becomes uncomfortable.

It is rare that a patient does not readily cooperate, but, if this should be the case, contact scanning conducted through the lids on A- or B-mode alone is used. In the examination of children, we prefer to use anesthesia up to the age of five years. Valium 10 mg one hour before the procedure has been useful for children five through eight years.

Index

Inflammation (*Continued*)
  orbital, 325–340
    changes with, 305–307, 306f
Inflammatory conditions and secondary
    retinal detachments, 203, 203f
Intensity, ultrasonic, 39, 41–43, 44f
Intensity modulated techniques, 106
Interfaces, acoustic, 13f
Internal echoes and orbital tumors, 303
Internal heterogeneity, 224f
Internal homogeneity, 224f
Internal reflection in choroidal tumors,
    222
Internal tissue characteristics, 157
Internal tissue texture, 75, 220, 225–
    226
Intervals, time, 13f, 14
Interval counter, electronic. *See*
    Electronic interval counter
Intracranial abnormalities, 289
Intraocular forceps, 153
Intraocular lenses, calculation of
    dioptric power of, 93, 123,
    158
Intraocular lens implant, 182, 182f
  and axial length measurement, 122–
    124
Intraocular tumors, 153. *See also*
    Specific tumors
Introduction to diagnostic ultrasound,
    143–151
Introductory discussion and
    background material of ocular
    diagnosis, 153–158
Iris, as problem in measurement, 108,
    123
  on normal B-scan, 162
Iris adherence, 174, 174f
Iris bombé, 179, 179f, 244
Iris coloboma, 244
Iris cyst, 178f, 179
Iris sphincter, 179
Iris tumors, 179
Isodensitometer, 78
Isometric displays, 148f. *See also* Color
    plates
  B-mode, 65, 78–79, 80f
Isometric scanning, in diagnosis of
    choroidal tumors, 214
Isometric viewing, 154
  and intraocular foreign bodies, 260

KERATOCONUS, 173
Keratometry, 123
Keratoplasty, 175
Keratoprosthesis, 175–177, 175f, 176f

and axial length measurement, 122–
    124
and determination of dioptric power,
    93, 158
Kinesis of tumor tissue, 220, 226f, 230
Kinetic scans, A-scans, 154
  in displacement of lens, 181f
  in retinitis proliferans, 188f, 188
  in optic nerve trauma, 345
  in orbital evaluation, 287, 288, 305
  in orbital tumor diagnosis, 314
  in traumatic retinal detachment, 253
  of vitreous hemorrhage, 186
  of vitreous veils, 186, 186f
Kretz amplifier, 222
Kuhnt-Junius. *See* Disciform macular
    degeneration

LACERATION, orbital, 342
Lacerating wounds, 248
Lacrimal gland tumors, 304, 324–325,
    325f
  contact examination of, 288
Lateral resolution. *See* Resolution,
    lateral
Lead-zirconate-titanate, 6
Leading edge of choroidal tumors, 222,
    223f
Leiomyoma, 316, 316f
Lens, abnormalities of, 180–182, 180f,
    181f, 182f
  acoustic, 4, 20, 36
  calcified, and attenuation of sound,
    171
  displacement of, 177, 180, 180f, 196,
    249–251, 249f, 250f, 251f
  intraocular. *See* Intraocular lens
  position of, 93
  reimaging, 40
  sclerotic. *See* Cataract
  sound transmission of, 111f
  subluxation of, 180, 180f. *See also*
    Lens, displacement of
  volume calculation of, 126
Lens capsule, traumatic rupture of, 253
Lens implant, intraocular, 182, 182f
Lens injuries, following perforating or
    lacerating injuries, 252–253, 253f
Lens remnant, prior to
    prosthokeratoplasty, 175
Lens thickness, measurement of, 93
Lesions, arteriovenous, 289
Lids, 101f
Light fixation, 102, 107f
Limbus, in axial measurement, 102,
    103f

Shallow anterior chamber, 174f, 175, 243
Shallow orbit, 301
Sighting aperture, 107f
Silicone membrane, 106f
SMD. *See* Disciform macular degeneration
Snell's law, 20, 22
"Snow," 59, 59f, 75, 166, 167f
Solid orbital tumors, 302, 302f, 304, 313–316, 314f, 315f, 316f
"Solid" retinoblastoma, 210–213, 210f
Solid vitreous, 186, 187, 253
Sound absorption, by lens, 163f. *See also* Artifacts, absorption
  by tumor tissue, 216f
  from lens in diascleral scans, 162
Sound transmission, 111f
  by intraocular foreign bodies, 259
  in orbital diagnosis, 300f, 302, 302f, 303
Sound velocity, in cataract, 123. *See also* Velocity(ies)
  in retinoblastoma, 212–213
  of orbital tissues, 288
Spectra, calibration, 85
Spectral configuration, 85
Spectrum analysis, ultrasonic, 83–87, 84f, 86f, 87f
Speculum, artifacts and, 297
Spindle cell malignant melanoma, 230
"Spontaneous movements," 225, 231f
Squamous carcinoma, lacrimal gland, 324
S-shaped curve, 60, 222
Standard block, 118, 118f
Standardization, of measurement system, 92
Standoff, membrane covered, 93
  water-bath, 143
Standoff probe, 101f
Standoff tips, 108f
Staphyloma, 164f, 172f, 173, 173f, 301
Sterile technique, in ocular trauma, 248
Steroids, 290
  in Graves' disease, 329, 329f
Streaming, 47
Subluxated lens, 180, 180f. *See also* Lens, displacement of
Subretinal space, examination of, 198
Sub-Tenon's space. *See* Tenon's space
Supplemental ultrasonic information, 157
Surgical intervention, 183
  evaluation during, 149
  for orbital exploration, 330
  for retinal detachment, 197

vitreous, 182. *See also* Vitrectomy
Surgical perforation of the sclera, 255f
Suspected malignant melanoma, 214
"Swiss cheese," 75, 77, 166, 168f, 297
Systems, A-mode, 51, 53–65, 54f, 56f, 57f, 58f, 59f, 61f, 62f, 63f, 64t
  B-mode, 51, 65–79, 66f, 67f, 70f, 71f, 73f, 74f, 76f, 77f, 72t
  Bragg visualization, 41
  M-mode, 51
  pulsed-echo, 4
  reflective, 4
  Schlieren, 40–41, 40f, 41f
  time marker, 117
  ultrasonic, 51–87
  ultrasonic biometric, 95–100
System calibration, 81–83
System operation, in spectrum analysis, 84–85, 84f

TANGENTIAL perspectives, 151
Target, calibration, 71f
Techniques, holographic, 39
  image-enhancement, 65
  of ocular diagnosis, 155–156
Television, as display, 146f
Tenon's space, 307
  and edema, 305
  and orbital hemorrhage, 344
  inflammation of, 333–334, 334f, 338f
Texture changes, in choroidal tumors, 229f
Texture enhancement, 76f, 77f
Therapy(ies), medical, 290
  steroid, in Graves' disease, 329, 329f
  surgical, 290
Thermography, 289
Thickening of the cornea, 174–175, 174f
Three-dimensional conceptualization, 151
Three dimensional display, 155
Threshold levels, 59, 99, 166
Through-transmission ultrasound, 39
Thyroid ophthalmopathy, spectral analysis of, 86
Thyroid-related disease, 306. *See also* Graves' disease
Thyrotropic exophthalmos. *See* Graves' disease
Tilting, 79
Time axis, horizontal, 65
Time base, 117
Time distance, 92
Time marker system, 117, 111f
Time sweep, 65